Advances in Colonoscopy

Editors

CHARLES J. KAHI
DOUGLAS K. REX

GASTROINTESTINAL ENDOSCOPY
CLINICS OF NORTH AMERICA

www.giendo.theclinics.com

Consulting Editor
CHARLES J. LIGHTDALE

April 2015 • Volume 25 • Number 2

ELSEVIER

1600 John F. Kennedy Boulevard • Suite 1800 • Philadelphia, Pennsylvania, 19103-2899

http://www.theclinics.com

GASTROINTESTINAL ENDOSCOPY CLINICS OF NORTH AMERICA Volume 25, Number 2
April 2015 ISSN 1052-5157, ISBN-13: 978-0-323-35974-0

Editor: Kerry Holland
Developmental Editor: Donald Mumford

Gastrointestinal Endoscopy Clinics of North America (ISSN 1052-5157) is published quarterly by Elsevier Inc., 360 Park Avenue South, New York, NY 10010-1710. Months of issue are January, April, July, and October. Business and Editorial Offices: 1600 John F. Kennedy Blvd., Suite 1800, Philadelphia, PA, 19103-2899. Periodicals postage paid at New York, NY and additional mailing offices. Subscription prices are $335.00 per year for US individuals, $486.00 per year for US institutions, $175.00 per year for US students and residents, $370.00 per year for Canadian individuals, $576.00 per year for Canadian institutions, $465.00 per year for international individuals, $576.00 per year for international institutions, and $245.00 per year for Canadian and foreign students/residents. To receive student/resident rate, orders must be accompanied by name of affiliated institution, date of term, and the *signature* of program/residency coordinator on institution letterhead. Orders will be billed at individual rate until proof of status is received. Foreign air speed delivery is included in all *Clinics* subscription prices. All prices are subject to change without notice. **POSTMASTER:** Send address change to *Gastrointestinal Endoscopy Clinics of North America*, Elsevier Health Sciences Division, Subscription Customer Service, 3251 Riverport Lane, Maryland Heights, MO 63043. **Customer Service: 1-800-654-2452 (US). From outside the United States, call 1-314-447-8871. Fax: 1-314-447-8029. E-mail: JournalsCustomerService-usa@elsevier.com (for print support) or JournalsOnlineSupport-usa@elsevier.com (for online support).**

Reprints. For copies of 100 or more, of articles in this publication, please contact the Commercial Reprints Department, Elsevier Inc., 360 Park Avenue South, New York, NY 10010-1710. Tel. 212-633-3874; Fax: 212-633-3820; E-mail: reprints@elsevier.com.

Gastrointestinal Endoscopy Clinics of North America is covered in *Excerpta Medica, MEDLINE/PubMed (Index Medicus), and MEDLINE/MEDLARS.*

Contributors

CONSULTING EDITOR

CHARLES J. LIGHTDALE, MD
Professor of Medicine, Division of Digestive and Liver Diseases, Columbia University Medical Center, New York, New York

EDITORS

CHARLES J. KAHI, MD, MSc
Associate Professor of Clinical Medicine, Indiana University School of Medicine; Gastroenterology Section Chief, Richard L. Roudebush VA Medical Center, Indianapolis, Indiana

DOUGLAS K. REX, MD
Distinguished Professor of Medicine, Division of Gastroenterology/Hepatology, Department of Medicine, Indiana University School of Medicine, Indiana University, Indianapolis, Indiana

AUTHORS

DOUGLAS G. ADLER, MD, FACG, AGAF, FASGE
Associate Professor of Medicine, Director of Therapeutic Endoscopy, Director, GI Fellowship Program, Gastroenterology and Hepatology, Huntsman Cancer Center, University of Utah School of Medicine, Salt Lake City, Utah

JOSEPH C. ANDERSON, MD
Department of Veterans Affairs Medical Center, Department of Medicine, White River Junction, Vermont; The Geisel School of Medicine at Dartmouth Medical, Department of Medicine, Hanover, New Hampshire

MICHAEL J. BARTEL, MD
Gastroenterology Fellow, Gastroentrology and Hepatology, Mayo Clinic, Jacksonville, Florida

ELIZABETH BIRD-LIEBERMAN, MRCP, PhD
Translational Gastroenterology Unit, John Radcliffe Hospital, Headington, Oxford, United Kingdom

MICHAEL J. BOURKE, MBBS, FRACPS
Director of Endoscopy, Department of Gastroenterology and Hepatology, Westmead Hospital, Professor of Medicine, University of Sydney, Sydney, Westmead New South Wales, Australia

LAWRENCE B. COHEN, MD
Clinical Professor of Medicine, Department of Medicine (Gastroenterology), Icahn School of Medicine at Mount Sinai, New York, New York

GUIDO COSTAMAGNA, MD, FACG
Professor, Director of Digestive Endoscopy Unit, Catholic University, Rome, Italy

EVELIEN DEKKER, MD, PhD
Professor, Department of Gastroenterology and Hepatology, Academic Medical Center, Amsterdam, The Netherlands

JAMES E. EAST, MD(res), FRCP
Translational Gastroenterology Unit, John Radcliffe Hospital, Headington, Oxford, United Kingdom

NABIL F. FAYAD, MD
Associate Professor of Clinical Medicine, Division of Gastroenterology and Hepatology, Department of Medicine, Indiana University School of Medicine; Endoscopy Director, Section of Gastroenterology and Hepatology, Medicine Department, Richard L. Roudebush VA Medical Center, Indianapolis, Indiana

IAN M. GRALNEK, MD, PhD, MSHS, FASGE
Department of Gastroenterology, Ha'Emek Medical Center, Afula, Israel; Rappaport Faculty of Medicine, Technion-Israel Institute of Technology, Haifa, Israel

CESARE HASSAN, MD
Gastroenterologist, Digestive Endoscopy Unit, Catholic University, Rome, Italy

DAVID G. HEWETT, MBBS, MSc, PhD, FRACP
Associate Professor and Director, Medical Leadership Program, School of Medicine, The University of Queensland; Department of Gastroenterology, Queen Elizabeth II Jubilee Hospital, Brisbane, Queensland, Australia

JOEP EVERT GODFRIED IJSPEERT, MD
Department of Gastroenterology and Hepatology, Academic Medical Center, Amsterdam, The Netherlands

CHARLES J. KAHI, MD, MSc
Associate Professor of Clinical Medicine, Indiana University School of Medicine; Gastroenterology Section Chief, Richard L. Roudebush VA Medical Center, Indianapolis, Indiana

SHARA NGUYEN KET, MBBS, FRACP
Translational Gastroenterology Unit, John Radcliffe Hospital, Headington, Oxford, United Kingdom

AMIR KLEIN, BSc, MD
Advanced Endoscopy Fellow, Department of Gastroenterology and Hepatology, Westmead Hospital, Sydney, Westmead New South Wales, Australia

JAN PAUL MEDEMA, PhD
Professor, Laboratory for Experimental Oncology and Radiobiology, Center for Experimental Molecular Medicine, Academic Medical Center (AMC), Amsterdam, The Netherlands

LEON M.G. MOONS, MD, PhD
Department of Gastroenterology and Hepatology, University Medical Center Utrecht, Utrecht, The Netherlands

MICHAEL F. PICCO, MD, PhD
Associate Professor, Gastroentrology and Hepatology, Mayo Clinic, Jacksonville, Florida

GOTTUMUKKALA S. RAJU, MD, FASGE
Professor of Medicine, Department of Gastroenterology, Hepatology and Nutrition, University of Texas MD Anderson Cancer Center, Houston, Texas

AMIT RASTOGI, MD
Associate Professor of Medicine, University of Kansas School of Medicine, University of Kansas, Department of Gastroenterology, Kansas City, Kansas; Veterans Affairs Medical Center, Department of Gastroenterology, Kansas City, Missouri

DOUGLAS K. REX, MD
Distinguished Professor of Medicine, Division of Gastroenterology/Hepatology, Department of Medicine, Indiana University School of Medicine, Indiana University, Indianapolis, Indiana

SHREYAS SALIGRAM, MD, MRCP
University of Kansas School of Medicine, University of Kansas, Department of Gastroenterology, Kansas City, Kansas; Veterans Affairs Medical Center, Kansas City, Missouri

BRIAN P. SAUNDERS, MD, FRCP
Consultant Gastroenterologist, Adjunct Professor of Endoscopy, Imperial College London, London; Director, Wolfson Unit for Endoscopy, St. Mark's Hospital, Harrow, Middlesex, United Kingdom

PETER D. SIERSEMA, MD, PhD, FASGE
Department of Gastroenterology and Hepatology, University Medical Center Utrecht, Utrecht, The Netherlands

CRISTIANO SPADA, MD
Gastroenterologist, Digestive Endoscopy Unit, Catholic University, Rome, Italy

SELVI THIRUMURTHI, MD, MS
Associate Professor of Medicine, Department of Gastroenterology, Hepatology and Nutrition, University of Texas MD Anderson Cancer Center, Houston, Texas

MICHAEL B. WALLACE, MD, MPH
Professor, Gastroentrology and Hepatology, Mayo Clinic, Jacksonville, Florida

ANA IGNJATOVIC WILSON, MD, MRCP
Consultant Gastroenterologist, Honorary Senior Lecturer, Imperial College London, London; Wolfson Unit for Endoscopy, St. Mark's Hospital, Harrow, Middlesex, United Kingdom

Contents

> Colorectal cancer (CRC) is a heterogeneous disease and each CRC possesses a unique molecular tumor profile. The main pathways of oncogenesis are the chromosomal instability, microsatellite instability and serrated neoplasia pathway. Sessile serrated adenomas/polyps (SSA/Ps) may be the precursor lesions of CRC arising via the serrated neoplasia pathway. This has led to a paradigm shift because all SSA/Ps should be detected and resected during colonoscopy. The ability to accurately detect and resect only those polyps with a malignant potential could result in safer and cost-effective practice. Optimization of the endoscopic classification systems is however needed to implement targeted prevention methods.

> Precolonoscopy bowel preparation is adequate to identify lesions larger than 5 mm about 70% to 75% of the time, but the opportunity for further improvement exists. The use of high-quality formulations with established efficacy rates of 90% or greater, identification of patients who are at increased risk of an inadequate preparation, as well as patient education and motivation to be invested in the process further improves the success of cleansing. Endoscopists should strive to achieve an adequate bowel preparation In 85% or more of patients. High-quality colonoscopy requires high-quality bowel cleansing.

> Performing high-quality colonoscopy is one of the important goals of gastroenterology practices and requires achieving a high level of bowel cleansing, performing good and safe polypectomy, and detecting all polyps present in the colon. This article summarizes currently available techniques and technologies to maximize mucosal visualization. Several maneuvers can be applied during insertion and withdrawal of the colonoscope to optimize mucosal visualization and decrease the number of missed polyps. Newly developed technologies support the endoscopist in the detection of polyps. Each technique is reviewed, with emphasis on the impact on colorectal polyp detection.

The successful intubation of the cecum during screening or surveillance colonoscopy is vital to ensure complete mucosal inspection of the colon on withdrawal. Even when performed by an experienced endoscopist, colonoscope insertion can sometimes be challenging. Water-aided colonoscopy can be used to assist the endoscopist in navigating colons with anatomies that may be challenging owing to severe angulation or redundancy. Water-assisted colonoscopy involves the infusion of water without air and subsequent suctioning during insertion (exchange) or withdrawal (immersion or infusion). This review discusses the technique, effectiveness, and safety of water-assisted colonoscopy as well as the application in sedationless endscopy.

Adenoma removal prevents colorectal cancer (CRC) development. Lower adenoma detection rates correlate with increased postcolonoscopy CRC. Chromoendoscopy it is not practical for routine use. It was hoped that electronic imaging techniques would offer effective alternatives to improve detection; however, meta-analyses in average-risk patients indicate no benefit. Narrow band imaging may be of benefit for high-risk surveillance. Combining electronic imaging techniques with molecular imaging probes may highlight dysplasia at a molecular level. In future colonoscopy is likely to rely on sensitive and specific, labeled molecular probes detected by electronic endoscopic imaging to enhance detection and reduce miss rates for premalignant lesions.

Chromoendoscopy techniques improve the visualization of mucosal structures. This article reviews and summarizes key studies addressing the impact of chromoendoscopy on colonic neoplasia detection and differentiation of neoplastic from non-neoplastic polyps in average and high-risk populations, including patients with colonic inflammatory bowel disease (IBD). In this context, there are convincing data that chromoendoscopy differentiates neoplastic from non-neoplastic polyps in average-risk populations with high accuracy. Moreover, dye-based chromoendoscopy improves neoplasia detection in colonic IBD surveillance.

Although removal of adenomatous polyps has been shown to decrease the risk of colon cancer, distal hyperplastic polyps are thought to not have malignant potential. Most polyps detected during colonoscopy are diminutive ($\leq$5 mm) and rarely harbor advanced histology, such as high-grade dysplasia or cancer. Therefore, predicting histology in real-time during colonoscopy can potentially decrease the enormous expenditure that ensues from universal histopathologic evaluation of polyps, and several novel imaging technologies have been developed and tested over the past decade for this purpose. Of these different technologies, electronic chromoendoscopy seems to strike a fair balance between accuracy, feasibility, and cost.

New Paradigms in Polypectomy: Resect and Discard, Diagnose and Disregard

Ana Ignjatovic Wilson and Brian P. Saunders

Polypectomy at colonoscopy has been shown to reduce the subsequent risk of colorectal cancer. With the advent of national screening programs, the number of colonoscopies performed has increased worldwide. In addition, the recent drive for quality improvement combined with advances in colonoscopic technology has resulted in increased numbers of polyps detected, resected, and sent for histopathology leading to spiraling costs associated with the procedure. Being able to diagnose small polyps in vivo (optical diagnosis) would allow for adenomas to be resected and discarded without the need to retrieve them or send them for formal histopathology.

Advanced Polypectomy and Resection Techniques

Amir Klein and Michael J. Bourke

Most colorectal cancer arises from adenomatous polyps. This gradual process may be interrupted by screening and treatment using colonoscopy and polypectomy. Advances in imaging platforms have led to classification systems that facilitate prediction of histologic type and both stratification for and prediction of the risk of invasion. Endoscopic treatment should be the standard of care even for extensive advanced mucosal neoplasm. Technique selection is influenced by lesion features, location, patient factors, and local expertise. Postprocedural complications are more common following advanced resection and endoscopists should be familiar with risk factors, early detection methods, and management.

Management of Polypectomy Complications

Selvi Thirumurthi and Gottumukkala S. Raju

The 2 most significant complications of colonoscopy with polypectomy are bleeding and perforation. Incidence rates for bleeding (0.1%–0.6%) and perforation (0.7%–0.9%) are generally low. Recognition of pertinent risk factors helps to prevent these complications, which can be grouped into patient-related, polyp-related, and technique/device-related factors. Endoscopists should be equipped to manage bleeding and perforation. Currently available devices and techniques are reviewed to achieve hemostasis and close colon perforations.

Colonic Strictures: Dilation and Stents

Douglas G. Adler

Colonic strictures, both benign and malignant, are commonly encountered in clinical practice. Benign strictures are most commonly treated by balloon dilation and less frequently with stents. Balloon dilation can help forestall or obviate surgery in some patients. Colonic strictures of malignant etiology generally need to be managed by stents and/or surgery.

GASTROINTESTINAL ENDOSCOPY CLINICS OF NORTH AMERICA

GASTROINTESTINAL ENDOSCOPY CLINICS
OF NORTH AMERICA

FORTHCOMING ISSUES

July 2015
Upper Gastrointestinal Bleeding
John Saltzman, Editor

October 2015
Advances in ERCP
Adam Slivka, Editor

RECENT ISSUES

October 2014
Esophageal Function Testing
John Pandolfino, Editor

July 2014
Nonpolypoid Colorectal Neoplasms in
Inflammatory Bowel Disease
Roy Soetikno and Tonya Kaltenbach,
Editors

ISSUE OF RELATED INTEREST

Gastroenterology Clinics of North America March 2014 (Vol 43, No 1)
Gastroesophageal Reflux Disease
Joel Richter, Editor

Foreword
Modern Colonoscopy Continues to Evolve and Improve

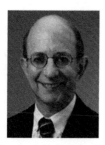

Charles J. Lightdale, MD
Consulting Editor

This is not your father's colonoscopy. A generation ago, it seemed that colonoscopy had probably peaked and couldn't get much better. Colonoscopy became the method of choice for colorectal cancer screening and prevention. The impact of colonoscopy on decreasing mortality from colorectal cancer was documented and proven. But, as the data accumulated, it also became clear that there were colon cancers diagnosed in a small percentage of patients who had negative colonoscopies in the recent past. Most of these cancers were in the right side of the colon. Fortunately, colonoscopy has changed to address these issues. A new generation of experts have set a higher bar for colonoscopy and have shown the ways that colonoscopy can improve and rise to greater levels of achievement.

If there could be an epicenter of modern colonoscopy, it would have to be placed in Indianapolis at Indiana University (IU). Drs Douglas Rex and Charles Kahi from IU have been without a doubt at the forefront of the revolution in colonoscopy with a focus on improving the prevention of colon cancer. They are the guest editors for this issue of the *Gastrointestinal Endoscopy Clinics of North America*, which is dedicated to "Advances in Colonoscopy." They have taken a comprehensive approach and have gathered a formidable group of international experts to cooperate in covering all the key topics that must be understood and mastered. From new insights into colon cancer biology and different polyp-cancer pathways, from descriptions of new techniques and technologies for detecting, diagnosing, and removing colon lesions, from better colon preps, to improving operator standards and quality, this issue has it all. For most gastrointestinal endoscopists, colonoscopy is the most important and

Gastrointest Endoscopy Clin N Am 25 (2015) xiii–xiv
http://dx.doi.org/10.1016/j.giec.2015.02.001
1052-5157/15/$ – see front matter © 2015 Elsevier Inc. All rights reserved.

giendo.theclinics.com

frequently performed endoscopic procedure. If you want to perform colonoscopy at the highest level, this issue of the *Gastrointestinal Endoscopy Clinics of North America* is essential reading.

Charles J. Lightdale, MD
Division of Digestive and Liver Diseases
Columbia University Medical Center
161 Fort Washington Avenue, Room 812
New York, NY 10032, USA

E-mail address:
CJL18@cumc.columbia.edu

Preface
Advances in Colonoscopy

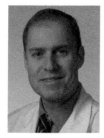 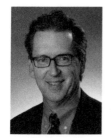

Charles J. Kahi, MD, MSc   Douglas K. Rex, MD
Editors

Colonoscopy is arguably the medical procedure with the most profound and lasting impact on patients' lives. High-quality colonoscopy with polypectomy prevents colorectal cancer and is the dominant colorectal screening modality in the United States. The effectiveness of colonoscopy is based on considerable observational data, which also show that the level of protection in the proximal colon is variable and operator-dependent. Reducing this operator dependence has become a research and quality improvement priority, and the past few years have witnessed extraordinary developments in the field of colonoscopy. These have included advances in our understanding of colorectal neoplasia pathways, new methods to achieve optimal bowel preparation, improvements in colonoscopy technique, novel technologies including paradigm-shifting ones that allow virtual histologic assessment of polyps, and advances in polypectomy and therapeutic colonoscopy.

This issue of *Gastrointestinal Endoscopy Clinics of North America* assembles a team of well-known international experts, who have devoted their careers to the fight against colorectal cancer, to provide an overview of the latest developments in the field of

Gastrointest Endoscopy Clin N Am 25 (2015) xv–xvi
http://dx.doi.org/10.1016/j.giec.2015.01.001
1052-5157/15/$ – see front matter © 2015 Published by Elsevier Inc.

giendo.theclinics.com

colonoscopy and polypectomy. We are indebted to them for sharing their time and expertise, and making this volume a reality. We hope you will find it informative, and of help in your practice.

Charles J. Kahi, MD, MSc
Indiana University School of Medicine
Indianapolis, IN 46202, USA

Richard L. Roudebush VA Medical Center
Indianapolis, IN 46202, USA

Douglas K. Rex, MD
Department of Medicine
Division of Gastroenterology/Hepatology
Indiana University School of Medicine
Indiana University
Indianapolis, IN 46202, USA

E-mail addresses:
ckahi2@iu.edu (C.J. Kahi)
drex@iupui.edu (D.K. Rex)

Colorectal Neoplasia Pathways: State of the Art

Joep Evert Godfried IJspeert, MD[a], Jan Paul Medema, PhD[b],
Evelien Dekker, MD, PhD[c],*

KEYWORDS

- Colorectal cancer • Chromosomal instability • Microsatellite instability
- Serrated neoplasia pathway • Colonoscopy • Colorectal polyps

KEY POINTS

- Colorectal cancer (CRC) is a very heterogeneous disease resulting from multiple over-arching neoplasia pathways, of which the chromosomal instability, the microsatellite instability, and the serrated neoplasia pathways are the most significant.
- Besides conventional adenomas, serrated polyps also seem to be precursor lesions of CRC, arising via the serrated neoplasia pathway.
- Accurate endoscopic characterization of premalignant colonic lesions would enable the implementation of targeted treatment in the near future, resulting in effective, safe, as well as cost-effective CRC prevention.

INTRODUCTION

Colorectal cancer (CRC) is a very heterogeneous disease with regards to tumor development as well as clinical tumor behavior. Due to the presence or absence of diverse genetic and epigenetic alterations, each CRC appears to possess a unique molecular tumor profile.[1] The oncogenesis of CRC is extensively evaluated compared to other solid tumors in the human body (**Fig. 1**). This is partly due to its high priority because CRC has high morbidity and mortality rates in the Western world.[2] Other factors are the slow progression of disease and the possibility to sample CRC precursor lesions, enabling the assessment of molecular changes in consecutive steps of tumorigenesis.[3]

Disclosure Statement and Competing Interests: For all authors, none to declare.
[a] Department of Gastroenterology and Hepatology, Academic Medical Center, Meibergdreef 9, Room C2-231, Amsterdam 1105 AZ The Netherlands; [b] Laboratory for Experimental Oncology and Radiobiology, Center for Experimental Molecular Medicine, Academic Medical Center (AMC), Meibergdreef 9, Room G2-131, Amsterdam 1105 AZ, The Netherlands; [c] Department of Gastroenterology and Hepatology, Academic Medical Center, Meibergdreef 9, Room C2-115, Amsterdam 1105 AZ, The Netherlands
* Corresponding author.
E-mail address: e.dekker@amc.uva.nl

Gastrointest Endoscopy Clin N Am 25 (2015) 169–182
http://dx.doi.org/10.1016/j.giec.2014.11.004
1052-5157/15/$ – see front matter © 2015 Elsevier Inc. All rights reserved.

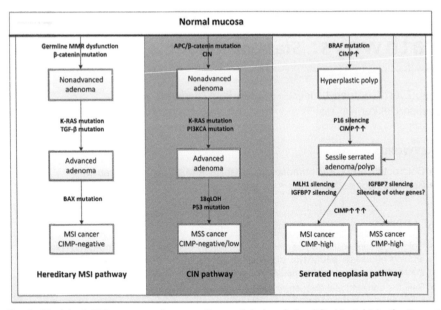

Fig. 1. Model of CRC oncogenesis presenting a global and simplified insight in the 3 most studied colorectal neoplasia pathways.

Until recently, conventional adenomas (further referred to as adenomas) were regarded as the only precursors of CRC, developing into cancer via the adenoma-carcinoma pathway.[4] A multistep molecular sequence responsible for the adenoma-carcinoma pathway was first described by Fearon and Vogelstein.[5] Although more recent literature has demonstrated that a minority of CRCs arise exactly via the pathway described by Fearon and Vogelstein,[5] the model has long been a prominent paradigm for research concerning the origin of CRC and other solid tumors.[6] Currently, multiple colorectal neoplasia pathways are distinguished, of which the chromosomal instability (CIN) pathway; the microsatellite instability (MSI) pathway; and the CpG island methylator pathway (CIMP), also referred to as the serrated neoplasia pathway, are the best studied.[7–9] Oncogenesis occurring via these pathways may, however, not be completely separated. Crossover, or even overlap, between the pathways is likely to exist. Serrated polyps (SPs), rather than adenomas, are suggested to be the precursor lesions of CRC arising via the serrated neoplasia pathway, responsible for approximately 15% to 30% of CRC.[10–12] This finding has led to an important paradigm shift in daily practice for colonoscopies because it has become apparent that adenomas as well as premalignant SP subtypes should be detected and resected to effectively prevent CRC.[13]

Only a small percentage of polyps seem to develop into CRC, whereas most polyps remain stable over time or even regress.[14,15] However, for adenomas as well as for SPs, it is unclear which molecular alterations induce the final transition toward invasive growth. As a result, it is still largely unknown which lesions will develop into CRC and which lesions will have a benign course. Profound knowledge of the colorectal neoplasia pathways is essential for each endoscopist to optimize current prevention strategies. Ongoing research could, it is hoped, lead toward the targeted resection of truly premalignant colorectal lesions in the near future.

FROM ADENOMA TO CARCINOMA

Histopathologically, every adenoma can be subdivided based on the severity of dysplasia (low-grade or high-grade) and presence and proportion of a villous component (tubular, tubulovillous or villous adenoma).[16] It is generally accepted that adenomas with high-grade dysplasia and/or villous components harbor an increased risk to develop into cancer compared with tubular adenomas with low-grade dysplasia. Studies that show the natural course of adenomas are, however, scarce.[14,15,17,18] Several decades ago, Muto and colleagues[17] demonstrated in an observational study that less than 5% of small tubular adenomas with low-grade dysplasia will eventually transform into CRC. This percentage increased significantly for adenomas with high-grade dysplasia and/or a villous component. In a more recent study, Brenner and colleagues[18] demonstrated that the 10-year cumulative risk of an advanced adenoma ($\geq$25% villous component, high-grade dysplasia or size $\geq$10 mm) to develop into cancer was increased from 25.4% at age 55 years to 42.9% at age 80 years in women, and from 25.2% at age 55 years to 39.7% at age 80 years in men. In this study, risk estimates were based on CRC incidence and the prevalence of advanced adenomas per age group. In an endoscopic study, Hofstad and colleagues[14] demonstrated that small adenomas (6–9 mm) left in situ may partly regress or partly increase in size, whereas 25% of polyps appeared unchanged after 3 years. In a computed tomography–colography study, Pickhardt and colleagues[15] demonstrated that small adenomas with a prominent villous component or high-grade dysplasia show a more rapid growth than small tubular adenomas with low-grade dysplasia. Polyps were acquired via polypectomy after a mean surveillance of 2.3 years. These studies strengthen the hypothesis that advanced adenomas possess a higher malignant potential than nonadvanced adenomas.

The Chromosomal Instability Pathway

The CIN pathway is the most evaluated sequence of colorectal carcinogenesis, arising from adenoma precursor lesions. It is suggested that around 70% of CRCs arise via the CIN pathway.[7,10] CIN refers to structural changes or numerical gains or losses of chromosomes that result in variability in the karyotype of individual cells (aneuploidy) and subsequent loss of heterozygosity (LOH) of genes.[19] Karyotype copy defects during cell mitosis are responsible for chromosome instability. The exact underlying cause of aneuploidy is unknown.[20] The total dwell time of tumor development via the CIN pathway is assumed to be approximately 10 to 15 years.[17]

Initiation of adenoma development

An important initiating mutation for early adenoma development is the mutation of the adenomatous polyposis coli (APC) tumor suppressor gene, which has a role in the Wnt pathway.[21] Familial adenomatous polyposis (FAP) has served as a valuable model to evaluate the exact function of the APC gene.[22] FAP patients have a germline mutation in the APC gene, which results in the phenotypic expression of hundreds of adenomas throughout the colorectum. The inactivation of APC will result in accumulation of β-catenin and a subsequent stimulation of T-cell factor-1 (TCF-1) and lymphoid enhancing factor-1 (LEF-1) transcription factors. This will result in increased proliferation of colorectal cells.[3,23] The Wnt pathway can also be triggered via a gain-of function mutation in β-catenin, which is present in up to 50% of CIN-tumors without an APC mutation.[24]

A second prevalent mutation in early adenoma development is the Kirsten-rat sarcoma 2 viral oncogene homolog (K-RAS) proto-oncogene mutation, which is involved in the mitogen-activated protein kinase (MAPK) cascade.[25] Point mutations are found in 30% to 40% of CRCs.[25] RAS proteins act as molecular switches that control intracellular signal transduction and are important for cell proliferation and apoptosis.[26] A K-RAS mutation can result in resistance to inhibition of surface receptors, such as the epidermal growth factor receptor, and will permit the cell to evade apoptosis.[3]

Progression of adenomas

A late event in colorectal tumorigenesis is a mutation in the p53 tumor suppressor gene, located on chromosome 17p.[27] p53 is often defined as the guardian of the genome, playing an essential role in its stability.[28] A mutation in p53 or 17p allelic loss has been reported in 4% to 26% of adenomas, in approximately 50% of adenomas with high-grade dysplasia, and in 50% to 75% of adenocarcinomas. This distribution of results has led to the belief that functional inactivation of p53 protein might be associated with the transition from adenoma to carcinoma, although it is unclear whether this mutation is absolutely required.[29]

LOH of chromosome 18q is a genetic alteration that occurs in approximately 70% of colorectal adenocarcinomas.[30] Many tumor suppressor genes are located on chromosome 18q of which deleted in colorectal carcinoma (DCC), SMAD 4, and SMAD 2 are important in regulation of controlled cell proliferation and apoptosis.[1] 18q loss is often co-occurring with the loss of p53. Combined loss occurs in 65% of CRC.[31]

Co-occurring events

Many other molecular events are described in the CIN pathway to CRC. For example, a mutation in the PI3K pathway is often seen, which can eventually result in accelerated cell growth.[3] Also, microRNAs may play a role in the tumorigenesis of CIN-derived CRCs. MicroRNAs are noncoding RNAs that regulate protein expression by inhibition of messenger RNA translation. The amount of microRNAs involved in CRC pathogenesis is large and expanding. MicroRNAs can be upregulated or downregulated in CRC, operating like oncogenes and tumor suppressor genes.[3]

The Microsatellite Instability Pathway

The second major colorectal neoplasia pathway in which adenomas are involved is the MSI pathway. Around 15% of CRCs possess genetic instability due to MSI.[10] Of these tumors, approximately 20% have a hereditary cause and arise in patients with a germline mutation in one of the mismatch repair genes, the Lynch syndrome.[32] The other 80% of MSI CRC seem to arise due to the hypermethylation of the promoter of the human MutL homologue (hMLH) 1, a specific mismatch repair gene.[9] The latter is a sporadic epigenetic alteration, which may exemplify a distinct pathway to colon cancer and is suggested to play an important role in the serrated neoplasia pathway (see later discussion). The pathophysiology of mismatch repair (MMR) system dysfunction and subsequent elevated cancer risk does, however, also account for tumors with a sporadic cause of MMR dysfunction.[11] Tumor development via the hereditary MSI pathway is assumed to be faster compared with CIN oncogenesis, resulting in CRC within approximately 3 to 5 years.[33]

Pathophysiology of MMR dysfunction

Microsatellites or simple sequence repeats are repeated nucleotide sequences of DNA made of base-pairs, prone to mutations and base-pair substitutions during replication.[34] The MMR system identifies and corrects errors that occur during the replication of DNA polymerase. MMR dysfunction will result in instability in the length of microsatellites, causing frame-shift mutations.[35] The mutation rate in the DNA of a colorectal mucosal cell is increased by a 100-fold when the MMR system is disabled, facilitating accelerated tumorigenesis.[36] A mutation in one of the MMR genes is an important factor in oncogenesis, but is not singly sufficient to develop CRC.[9]

Other molecular alterations in the hereditary microsatellite instability pathway
Activation of the Wnt pathway is an important factor in early adenoma development in the hereditary MSI pathway, although not always observed. However, compared with the CIN pathway, Wnt pathway activation is more often due to a mutation in β-catenin than in the APC gene.[37] In addition, alterations in the MAPK pathway seem to play a role in CRC development in patients with Lynch syndrome. K-RAS is often mutated in these patients.[9] Another role is reserved for transforming growth factor-β, which is an inhibitor of epithelial cell growth. More than 80% of tumors derived via the hereditary MSI pathway harbor a mutation in this gene.[38]

Transition to CRC seems to occur by influence of a mutation in the human BAX gene, which is normally activated by p53.[39] A mutation in the BAX gene will result in an escape from intrinsic cell apoptosis, equal to a p53 gene mutation. A study demonstrated that 54.2% of Lynch syndrome CRCs showed a BAX-gene mutation, while only 4.2% of tumors showed a p53 mutation.[40]

SERRATED POLYPS, AN ALTERNATIVE ROUTE TO COLORECTAL CANCER

Historically, colonic polyps were mainly subdivided into adenomas and hyperplastic (or metaplastic) polyps (HPs).[17] Whereas adenomas were considered premalignant, HPs were regarded as harmless, not harboring any neoplastic potential. Research from the last decades, however, has changed these views. The recent classification of the World Health Organization has reorganized HPs into an overarching group of SPs, histopathologically characterized by a saw-tooth infolding of the crypt epithelium.[16] SPs are subdivided into HPs, sessile serrated adenomas/polyps (SSA/Ps) and traditional serrated adenomas (TSAs). HPs can be further subdivided into a microvesicular-type HP (MVHP), a goblet cell–type HP, and a mucin-poor–type HP.[16] It is suggested that SSA/Ps are the main precursors of CRC developing via the serrated neoplasia pathway, responsible for approximately 15% to 30% of CRCs.[10–12] TSAs are also considered premalignant; however, oncogenesis is indistinct and TSAs seem to be very rare in asymptomatic patient cohorts.[41,42]

Several studies have compared the molecular profile of conventional adenomas, SPs, and CRCs, and detected a high correlation between SPs and a subset of CRCs.[43–45] This has led to the proposal of a colonic mucosa→MVHP→SSA/P→SSA/P with dysplasia→CRC sequence.[46] In this pathway, it is yet unclear if SSA/Ps could also directly originate from colonic mucosa without HPs as an intermediate stage. The natural course of SSA/Ps, as well as HPs, however, is indistinct and no proper studies have been performed that demonstrate the actual cancer risk of individual SPs.[47] In one study, subjects diagnosed with a single SSA/P were prospectively followed for a median of 7.2 years. In total, 12.5% of these subjects developed cancer, compared with 1.8% for matched subjects diagnosed with an HP or tubular adenoma.[48] In a recent study based on genome-wide profiling of gene expression, a subset of CRCs showed close molecular similarities to SSA/P and had an unfavorable prognosis.[49] Therefore, it seems important that all SSA/Ps are detected and radically resected during colonoscopy to prevent CRC.

The Serrated Neoplasia Pathway

The existence of the serrated neoplasia pathway as a distinct sequence to CRC was first described approximately 15 years ago and is characterized by hypermethylation and subsequent silencing of tumor-suppressor genes as well as a mutation in the BRAF-oncogene.[10,46,50] Much is learned from patients with serrated polyposis syndrome to gain a better understanding of the molecular changes found in the serrated neoplasia pathway.[51] However, the total dwell time of tumorigenesis is largely unknown. A relatively rapid development of CRC is suggested in the literature, comparable with carcinogenesis in patients with Lynch syndrome.[52] A relatively slow progression of disease is also proposed based on a cross-sectional study using computerized algorithms, showing a median transition time of 15 years from SSA/P to CRC.[53]

Key features of the serrated neoplasia pathway

The key feature of oncogenesis via the serrated neoplasia pathway is the hypermethylation of CpG islands on the promoter regions of tumor suppressor genes, resulting in subsequent silencing of these genes.[12] The CIMP is a common way to describe the methylation status of a lesion, which can be expressed as a CIMP-high, CIMP-low, or CIMP-negative phenotype.[54] In 2 recent studies, the CIMP-high phenotype was found in 20% to 26% of SPs, which increased to 63% for proximal SSA/Ps.[44,45] The CIMP-high phenotype was detected in approximately 1% of adenomas, indicating an association between SPs and CIMP-high CRC. For this reason, the serrated neoplasia pathway is also often referred to as the CIMP pathway. It is also plausible that a small subset of CIMP-high CRCs arise from adenomas rather than from SPs. Similarly, some SPs may develop into CRCs without CIMP.

Hypermethylation and subsequent silencing of hMLH1 is an important step for oncogenesis in CIMP-high tumors and will lead to a dysfunction of the MMR system and subsequent MSI, comparable with a germline mutation in hMLH1 as seen in Lynch syndrome.[55] Although silencing of MLH1 is a major and accelerating step in oncogenesis via the serrated neoplasia pathway, it is not obligatory. Jass[10] showed that, in a cohort of subjects with CRC, 12% of tumors had a CIMP-high MSI phenotype, whereas 8% had a CIMP-high microsatellite stable (MSS) phenotype, both highly correlated to SPs.

Other well-described molecular alterations are the silencing of tumor suppressor genes p16 and IGFB7. P16 is a cell cycle inhibitor and dysfunction will result in senescence of the lesion and progression from nonadvanced to more advanced precursor lesions.[56] IGFBP7 functions downstream of p53 and silencing of this gene can mimic the inactivation of p53 associated to the progression from advanced precursor lesions to CRC.[57]

A mutation in the BRAF-oncogene seems to be another key feature in the serrated neoplasia pathway.[58] BRAF has a role in the MAPK cascade and is regulated by the activity of K-RAS. A point mutation in BRAF will result in uncontrolled cell proliferation, comparable with the effect of a K-RAS mutation, often seen in adenomas.[59] In 2 large recent studies the presence of a BRAF mutation was found in 50% to 72% of MVHPs, 70% to 80% of SSA/Ps, and only 1% of adenomas.[45,60] Another study showed a strong correlation between the presence of a BRAF mutation and a CIMP-high phenotype in CRC. A BRAF mutation was found in 77% of CIMP-high tumors, 18% of CIMP-low, and 0% of CIMP-negative CRCs.[58] These results strengthen the hypothesis of a distinct serrated neoplasia pathway arising from SPs and resulting in CIMP-high, BRAF-mutant CRCs.

CLINICAL IMPLICATIONS: WHICH POLYPS TO RESECT?

It has been demonstrated that resecting all polyps during colonoscopy reduces CRC incidence.[61] This strategy is, however, related to an increased duration of the colonoscopy procedure, an increased risk of adverse events, and a substantial increase in costs.[62,63] Ideally, only those polyps with a truly increased risk to develop into cancer would be resected during colonoscopy, whereas lesions with a benign natural history would be left in situ. Several difficulties hamper the implementation of targeted polyp resection in daily practice. First, for adenomas, as well as for SPs, it is still unknown exactly which lesions will eventually evolve into cancer. Second, for such a strategy, accurate endoscopic, as well as pathologic, characterization of lesions with an increased malignant potential is important but difficult. Great progress has been made in recent years. Representative images of several polyp subtypes are shown in **Fig. 2**.

Endoscopic Characterization of High-Risk Adenomas

A great amount of research has been performed to enable the characterization of adenomas with an increased malignant potential during colonoscopy. Several endoscopic features are characterized, of which the most important seems to be polyp size. In a systematic review using data from 4 studies with 20,562 screening colonoscopies, Hassan and colleagues[64] showed that presence of an equal to or greater than 25% villous component and/or high-grade dysplasia was detected in 4.6% (95% CI 3.4–5.8) of diminutive, 7.9% (95% CI 6.3–9.4) of small, and 87.5% (95% CI 86–89.4) of large polyps. For this reason, adenoma size equal to or greater than 10 mm is taken into account in the definition of an advanced adenoma.[65]

Adenoma morphology might also help identify adenomas with an increased risk. In a large cross-sectional study, Soetikno and colleagues[66] showed that approximately 15% of adenomas have a nonpolypoid (flat or depressed) morphology. These lesions were more likely to contain carcinoma compared with polypoid lesions, irrespective of size (odds ratio, 9.78; 95% CI 3.93–24.4). To warrant universal practice for the assessment of polyp morphology, the Paris classification was designed. In the Paris classification, Japanese, European, and American classification systems were combined to facilitate the characterization of adenomas with an increased cancer risk.[67] A recent study, however, showed that the interobserver variability among endoscopists using the Paris classification for the assessment of polyp morphology was very high.[68] A simplified classification system might, therefore, be helpful to increase homogeneity in the assessment of polyp morphology.

A third characteristic that could help differentiate between advanced and nonadvanced adenomas is the polyp pit pattern. Kudo and colleagues[69] were the first to describe a classification system based on pit pattern that enables characterization of HPs, tubular adenomas, adenomas with a villous component, and adenomas with a component of invasive growth. This validated classification system showed high accuracy when used by expert gastroenterologists.[70] Other current classification systems, such as the narrow-band imaging (NBI) international colorectal endoscopic (NICE) criteria, do not differentiate between subtypes of adenomas.

Endoscopic Characterization of High-Risk Serrated Polyps

Several endoscopic characteristics enable the differentiation of SP subtypes, although difficult. First, polyp location could help to characterize SPs with an increased malignant potential. Approximately 75% of HPs are found in the left-side colon, whereas SSA/P are more often proximally located.[46,71] Recent literature however showed that the proportion of distally located SSA/Ps (40%) was reasonably large and that SSA/Ps with dysplasia might even be equally divided throughout the colorectum.[42,72]

Second, polyp size could help to identify SSA/Ps. Hazewinkel and colleagues[42] showed that in an average-risk population the median size of HPs is 3 mm, whereas median size of SSA/Ps is 5 mm, increasing to 7 mm in the right-side colon. Bouwens and colleagues,[72] however, showed that SSA/Ps with or without dysplasia do not

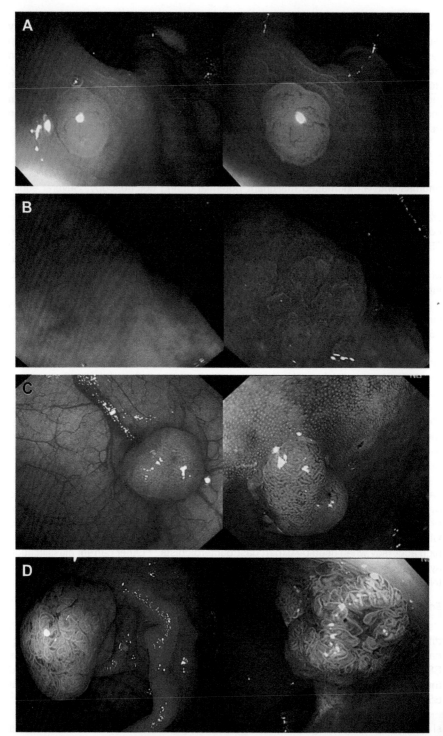

Fig. 2. Representative high-resolution white light endoscopy image and NBI image of several polyp subtypes: (*A*) HP; (*B*) SSA/P; (*C*) tubular adenoma; (*D*) villous adenoma.

differ in size. Rosty and colleagues[71] showed that the mean size of SSA/P with an associated malignant component is also small, with a median size of 9 mm.

Tadepalli and colleagues[73] described 7 endoscopic characteristics to characterize SSA/Ps. The most prevalent visual descriptors were the presence of a mucus cap (63.9%), rim of debris or bubbles (51.9%), alteration of the contour of a fold (37.3%), and interruption of the underlying mucosal vascular pattern (32.3%).[73] In a recent study, no differences could be found between SSA/P with or without dysplasia using these visual descriptors, except for a dome-shaped presentation.[72] Hazewinkel and colleagues[74] also described endoscopic features to characterize SSA/Ps using NBI. The presence of a clouded surface, indistinct borders, irregular shape, and dark spots inside the crypts were individually associated with SSA/Ps in a multivariate regression analysis compared with HPs.

Histopathologic Differentiation of Serrated Polyps

Besides the endoscopic difficulties differentiating SP subtypes, the histopathological differentiation of SSA/Ps and HPs is also difficult. Histopathologically, the presence of at least 2 irregular dilated crypts, including dilatation of the base of the crypts, is suggestive for SSA/P.[16] Identification of these dilated crypts is subjective and the interobserver agreement between pathologists in the differentiation of SSA/Ps and HPs is, therefore, poor.[75] Consequently, histopathologic assessment of SPs is preferably performed by pathologists with expertise in the gastrointestinal tract. Comprehensive training of pathologists is necessary to achieve universal practice in the near future.

Toward Targeted Polyp Resection

Based on current knowledge, several classification systems have been developed to endoscopically differentiate between neoplastic and non-neoplastic colonic polyp subtypes, of which the Kudo classification and the NICE classification are the most significant.[69,76] The above described Kudo classification is validated using both chromoendoscopy and magnifying endoscopy and has been proven to be highly accurate among experts.[70] The simpler NICE classification is validated for the differentiation of small and diminutive adenomas, HPs, and submucosal invasive carcinoma.[76,77] This classification system makes use of the increased vascularization of adenomas compared with HPs to differentiate both polyp subtypes. A major drawback of the Kudo, as well as the NICE classification, is that the characterization of premalignant SSA/Ps is not facilitated, causing premalignant SSA/Ps to be diagnosed as neoplastic or as non-neoplastic polyp equally often.[78] Implementation of targeted polyp resection based on these classification systems seems hindered at this time. The development of an integrative system that enables the characterization of all prevalent polyp subtypes, including SSA/Ps, should be developed and validated. Such a system could contribute to the implementation of more balanced CRC prevention strategies in the near future.

SUMMARY

CRC is a very common and heterogeneous disease in which the accumulation of genetic and epigenetic alterations via overarching pathways will result in tumors with a unique molecular profile. The molecular comparison of CRC and polyps has led to the designation of neoplastic as well as non-neoplastic lesions, which is of interest in the context of preventive strategies. The ability to accurately detect and resect only those polyps with a malignant potential could result in a safer as well as more cost-effective practice in the near future. Promising research has been performed to achieve these goals. Optimization of the current classification systems is necessary to ensure safe implementation. This could result in well-balanced practice to prevent CRC, based on the current knowledge on the different colorectal neoplasia pathways.

REFERENCES

1. Sideris M, Papagrigoriadis S. Molecular biomarkers and classification models in the evaluation of the prognosis of colorectal cancer. Anticancer Res 2014;34(5): 2061–8.
2. Siegel R, Naishadham D, Jemal A. Cancer statistics, 2013. CA Cancer J Clin 2013;63(1):11–30. http://dx.doi.org/10.3322/caac.21166.
3. Colussi D, Brandi G, Bazzoli F, et al. Molecular pathways involved in colorectal cancer: implications for disease behavior and prevention. Int J Mol Sci 2013; 14:16365–85. http://dx.doi.org/10.3390/ijms140816365.
4. Jackman R, Mayo C. The adenoma-carcinoma sequence in cancer of the colon. Surg Gynecol Obstet 1951;93(3):327–30.
5. Fearon EF, Vogelstein B. A genetic model for colorectal tumorigenesis. Cell 1990; 61:759–67.
6. Fearon ER. Molecular genetics of colorectal cancer. Annu Rev Pathol 2011;6: 479–507. http://dx.doi.org/10.1146/annurev-pathol-011110-130235.
7. Pino MS, Chung DC. The chromosomal instability pathway in colon cancer. Gastroenterology 2010;138(6):2059–72. http://dx.doi.org/10.1053/j.gastro.2009. 12.065.
8. Leggett B, Whitehall V. Role of the serrated pathway in colorectal cancer pathogenesis. Gastroenterology 2010;138:2088–100. http://dx.doi.org/10.1053/j.gastro. 2009.12.066.
9. Boland CR, Goel A. Microsatellite instability in colorectal cancer. Gastroenterology 2010;138. http://dx.doi.org/10.1053/j.gastro.2009.12.064.
10. Jass JR. Classification of colorectal cancer based on correlation of clinical, morphological and molecular features. Histopathology 2007;50(1):113–30. http://dx.doi.org/10.1111/j.1365-2559.2006.02549.x.
11. Snover DC. Update on the serrated pathway to colorectal carcinoma. Hum Pathol 2011;42(1):1–10. http://dx.doi.org/10.1016/j.humpath.2010.06.002.
12. Toyota M, Ahuja N, Ohe-Toyota M, et al. CpG island methylator phenotype in colorectal cancer. Proc Natl Acad Sci U S A 1999;96:8681–6. http://dx.doi.org/10. 1073/pnas.96.15.8681.
13. Torlakovic E, Skovlund E, Snover DC, et al. Morphologic reappraisal of serrated colorectal polyps. Am J Surg Pathol 2003;27(1):65–81. Available at: http://www. ncbi.nlm.nih.gov/pubmed/12502929.
14. Hofstad B, Vatn MH, Andersen SN, et al. Growth of colorectal polyps: redetection and evaluation of unresected polyps for a period of three years. Gut 1996;39(3): 449–56.
15. Pickhardt PJ, Kim DH, Pooler BD, et al. Assessment of volumetric growth rates of small colorectal polyps with CT colonography: a longitudinal study of natural history. Lancet Oncol 2013;14:711–20. http://dx.doi.org/10.1016/S1470-2045(13)70216-X.
16. Bosman FT, Carneiro F, Hruban R. World Health Organization classification of tumours of the digestive system. Lyon (France): IARC Press; 2010. p. 160–5.
17. Muto T, Bussey HJ, Morson B. The evolution of cancer of the colon and rectum. Cancer 1975;6(36):2251–70.
18. Brenner H, Hoffmeister M, Stegmaier C, et al. Risk of progression of advanced adenomas to colorectal cancer by age and sex: estimates based on 840,149

screening colonoscopies. Gut 2007;56:1585–9. http://dx.doi.org/10.1136/gut. 2007.122739.

19. Lengauer C, Kinzler KW, Vogelstein B. Genetic instabilities in human cancers. Nature 1998;396:643–9. http://dx.doi.org/10.1038/25292.

20. Decordier I, Cundari E, Kirsch-Volders M. Mitotic checkpoints and the maintenance of the chromosome karyotype. Mutat Res 2008;651:3–13. http://dx.doi.org/10.1016/j.mrgentox.2007.10.020.

21. Powell SM, Zilz N, Beazer-Barclay Y, et al. APC mutations occur early during colorectal tumorigenesis. Nature 1992;359:235–7. http://dx.doi.org/10.1038/359235a0.

22. Bodmer W, Bailey C, Bodmer J, et al. Localization of the gene for familial adenomatous polyposis on chromosome 5. Nature 1987;328(6131):614–6.

23. Sierra J, Yoshida T, Joazeiro CA, et al. The APC tumor suppressor counteracts beta-catenin activation and H3K4 methylation at Wnt target genes. Genes Dev 2006;20:586–600. http://dx.doi.org/10.1101/gad.1385806.

24. Morin PJ, Sparks AB, Korinek V, et al. Activation of beta-catenin-Tcf signaling in colon cancer by mutations in beta-catenin or APC. Science 1997;275:1787–90. http://dx.doi.org/10.1126/science.275.5307.1787.

25. Church D, Midgley R, Kerr D. Biomarkers in early-stage colorectal cancer: ready for prime time? Dig Dis 2012;30(Suppl 2):27–33. http://dx.doi.org/10.1159/000341890.

26. Pruitt K, Der CJ. Ras and Rho regulation of the cell cycle and oncogenesis. Cancer Lett 2001;171:1–10. http://dx.doi.org/10.1016/S0304-3835(01)00528-6.

27. Baker SJ, Preisinger AC, Jessup JM, et al. p53 gene mutations occur in combination with 17p allelic deletions as late events in colorectal tumorigenesis. Cancer Res 1990;50:7717–22.

28. Bálint EE, Vousden KH. Activation and activities of the p53 tumour suppressor protein. Br J Cancer 2001;85:1813–23. http://dx.doi.org/10.1054/bjoc.2001.2128.

29. Leslie A, Carey FA, Pratt NR, et al. The colorectal adenoma-carcinoma sequence. Br J Surg 2002;89(7):845–60. http://dx.doi.org/10.1046/j.1365-2168.2002.02120.x.

30. Vogelstein B, Fearon ER, Hamilton SR, et al. Genetic alterations during colorectal-tumor development. N Engl J Med 1988;319:525–32. http://dx.doi.org/10.1097/00043764-198910000-00001.

31. Lanza G, Matteuzzi M, Gafá R, et al. Chromosome 18q allelic loss and prognosis in stage II and III colon cancer. Int J Cancer 1998;79:390–5 pii:10.1002/(SICI)1097-0215(19980821)79:4<390::AID-IJC14>3.0.CO;2–9.

32. Lynch HT, Smyrk T, Lynch JF. Overview of natural history, pathology, molecular genetics and management of HNPCC (Lynch syndrome). Int J Cancer 1996;69:38–43 pii:10.1002/(SICI)1097-0215(19960220)69:1<38::AID-IJC9>3.0.CO;2-X.

33. Edelstein DL, Axilbund J, Baxter M, et al. Rapid development of colorectal neoplasia in patients with lynch syndrome. Clin Gastroenterol Hepatol 2011;9:340–3. http://dx.doi.org/10.1016/j.cgh.2010.10.033.

34. Lee JK, Chan AT. Molecular prognostic and predictive markers in colorectal cancer: current status. Curr Colorectal Cancer Rep 2011;7:136–44. http://dx.doi.org/10.1007/s11888-011-0091-4.

35. Perez-Cabornero L, Sanz MI, Sampedro EV, et al. Frequency of rearrangements in lynch syndrome cases associated with MSH2: characterization of a new deletion involving both EPCAM and the 5' part of MSH2. Cancer Prev Res (Phila) 2011;4:1556–62. http://dx.doi.org/10.1158/1940-6207.CAPR-11-0080.

36. North P, Thomas DC, Umar A, et al. Microsatellite instability and mismatch repair defects in cancer cells. Mutat Res 1996;350:201–5.

37. Miyaki M, Iijima T, Kimura J, et al. Frequent mutation of beta-catenin and APC genes in primary colorectal tumors from patients with hereditary nonpolyposis colorectal cancer. Cancer Res 1999;59:4506–9.

38. Markowitz S, Wang J, Myeroff L, et al. Inactivation of the type II TGF-beta receptor in colon cancer cells with microsatellite instability. Science 1995;268:1336–8. http://dx.doi.org/10.1126/science.7761852.

39. Miyashita T, Reed JC. Tumor suppressor p53 is a direct transcriptional activator of the human bax gene. Cell 1995;80:293–9. http://dx.doi.org/10.1016/0092-8674(95)90412-3.

40. Yagi OK, Akiyama Y, Nomizu T, et al. Proapoptotic gene BAX is frequently mutated in hereditary nonpolyposis colorectal cancers but not in adenomas. Gastroenterology 1998;114:268–74. http://dx.doi.org/10.1016/S0016-5085(98)70477-9.

41. Abdeljawad K, Vemulapalli KC, Kahi CJ, et al. Sessile serrated polyp prevalence determined by a colonoscopist with a high lesion detection rate and an experienced pathologist. Gastrointest Endosc 2014. http://dx.doi.org/10.1016/j.gie.2014.04.064.

42. Hazewinkel Y, de Wijkerslooth TR, Stoop EM, et al. Prevalence of serrated polyps and association with synchronous advanced neoplasia in screening colonoscopy. Endoscopy 2014;46(3):219–24. http://dx.doi.org/10.1055/s-0033-1358800.

43. O'Brien MJ, Yang S, Mack C, et al. Comparison of microsatellite instability, CpG island methylation phenotype, BRAF and KRAS status in serrated polyps and traditional adenomas indicates separate pathways to distinct colorectal carcinoma end points. Am J Surg Pathol 2006;30:1491–501. http://dx.doi.org/10.1097/01.pas.0000213313.36306.85.

44. Burnett-Hartman AN, Newcomb PA, Potter JD, et al. Genomic aberrations occurring in subsets of serrated colorectal lesions but not conventional adenomas. Cancer Res 2013;73:2863–72. http://dx.doi.org/10.1158/0008-5472.CAN-12-3462.

45. Fernando WC, Miranda MS, Worthley DL, et al. The CIMP phenotype in BRAF mutant serrated polyps from a prospective colonoscopy patient cohort. Gastroenterol Res Pract 2014;2014:374926. http://dx.doi.org/10.1155/2014/374926.

46. Rex DK, Ahnen DJ, Baron JA, et al. Serrated lesions of the colorectum: review and recommendations from an expert panel. Am J Gastroenterol 2012;107:1315–29. http://dx.doi.org/10.1038/ajg.2012.161 [quiz: 1314, 1330].

47. Hoff G. New polyps, old tricks: controversy about removing benign bowel lesions. Br Med J 2013;347:f5843. http://dx.doi.org/10.1136/bmj.f5843.

48. Lu FI, van Niekerk DW, Owen D, et al. Longitudinal outcome study of sessile serrated adenomas of the colorectum: an increased risk for subsequent right-sided colorectal carcinoma. Am J Surg Pathol 2010;34:927–34. http://dx.doi.org/10.1097/PAS.0b013e3181e4f256.

49. De Sousa E Melo F, Wang X, Jansen M, et al. Poor-prognosis colon cancer is defined by a molecularly distinct subtype and develops from serrated precursor lesions. Nat Med 2013;19(5):614–8. http://dx.doi.org/10.1038/nm.3174.

50. Iino H, Jass JR, Simms LA, et al. DNA microsatellite instability in hyperplastic polyps, serrated adenomas, and mixed polyps: a mild mutator pathway for colorectal cancer? J Clin Pathol 1999;52:5–9. http://dx.doi.org/10.1136/jcp.52.1.5.

51. Boparai KS, Dekker E, Polak MM, et al. A serrated colorectal cancer pathway predominates over the classic WNT pathway in patients with hyperplastic polyposis syndrome. Am J Pathol 2011;178(6):2700–7. http://dx.doi.org/10.1016/j.ajpath.2011.02.023.

52. Edelstein DL, Axilbund JE, Griffin CA, et al. Serrated polyposis: rapid and relentless development of colorectal neoplasia. Gut 2013;62(3):404–8. http://dx.doi.org/10.1136/gutjnl-2011-300514.

53. Lash RH, Genta RM, Schuler CM. Sessile serrated adenomas: prevalence of dysplasia and carcinoma in 2139 patients. J Clin Pathol 2010;63(8):681–6. http://dx.doi.org/10.1136/jcp.2010.075507.

54. Chan AO, Issa JP, Morris JS, et al. Concordant CpG island methylation in hyperplastic polyposis. Am J Pathol 2002;160:529–36. http://dx.doi.org/10.1016/S0002-9440(10)64872-9.

55. Yamamoto H, Min Y, Itoh F, et al. Differential involvement of the hypermethylator phenotype in hereditary and sporadic colorectal cancers with high-frequency microsatellite instability. Genes Chromosomes Cancer 2002;33:322–5. http://dx.doi.org/10.1002/gcc.10010.

56. Kriegl L, Neumann J, Vieth M, et al. Up and downregulation of p16(Ink4a) expression in BRAF-mutated polyps/adenomas indicates a senescence barrier in the serrated route to colon cancer. Mod Pathol 2011;24(7):1015–22. http://dx.doi.org/10.1038/modpathol.2011.43.

57. Wajapeyee N, Serra RW, Zhu X, et al. Oncogenic BRAF induces senescence and apoptosis through pathways mediated by the secreted protein IGFBP7. Cell 2008;132:363–74. http://dx.doi.org/10.1016/j.cell.2007.12.032.

58. Kambara T, Simms LA, Whitehall VL, et al. BRAF mutation is associated with DNA methylation in serrated polyps and cancers of the colorectum. Gut 2004;53:1137–44. http://dx.doi.org/10.1136/gut.2003.037671.

59. Rajagopalan H, Bardelli A, Lengauer C, et al. Tumorigenesis: RAF/RAS oncogenes and mismatch-repair status. Nature 2002;418:934. http://dx.doi.org/10.1038/418934a.

60. Burnett-Hartman AN, Passarelli MN, Adams SV, et al. Differences in epidemiologic risk factors for colorectal adenomas and serrated polyps by lesion severity and anatomical site. Am J Epidemiol 2013;177(7):625–37. http://dx.doi.org/10.1093/aje/kws282.

61. Winawer SJ, Zauber AG, Ho MN, et al. Prevention of colorectal cancer by colonoscopic polypectomy. The National Polyp Study Workgroup. N Engl J Med 1993;329:1977–81. http://dx.doi.org/10.1056/NEJM199312303292701.

62. Heldwein W, Dollhopf M, Meining A, et al. The Munich Polypectomy Study (MUPS): prospective analysis of complications and risk factors in 4000 colonic snare polypectomies. Endoscopy 2005;37(11):1116–22. http://dx.doi.org/10.1055/s.

63. Hassan C, Pickhardt PJ, Rex DK. A resect and discard strategy would improve cost-effectiveness of colorectal cancer screening. Clin Gastroenterol Hepatol 2010;8(10):865–9. http://dx.doi.org/10.1016/j.cgh.2010.05.018.

64. Hassan C, Pickhardt PJ, Kim DH, et al. Systematic review: distribution of advanced neoplasia according to polyp size at screening colonoscopy. Aliment Pharmacol Ther 2010;31:210–7. http://dx.doi.org/10.1111/j.1365-2036.2009.04160.x.

65. Winawer SJ, Zauber AG. The advanced adenoma as the primary target of screening. Gastrointest Endosc Clin N Am 2002;12:1–9. http://dx.doi.org/10.1016/S1052-5157(03)00053-9.

66. Soetikno RM, Kaltenbach T, Rouse RV, et al. Prevalence of nonpolypoid (flat and depressed) colorectal neoplasms in asymptomatic and symptomatic adults. JAMA 2008;299:1027–35. http://dx.doi.org/10.1016/S0739-5930(08)79073-1.

67. Lambert R, Lightdale CJ. The Paris endoscopic classification of superficial neoplastic lesions: esophagus, stomach, and colon - Paris, France November 30 to December 1, 2002: foreword. Gastrointest Endosc 2003;58. http://dx.doi.org/10.1016/S0016-5107(03)02168-0.

68. Van Doorn S, Hazewinkel Y, East J, et al. Polyp morphology: an interobserver evaluation for the Paris classification among international experts. Am J Gastroenterol 2014. [Epub ahead of print].

69. Kudo S, Tamura S, Nakajima T, et al. Diagnosis of colorectal tumorous lesions by magnifying endoscopy. Gastrointest Endosc 1996;44(1):8–14.

70. Su MY, Ho YP, Chen PC, et al. Magnifying endoscopy with indigo carmine contrast for differential diagnosis of neoplastic and nonneoplastic colonic polyps. Dig Dis Sci 2004;49:1123–7. http://dx.doi.org/10.1023/B: DDAS.0000037798.55845.f7.

71. Rosty C, Hewett DG, Brown IS, et al. Serrated polyps of the large intestine: current understanding of diagnosis, pathogenesis, and clinical management. J Gastroenterol 2013;48(3):287–302. http://dx.doi.org/10.1007/s00535-012-0720-y.

72. Bouwens MW, van Herwaarden YJ, Winkens B, et al. Endoscopic characterization of sessile serrated adenomas/polyps with and without dysplasia. Endoscopy 2014;46(3):225–35. http://dx.doi.org/10.1055/s-0034-1364936.

73. Tadepalli US, Feihel D, Miller KM, et al. A morphologic analysis of sessile serrated polyps observed during routine colonoscopy (with video). Gastrointest Endosc 2011;74(6):1360–8. http://dx.doi.org/10.1016/j.gie.2011.08.008.

74. Hazewinkel Y, López-Cerón M, East JE, et al. Endoscopic features of sessile serrated adenomas: validation by international experts using high-resolution white-light endoscopy and narrow-band imaging. Gastrointest Endosc 2013; 77(6):916–24. http://dx.doi.org/10.1016/j.gie.2012.12.018.

75. Farris AB, Misdraji J, Srivastava A, et al. Sessile serrated adenoma: challenging discrimination from other serrated colonic polyps. Am J Surg Pathol 2008;32: 30–5. http://dx.doi.org/10.1097/PAS.0b013e318093e40a.

76. Hewett DG, Kaltenbach T, Sano Y, et al. Validation of a simple classification system for endoscopic diagnosis of small colorectal polyps using narrow-band imaging. Gastroenterology 2012;143(3):599–607.e1. http://dx.doi.org/10.1053/j.gastro.2012.05.006.

77. Hayashi N, Tanaka S, Hewett DG, et al. Endoscopic prediction of deep submucosal invasive carcinoma: validation of the narrow-band imaging international colorectal endoscopic (NICE) classification. Gastrointest Endosc 2013;78:625–32. http://dx.doi.org/10.1016/j.gie.2013.04.185.

78. Kumar S, Fioritto A, Mitani A, et al. Optical biopsy of sessile serrated adenomas: do these lesions resemble hyperplastic polyps under narrow-band imaging? Gastrointest Endosc 2013;78(6):902–9. http://dx.doi.org/10.1016/j.gie.2013.06.004.

Advances in Bowel Preparation for Colonoscopy

Lawrence B. Cohen, MD

KEYWORDS

- Bowel preparation • Colonoscopy • Endoscopy • Bowel cleaning

KEY POINTS

- Selection of a bowel preparation agent should be tailored to the needs of each patient with particular attention to individuals with chronic constipation, multiple comorbid conditions, or an inadequate preparation during prior colonoscopy.
- Patient education and willingness to participate in the preparation process can improve the outcome of bowel cleansing.
- Endoscopists should be prepared to spend time during each procedure cleaning the colon. The quality of bowel preparation should be assessed during scope withdrawal when cleaning efforts have been completed.
- An adequate preparation permits the detection of lesions greater than 5 mm in size and is defined as one that enables the examiner to adhere to current guidelines for colorectal cancer screening and surveillance.
- Practitioners should benchmark the proportion of their colonoscopies with an adequate preparation and should aim to meet or exceed a threshold rate of 85%.

INTRODUCTION

Despite its straightforward purpose and unpretentious name, bowel cleansing for colonoscopy remains a challenge for endoscopists and patients alike. Its objective to remove all solid and liquid debris from the colon lumen in order to make it possible for the operator to perform a thorough examination of the mucosal surface seems simple enough. Nonetheless, roughly 1 in 4 colonoscopies performed in the United States and western Europe are considered to have an inadequate-quality preparation.[1,2] Even a thin film of mucus or chyme coating the mucosa may obscure a clinically important lesion. The introduction of split-dose regimens has significantly enhanced the ability to achieve high-quality cleansing, especially within the proximal

Department of Medicine (Gastroenterology), Icahn School of Medicine at Mount Sinai, 1112 Park Avenue, 1A, New York, NY 10128, USA
E-mail address: lawrence.cohen@digestivecarenyc.com

Gastrointest Endoscopy Clin N Am 25 (2015) 183–197
http://dx.doi.org/10.1016/j.giec.2014.11.003
1052-5157/15/$ – see front matter © 2015 Elsevier Inc. All rights reserved.

giendo.theclinics.com

colon, and has improved the detection rate of flat polyps that may be readily obscured by mucosal staining or a small pool of fluid.[3,4]

Coincident with efforts to design a more effective dosing schema have been attempts to develop effective purgatives that are more acceptable to patients. Several lower-volume preparations have recently been approved in the United States. Notwithstanding these efforts, conventional 4-L polyethylene glycol (PEG) with electrolytes remains the benchmark by which the efficacy of other preparations should be compared.[5]

In an effort to improve the overall quality of bowel preparation, and consequently the quality and effectiveness of colonoscopy, the US Multi-Society Task Force (MSTF) on colorectal cancer (CRC) now recommends that clinicians meet or exceed a target rate of 85% for adequate bowel preparation.[6] While acknowledging that rates of adequate preparation are related, in part, to a variety of patient factors such as age, gender, comorbid disease, and socioeconomic status, and that differences in these and other variables from practice to practice can significantly affect the proportion of patients with an adequate preparation, the gastrointestinal professional societies think that it is possible for most practitioners in the United States to achieve this goal. However, for some endoscopists it will require a reformulation of their approach to bowel preparation with greater emphasis on patient education, increased patient activation, adoption of preparation agents that have track records for high rates of success, and the implementation of split-dose regimens. This article reviews recent updates to bowel preparation guidelines and the evidence supporting these recommendations.

BOWEL PREPARATION AND ITS IMPACT ON COLONOSCOPY QUALITY

The quality of bowel cleansing at colonoscopy should be assessed during scope withdrawal, after all efforts at washing and suctioning fluid and debris from the lumen have been completed.[6] Such an approach to grading largely discounts the presence of retained fluid and small bits of stool, because these can usually be removed during the procedure. Given its importance in improving the quality of colonoscopy, the time required for adequate washing should not be minimized. A recent prospective study found that the mean time spent washing/suctioning during colonoscopy was 4.1 minutes.[7] As anticipated, the time and the volume of instilled fluid were inversely proportional to the baseline preparation grade, ranging from 2.7 to 9.2 minutes and 167 to 807 mL for excellent to poor preparations, respectively. In 33 (6%) patients, the quality of preparation was substantially improved, from fair/poor to good/excellent (or inadequate to adequate). This finding shows that intraprocedural washing and cleaning are integral components of the examination and can have an appreciable impact on the quality and cost-effectiveness of colonoscopy. The time allotted for each procedure should therefore be sufficient for the endoscopist to thoroughly cleanse those segments of the bowel that are not adequately prepared during the preprocedure period.

The quality of the bowel preparation should be recorded in a written report generated after each colonoscopy. Many clinicians use a nonstandardized 4-point scale (excellent, good, fair, and poor) to describe the quality of bowel cleansing, often without a precise definition of each grade. As a result, a preparation rated good by one endoscopist may be considered fair by another. Further, the adequacy of a fair preparation, in terms of adenoma detection, has yet to be fully defined. Nonetheless, many endoscopists shorten the interval between examinations when the quality of the bowel preparation is considered inadequate. For example, a retrospective review of more than 16,000 colonoscopies performed at an academic medical center found that nearly 60% of average-risk patients with normal colonoscopy results underwent early repeat examination because of a preparation quality rated as fair.[8] A recent systematic review and meta-analysis of 11 studies observed no difference in adenoma detection rate (ADR) between examinations with intermediate-quality (fair) compared with those with high-quality preparation (good or excellent) (odds ratio [OR], 0.94; 95% confidence interval [CI], 0.80, 1.10).[9] In contrast, ADRs were significantly higher with both intermediate-quality (OR, 1.39; 95% CI, 1.08, 1.79) and high-quality preparations (OR, 1.41; 95% CI, 1.21, 1.64) compared with low-quality (poor) preparations. Similar findings were observed in an analysis of 13,000 colonoscopies within a statewide registry, with comparable ADRs in examinations with fair-quality versus optimal-quality preparation.[10] If confirmed by other investigators, these findings indicate that a fair-quality preparation could be sufficient for the detection of adenomas during screening and surveillance colonoscopy.

The current emphasis is on classifying a bowel preparation as either adequate or inadequate. An adequate preparation is one that allows the detection of lesions greater than 5 mm in size.[11] As such, the term adequate implies that bowel cleansing is sufficiently good for the examiner to identify clinically important lesions. The US MSTF guidelines define an adequate preparation as one that enables the endoscopist to follow the recommended screening and surveillance guidelines.[6]

IMPLICATIONS OF AN INADEQUATE BOWEL PREPARATION

Adenoma detection is currently the most important measure of colonoscopy quality (**Box 1**).[12] Data from a national endoscopic database indicated that an adequate-quality preparation resulted in a higher detection rate for adenomas of all sizes (OR, 1.21; 95% CI, 1.16, 1.25) compared with an inadequate preparation.[1] Similar findings were observed in a prospective, multicenter European trial in which all polyps (OR, 1.46; 95% CI, 1.11, 1.93) as well as larger (>10 mm) polyps (OR, 1.72; 95% CI, 1.11, 2.67) were detected more often with a high-quality compared with a low-quality preparation.[2] Flat lesions within the proximal colon are also more likely to be detected when the preparation quality is rated as good. For example, a single-center study reported significantly more flat polyps detected with a higher-quality (same-day) versus a lower-quality (day-before) preparation (21.6% vs 9%; $P = .02$).[4]

In contrast, poor-quality bowel preparation leads to lower detection rates, which means more missed lesions. Two single-center studies from academic medical

---

Box 1
Adverse consequences of inadequate bowel preparation for colonoscopy

Lower detection rate of adenomas (all sizes)

Lower detection rate of flat lesions (proximal colon)

Prolonged cecal intubation time

Lower cecal intubation rate

Increased time washing and suctioning debris

Prolonged withdrawal time

Increased costs of CRC prevention

Patient dropout of CRC prevention program

centers examined the rate of missed lesions with an inadequate bowel preparation on the index examination, based on the results of a follow-up procedure performed within 3 years of the baseline study.[13,14] The overall adenoma miss rates were, respectively, 42% and 47.9%. Although the absolute numbers may differ from one center to another, these rates show that significant numbers of polyps, both large and small, are missed with an inadequate preparation.

Operational efficiency is also affected by the quality of bowel preparation.[15] European investigators observed that cecal intubation time (11.9 vs 16.1 minutes; $P<.001$), instrument withdrawal time (9.8 vs 11.3 minutes; $P<.001$), and cecal intubation rates (90.4% vs 71.1%; OR, 3.33; 95% CI, 2.36, 4.70) were all better with high-quality than low-quality preparations.[2] As indicated earlier, the intraprocedural time washing the bowel was prolonged with poor-quality preparations.[7]

Endoscopists have long struggled to find the most appropriate follow-up strategy when the quality of bowel preparation is suboptimal. There is evidence of surveillance overuse in low-risk patients and well as underuse in high-risk patients.[16,17] For example, a review of practice patterns among 152 physicians from 55 practices indicated that more aggressive surveillance strategies were recommended when the preparation quality was good/fair/poor compared with those rated excellent.[16] In an effort to provide better guidance to clinicians, the 2012 MSTF guidelines state that, "If the bowel preparation is poor, the MSTF recommends that in most cases the examination should be repeated within 1 year. … If the bowel preparation is fair but adequate (to detect lesions >5 mm) and if small (<10 mm) tubular adenomas are detected, follow-up at 5 years should be considered."[18] In order to improve compliance with clinical practice guidelines, both governmental and commercial payers are developing quality measures for colonoscopy that reflect clinicians' adherence with screening and surveillance guidelines. For example, the Physician Quality Reporting System, developed by Medicare, will begin using payment adjustments in 2015 to encourage physicians to report on specific measures related to follow-up intervals for screening and surveillance examinations.[19] The message is clear: consistent high-quality bowel cleaning is a necessary element of effective and efficient colonoscopy. A rate of 85% has been proposed by the MSTF on CRC as a benchmark for adequate preparation on a per-physician basis.[6]

DIFFICULT-TO-PREPARE PATIENTS

Several patient-related characteristics, including age, gender, body mass index (BMI), and hospital inpatient status, have been associated with the quality of preparation (**Box 2**). The association with higher age and male gender has a low predictability level and is not consistently observed across all studies.[6] In contrast, a large study of 1588 patients found that BMI greater than 25 was an independent predictor of inadequate preparation, with each unit increase in BMI more than 25 increasing the likelihood of inadequate preparation by 2.1%.[20] Further, additional independent predictors of inadequate preparation, combined with high BMI, exponentially increased the risk of a suboptimal preparation.

Various medical conditions and medications are also associated with an increased likelihood of inadequate preparation. The list of conditions includes stroke and Parkinson disease, impaired mobility, diabetes mellitus, spinal cord injury, and prior gastrointestinal resection. The medications that have been implicated include narcotics and tricyclic antidepressants. Although the OR for any of these conditions alone adversely affecting the preparation is low, ranging from 1.1 to 3.2, a cumulative effect has been observed so that elderly patients with multiple comorbid diseases have a significantly

Box 2
Risk factors for inadequate preparation
Patient characteristics
Older age
Male gender
Higher body mass index
Inpatient status
Health conditions/medication usage
Multiple comorbid conditions
Neurologic conditions (stroke, Parkinson)
Impaired mobility
Prior gastrointestinal surgical resection
Diabetes mellitus
Spinal cord injury
Medications associated with constipation as side effect
Social/behavioral characteristics
Reduced health literacy
Lower patient activation

increased likelihood of having an inadequate preparation. Several investigators have attempted to develop a predictive model using a composite score to increase the success in identifying individuals at risk.[20,21] One such model had only modest ability to predict an inadequate preparation (area under the curve, 0.63), and its utility in clinical practice seems limited at present.[21]

Additional predictors of inadequate preparation include health literacy and patient activation.[22–25] Although other variables, such as health insurance status, socioeconomic status, and educational level, have also been observed to predict suboptimal bowel preparation in earlier studies, it is likely that the common denominator is reduced health literacy, which can lead to difficulty or inability to read the educational materials and instructions provided before colonoscopy, failure to comprehend the importance of bowel preparation in the overall success of colonoscopy, or lack of understanding regarding preventive health measures. Patient activation refers to the motivation or mind-set of a patient to participate, or be engaged, in their health care.[26] Although seemingly interrelated, health literacy and patient activation are independent variables as predictors of inadequate preparation. In a recent study of nearly 500 outpatients followed either at an academic medical center clinic or a federally qualified health center, low levels of patient activation (OR, 2.12; 1.3–3.45), but not health literacy (OR, 0.76; 0.38–1.52), was an independent predictor of inadequate preparation.[25] The solution to this problem, put succinctly in a recent editorial, is "education, motivation, and reminders."[27] This can be in the form of 1:1 teaching sessions, bowel preparation classes, instructional videos, online tutorials, or in some cases patient navigators. More research is needed to develop better methods for improving patient understanding and willingness to become actively involved in the preparation process.

SELECTING A BOWEL PREPARATION AGENT

Prescription Agents

Bowel cleaning agents for precolonoscopy preparation have evolved from large-volume (7–12 L) solutions with hypertonic saline to osmotically balanced solutions containing PEG and electrolytes. Originally formulated as a 4-L preparation, a lower-volume PEG regimen combined with an adjunctive agent (MoviPrep, Salix Pharmaceutical, Raleigh, NC) was subsequently developed in order to improve patient tolerance. Sodium phosphate solution, another popular preparation that was available for almost 20 years, was withdrawn from the US market in December 2008 because of concern over phosphate-induced renal insufficiency. However, a tablet formulation of sodium phosphate (OsmoPrep; Salix Pharmaceuticals, Raleigh, NC) remains available by physician prescription. In addition, oral sodium sulfate (SUPREP, Braintree Laboratories, Braintree, MA), sodium picosulfate/magnesium citrate (Prepopik, Ferring Pharmaceuticals, Inc, Parsippany, NJ), and a combination preparation that includes PEG plus sodium sulfate (Suclear, Braintree Laboratories, Braintree, MA) were all approved in the United States in the last several years. In addition to these prescriptive agents, several over-the counter (OTC) products are used, the most common of which are PEG-3350 powder, magnesium citrate, and bisacodyl tablets.

Bowel preparation formulations are assessed based on 3 criteria: efficacy, safety, and tolerability. We assume that important differences in safety among the most widely used prescriptive agents, which would influence our prescribing pattern, do not exist. The choice among agents therefore rests on their relative efficacy, tolerability, and in some instances cost. The comparative efficacy of bowel cleansing regimens before colonoscopy has been assessed and quantified in countless clinical trials, systematic reviews, and meta-analyses. Differences in dosing regimens, dietary restrictions, patient populations, use of adjunctive agents, and methods for assessing outcomes among studies have sometimes led to conflicting results. A 2014 US MSTF guideline concluded that split-dose 4-L PEG with electrolytes provides high-quality bowel cleansing.[6] The guideline also indicates that a lower-volume PEG formulation (2 L) achieves bowel cleansing in healthy nonconstipated individuals that is not inferior to that of a 4-L formulation. This conclusion was supported by a recent meta-analysis of 11 trials, representing 3443 patients, which compared 2-L PEG plus ascorbate with 4-L PEG.[28] The pooled OR for preparation efficacy was 1.08 (95% CI, 0.98–1.28; $P = .34$). Tolerability was superior with 2-L PEG with ascorbate compared with 4-L PEG (OR, 2.23; 95% CI, 1.67–2.98; $P<.00001$).

The efficacy and tolerability of oral sodium sulfate (OSS) have been evaluated in at least 4 unique multicenter trials against a variety of other agents. In a study of 923 patients, representing the combined results of 2 parallel studies, OSS was not inferior to 2-L PEG with ascorbate (OR, 1.12, 0.77–1.62).[29] Another study of OSS compared sodium sulfate in a split-dose with 4-L PEG taken the day before.[30] The superiority of OSS (98.4% vs 89.6%; $P<.04$) reflected both the efficacy of the agent and the benefits of split dosing. A multicenter trial of 338 randomized patients resulted in a higher proportion of successful preparations (excellent or good) with OSS compared with sodium picosulfate plus magnesium citrate (94.7% vs 85.7%; $P = .006$) when both preparations were given in split doses.[31] Another multicenter trial compared a new hybrid preparation, consisting of a reduced dose of OSS plus 2 L of sulfate-free (SF) PEG with electrolytes versus 2 different 2-L PEG preparations.[32] Study 1, which compared split-dose OSS plus SF-PEG with 2-L PEG with ascorbate, found identical rates of excellent or good bowel preparation (93.5%) in both arms. Study 2, which compared OSS plus SF-PEG versus 2-L PEG plus 10 mg of bisacodyl, both taken the evening before colonoscopy, resulted in successful preparation in 89.8% and 83.5%, respectively. With respect to patient tolerability, vomiting was more frequent with OSS plus SF-PEG, whereas bloating was worse with PEG with ascorbate.

Sodium picosulfate combined with magnesium salts was approved by the US Food and Drug Administration for bowel cleansing before colonoscopy in 2012, after achieving considerable acceptance in Canada, Europe, and Australia. An analysis of 10 trials comparing sodium picosulfate combined with either magnesium oxide or magnesium citrate showed no significant difference in efficacy compared with PEG with electrolytes (OR, 0.92, 0.63–1.36).[6] One trial of 250 intention-to-treat patients compared picosulfate split-dose versus picosulfate taken either the day before or the same day. The split-dosing regimen had a significantly higher proportion of adequate preparations compared with day before or same day (OR, 3.54, 1.95–6.45).[33] A large multicenter trial of 862 patients, which randomized 2:1 split-dose versus day-before dosing of picosulfate plus magnesium citrate, observed 85.8% adequate preparation with split dosing compared with 69.8% in the group receiving the preparation the day before colonoscopy.[34]

Issues regarding the safety of oral sodium phosphate preparations have been raised in recent years, because of concerns about the risk of major fluid and electrolyte shifts as well as chronic kidney disease resulting from acute phosphate nephropathy.[35] Risk factors that predispose patients to acute phosphate nephropathy include renal insufficiency (as reflected in a reduced creatinine clearance rate), inadequate hydration during bowel preparation, reduced time interval between the 2 doses of sodium phosphate (less than 12 hours), hypertension with renal arteriolar sclerosis, and certain medications (diuretics, nonsteroidal antiinflammatory drugs, and renin-angiotensin inhibitors).[36] In addition, heart failure, cirrhosis, and advanced age may also be risk factors for acute phosphate nephropathy. The risks associated with the use of sodium phosphate are now thought to make its use as a first-line agent for precolonoscopy bowel preparation unsuitable. Appropriate cautions, as indicated in the product label, should be exercised when using this agent for bowel preparation before colonoscopy.

Over-the-counter Agents

Several OTC laxative agents have been adapted for use during bowel cleansing before colonoscopy. In the United States, the 2 most widely used compounds are PEG-3350 powder and magnesium citrate. Although these products are generally safe when used for their intended purpose, their safety as well as their efficacy for preprocedure bowel cleansing is largely unknown.

The most frequently used formula for PEG powder consists of 1 bottle of PEG-3350 (238 g) mixed with 1890 mL (64 ounces) of Gatorade (PepsiCo, Chicago, IL) to create a 2-L PEG preparation. Bisacodyl tablets or magnesium citrate are sometimes given in combination with the PEG solution. A meta-analysis of 5 studies, comprising 1418 patients, assessed the efficacy and tolerability of PEG powder with Gatorade compared with standard PEG with electrolytes (3.8–4 L).[37] PEG-3350 powder was associated with fewer satisfactory bowel preparations compared with larger-volume PEG plus electrolytes (OR, 0.65; 95% CI, 0.43–0.98; $P = .04$). However, no difference in polyp detection was observed between treatment groups. Patient willingness to repeat their preparation was superior with PEG powder compared with larger-volume PEG (OR, 7.32; 95% CI, 4.88–10.98; $P<.01$).

The use of magnesium citrate, an OTC laxative packaged in a 300-mL (10-ounce) bottle, has achieved significant market share in the United States, according to anecdotal reports. When used at a dose of 300 mL times 3, it produced excellent or good-quality bowel cleansing in 94% and 97% of cases in the right and left colon, respectively.[38] Transient hypermagnesemia has been reported, although clinically important adverse events have not been observed in healthy persons. The use of magnesium-based agents should be avoided in patients with chronic kidney disease.

Adjunctive Agents

A variety of adjunctive agents designed to improve evacuation, mucosal cleansing, and/or patient tolerability have been assessed. The list of such compounds, although not exhaustive, includes senna, bisacodyl, menthol, olive oil, promotility agents, sodium ascorbate, sodium sulfate, probiotics, spasmolytics, and simethicone. However, no adjunctive agent has been established to consistently improve the efficacy of colonoscopy or the tolerability for bowel preparation. This conclusion is supported by both the US and European guidelines.[6,39] Nevertheless, clinicians sometimes find benefit in the use an adjunctive agent. For example, the use of simethicone to eliminate bubbles or foam seems sensible despite the absence of scientific evidence supporting its utility. A thorough review of this subject is beyond the scope of this article and interested readers are referred to a recent review article on the subject.[40]

Strategies for Hard-to-prepare Patients

Individuals with 1 or more risk factors for an inadequate bowel preparation, in particular those with a history of chronic constipation, multiple comorbid conditions, or an inadequate bowel preparation previously, need a more intensive bowel cleansing regimen. In such cases, a 4-L PEG preparation with electrolytes seems to be preferable to a 2-L PEG preparation. Although there are no published studies to support this statement, it seems to be intuitive and is supported by expert opinion.[27] Another approach is the addition of an adjunctive agent such as 300 mL (10 ounces) of magnesium citrate or 10 mg of bisacodyl to a standard 2-L or 4-L PEG. Again, there is only anecdote to support these approaches because published data on bowel preparation in these patient subgroups are absent.

However, what is known is that a sizable proportion of patients (23%) with an inadequate preparation at their first examination will have an inadequate preparation on repeat examination.[41] An exception to this is next-day (salvage) colonoscopy, for which the odds of repeat failure are significantly reduced (OR, 0.31; 95% CI, 0.1–0.92). In another study of patients with an inadequate preparation after 4-L PEG, 20-mg oral bisacodyl combined with 4-L PEG was associated with a salvage rate of 80% on repeat procedure.[42] Even more successful was an intensive regimen that included a low-residue diet for 72 hours followed by liquids for 24 hours, combined with 10 mg of oral bisacodyl plus 1.5 L of PEG with electrolytes the evening before procedure, and another 1.5-L PEG with electrolytes on the day of colonoscopy. Ninety percent of patients had an adequate preparation as assessed using the Boston Bowel Preparation Scale (BBPS).[43]

DIET AND DOSING RECOMMENDATIONS
Diet

Bowel cleansing preparations have traditionally included a clear liquid diet for 24 hours before colonoscopy. However, there is a growing body of literature indicating that less stringent dietary restriction improves patient tolerance for bowel cleaning with no adverse effect on the quality of bowel preparation.[44–48] In most of these studies, the dietary regimen consisted of a low-residue diet until the evening before examination.

A recent multicenter trial went 1 step further by permitting patients to consume a regular diet. This randomized, investigator-blinded study of 801 healthy Korean outpatients undergoing afternoon colonoscopy compared clear liquid with regular diet on the day before examination followed by 4-L PEG on the morning of examination.[49] There was no difference in the proportion of patients with excellent or good preparation between the two groups, and detection rates for polyp and adenoma were similar as well. Patient compliance with bowel preparation was higher in the group receiving regular diet.

The US MSTF on CRC supports the use of either low-residue or full liquid diet until the evening before colonoscopy.[6] In contrast, the European Society of Gastrointestinal Endoscopy (ESGE) recommends a low-fiber diet on the day preceding colonoscopy.[39] Neither the US nor the European dietary guidelines take into consideration the agents selected for cleaning or the medical status of the patient. A compromise approach, albeit not supported by rigorous controlled trials, would be to permit a low-residue diet through lunch for patients receiving a 2-L PEG or other low-volume preparation and a low-residue diet until evening when using a 4-L PEG formulation. Prudence would dictate that patients with chronic constipation, multiple comorbid conditions, or a history of inadequate preparation previously receive at least 24-hours of clear liquid diet, perhaps accompanied by a low-residue diet for 24 to 48 hours before that time. Additional research in this field is necessary.

Preparation Dosing Strategies

A split-dose regimen is a dosing schema for bowel cleansing in which roughly half of the preparation is consumed on the day of the examination. The ideal time interval between the last dose of laxative and the start of colonoscopy remains subject to debate, and probably differs from person to person depending upon the oral-cecal transit rate. The US MSTF on CRC indicates that the second dose should begin 4 to 6 hours before colonoscopy, whereas the ESGE guideline states that this interval should be no longer than 4 hours.[6,39] The principle underlying dose splitting is that chyme and small bowel effluent begin to reaccumulate in the proximal colon within several hours after the first dose of laxative has flushed the colon. Pharmacokinetic studies show that the ideal window between the second dose of purgative and colonoscopy is 3 to 4 hours.[50] However, there are additional factors that must be weighed when selecting the optimal time for the second dose. These factors include the preprocedure fasting guidelines in effect at a particular endoscopy center and the patient's travel time from home to the endoscopy center.

The evidence supporting the benefits of a split-dose regimen compared with a 1-day regimen taken the day before colonoscopy is overwhelming.[3,51] A recent series of meta-analyses comparing split versus nonsplit dosing regimens for various laxative agents supports the overall superiority of split dosing, with an adequate preparation rate of 85% compared with 63% in the split and nonsplit groups, respectively.[52] Split-dose preparations have also been shown to improve ADR, providing validation of the split-dose regimen.[53,54] A survey of US endoscopy units participating in the American Society for Gastrointestinal Endoscopy Endoscopy Unit Recognition Program indicates that 82% offered split dosing, although nonexclusively in 39%.[55]

Same-day preparation represents a variation on the concept of split dosing. In the United States, it has been used almost exclusively for patients scheduled to undergo afternoon procedures.[56,57] In parts of Asia, same-day dosing has also been used for procedures beginning earlier in the day. In such cases, patients begin to consume preparation at around 6 AM and complete their preparation within 2 to 4 hours. A 2-hour minimum period of fasting is required between completion of the preparation and the initiation of sedation. The advantages of same-day preparation include the lack of disruption of normal activities on the day before colonoscopy; less interruption of sleep; and, in some cases, an unrestricted diet during the day before examination. Patient satisfaction with same-day preparation is often reported to be comparable or superior to standard dosing regimens.

SCORING PREPARATION QUALITY

Assessing and recording the quality of bowel preparation is an important element of every colonoscopy report. Most electronic endowriters prompt the endoscopist to rate the quality of preparation by providing a field or pull-down menu. Grading systems vary from one system to another, with some using a 4-point scale (excellent, good, fair, and poor) and others indicating adequate or inadequate. However, most endowriters do not define these terms and endoscopists are left to develop their own definitions for each descriptor. Clinicians using a free-form or preprinted paper reporting system have the same issues faced by users of endowriters except that they may not be prompted to enter a score and they must remember to enter the rating when preparing their reports.

Regardless of the method employed, the language for reporting the quality of bowel cleansing should be standardized. A rating of fair from one examiner should match the grade assigned by another examiner looking at the same colon. This principle is termed interobserver reliability. Further, the scale should be valid, meaning that it measures what it was designed to measure. Several bowel preparation scales have been used for clinical research, including the Aronchick,[58] Ottawa,[59] and Harefield[60] scales, and the BBPS.[61]

The Aronchick and Ottawa scales have been used widely in industry-sponsored clinical trials, in which the primary end point was effectiveness of the laxative as opposed to overall colon cleansing after washing/suctioning.[58,59] Both scales rate the quality of preparation before efforts are made by the endoscopist to improve visualization. The Harefield scale was also developed and validated for use in clinical research.[60] It is the most detailed scale proposed to date, rating each of 5 colon segments (rectum, sigmoid, descending, transverse, and ascending/cecum) on a 5-point scale. The results can be expressed on a segment-by-segment basis, assigned an overall score (A, B, C, or D), or rated as adequate versus inadequate. Ratings are all assigned after washing and suctioning have been completed. In my opinion, the Harefield scale is too complicated for general use by practicing endoscopists.

The BBPS is the most thoroughly studied scale.[61–64] During withdrawal of the colonoscope, 3 regions of the colon (ascending, transverse, and sigmoid) are each graded on a 3-point scale and the numbers summed so that 9 is a perfect score (**Box 3**). The developers originally proposed that scores less than 5 corresponded with an inadequate preparation. Recent analysis of a national endoscopic database showed that a BBPS greater than or equal to 6 (score of 2 or more in all 3 segments) was associated with recommendations for follow-up that were consistent with guidelines in 90% of cases. When the BBPS was 3 to 5, recommendations for follow-up were variable, whereas scores between 0 and 2 were almost uniformly considered to be poor and repeat examination recommended within 1 year in 96% of cases. The reliability of these findings across 74 endoscopists and multiple sites further supports the reliability of this scale.

Box 3
BBPS

1. Grading is performed during instrument withdrawal after all efforts at cleansing/washing have been completed.
2. Right, transverse, and left colon are each assigned a score from 0 to 3. The sum of the 3 segmental scores equals the total BBPS.
3. Scoring system:

   0, unprepped with solid stool obscuring the mucosa.

   1, portion of the mucosa seen, but other areas are not well seen because of residual stool or chyme.

   2, minor amount of residual stool, chime, or fluid but mucosa is seen well.

   3, entire mucosa is well seen, with no residual stool, liquid, or chyme.

4. Adequate preparation defined as total score greater than or equal to 6 and/or greater than or equal to 2 in all 3 segments.

SUMMARY

Precolonoscopy bowel preparation is adequate to identify lesions larger than 5 mm about 70% to 75% of the time. Recent improvement in the understanding of dosing schema and the widespread adoption of split-dose regimens in the United States have improved the overall quality of preparations, regardless of which purgative is used. However, the opportunity for further improvement does exist. The use of high-quality formulations with established efficacy rates of 90% or greater, identification of patients who are at increased risk of an inadequate preparation, as well as patient education and motivation to be invested in the process further improves the success of cleansing. Endoscopists should strive to achieve an adequate bowel preparation in 85% or more of patients. This is attainable by implementing the principles of bowel preparation reviewed in this chapter. High-quality colonoscopy requires high-quality bowel cleansing.

REFERENCES

1. Harewood GC, Sharma VK, de Garmo P. Impact of colonoscopy preparation quality on detection of suspected colonic neoplasia. Gastrointest Endosc 2003; 58(1):76–9.
2. Froehlich F, Wietlisbach V, Gonvers JJ, et al. Impact of colonic cleansing on quality and diagnostic yield of colonoscopy: the European Panel of Appropriateness of Gastrointestinal Endoscopy European multicenter study. Gastrointest Endosc 2005;61(3):378–84.
3. Cohen LB. Split-dosing of bowel preparations for colonoscopy: an analysis of its efficacy, safety, and tolerability. Gastrointest Endosc 2010;72:406–12.
4. Parra-Blanco A, Nicolas-Perez D, Gimeno-Garcia A, et al. The timing of bowel preparation before colonoscopy determines the quality of cleansing, and is a significant factor contributing to the detection of flat lesions: a randomized study. World J Gastroenterol 2006;12(38):6161–6.
5. Enestvedt BK, Tofani C, Laine LA, et al. 4-Liter split-dose polyethylene glycol is superior to other bowel preparations, based on systematic review and meta-analysis. Clin Gastroenterol Hepatol 2012;10(11):1225–31.

6. Johnson DA, Barkun AN, Cohen LB, et al. Optimizing adequacy of bowel cleansing for colonoscopy: recommendations from the U.S. Multi-Society Task Force on Colorectal Cancer. Gastrointest Endosc 2014;80(4):543–62.

7. MacPhail ME, Hardacker KA, Tiwari A, et al. Intraprocedural cleansing work during colonoscopy and achievable rates of adequate preparation in an open-access endoscopy unit. Gastrointest Endosc 2014. [Epub ahead of print].

8. Menees SB, Kim HM, Elliott EE, et al. The impact of fair colonoscopy preparation on colonoscopy use and adenoma miss rates in patients undergoing outpatient colonoscopy. Gastrointest Endosc 2013;78(3):510–6.

9. Clark BT, Rustagi T, Laine L. What level of bowel prep quality requires early repeat colonoscopy: systematic review and meta-analysis of the impact of preparation quality on adenoma detection rate. Am J Gastroenterol 2014;109(11):1714–23.

10. Anderson JC, Butterly LF, Robinson CM, et al. Impact of fair bowel preparation quality on adenoma and serrated polyp detection: data from the New Hampshire Colonoscopy Registry by using a standardized preparation-quality rating. Gastrointest Endosc 2014;80(3):463–70.

11. Rex DK, Bond JH, Winawer S, et al. Quality in the technical performance of colonoscopy and the continuous quality improvement process for colonoscopy: recommendations of the U.S. Multi-Society Task Force on Colorectal Cancer. Am J Gastroenterol 2002;97(6):1296–308.

12. Rex DK, Petrini JL, Baron TH, et al. Quality indicators for colonoscopy. Am J Gastroenterol 2006;101:873–85.

13. Lebwohl B, Kastrinos F, Glick M, et al. The impact of suboptimal bowel preparation on adenoma miss rates and the factors associated with early repeat colonoscopy. Gastrointest Endosc 2011;73:1207–14.

14. Chokshi RV, Hovis CE, Hollander T, et al. Prevalence of missed adenomas in patients with inadequate bowel preparation on screening colonoscopy. Gastrointest Endosc 2012;75(6):1197–203.

15. Rex DK, Imperiale TF, Latinovich DR, et al. Impact of bowel preparation on efficiency and cost of colonoscopy. Am J Gastroenterol 2002;7(7):1696–700.

16. Ransohoff DF, Yankaskas B, Gizlice Z, et al. Recommendations for post polypectomy surveillance in community practice. Dig Dis Sci 2011;56:2623–30.

17. Schoen RE, Pinsky PF, Weissfeld JL, et al. Utilization of surveillance colonoscopy in community practice. Gastroenterology 2011;138:73–81.

18. Lieberman DA, Rex DK, Winawer SJ, et al. Guidelines for colonoscopy surveillance after screening and polypectomy: a consensus update by the US Multi-Society Task Force on Colorectal Cancer. Gastroenterology 2012;143(3):844–57.

19. Available at: http://www.cms.gov/Medicare/Quality-Initiatives-Patient-Assessment-Instruments/PQRS/Downloads/2013MLNSE13__AvoidingPQRSPaymentAdjustment_083013.pdf. Accessed September 18, 2014.

20. Borg BB, Gupta NK, Zuckerman GR, et al. Impact of obesity on bowel preparation for colonoscopy. Clin Gastroenterol Hepatol 2009;7(6):670–5.

21. Hassan C, Fuccio L, Bruno M, et al. A predictive model identifies patients most likely to have inadequate bowel preparation for colonoscopy. Clin Gastroenterol Hepatol 2012;10(5):501–6.

22. Chan WK, Saravanan A, Manikam J, et al. Appointment waiting times and education level influence the quality of bowel preparation in adult patients undergoing colonoscopy. BMC Gastroenterol 2011;11(1):86.

23. Nguyen DL, Wieland M. Risk factors predictive of poor quality preparation during average risk colonoscopy screening: the importance of health literacy. J Gastrointestin Liver Dis 2010;19(4):369–72.

24. Lebwohl B, Wang TC, Neugut AI. Socioeconomic and other predictors of colonoscopy preparation quality. Dig Dis Sci 2010;55(7):2014–20.
25. Serper M, Gawron AJ, Smith SG, et al. Patient factors that affect quality of colonoscopy preparation. Clin Gastroenterol Hepatol 2014;12:451–7.
26. Smith SS, Curtis LM, Wardle J, et al. Skill set or mind set? Associations between health literacy, patient activation and health. PLoS One 2013;8(9):e74373.
27. Rex DK. Bowel preparation for colonoscopy: entering an era of increased expectations for efficacy. Clin Gastroenterol Hepatol 2014;12(3):458–62.
28. Xie Q, Chen L, Zhao F, et al. A meta-analysis of randomized controlled trials of low-volume polyethylene glycol plus ascorbic acid versus standard-volume polyethylene glycol solution as bowel preparations for colonoscopy. PLoS One 2014;9(6):399092.
29. Di Palma JA, Rodriguez R, McGowan J, et al. A randomized clinical study evaluating the safety and efficacy of a new, reduced-volume, oral sulfate colon-cleansing preparation for colonoscopy. Am J Gastroenterol 2009;104(9): 2275–84.
30. Rex DK, Di Palma JA, Rodriguez R, et al. A randomized clinical study comparing reduced-volume oral sulfate solution with standard 4-liter sulfate-free electrolyte lavage solution as preparation for colonoscopy. Gastrointest Endosc 2010; 72(2):328–36.
31. Rex DK, DiPalma JA, McGowan J, et al. A comparison of oral sulfate solution with sodium picosulfate: magnesium citrate in split doses as bowel preparation for colonoscopy. Gastrointest Endosc 2014;80:1113–23.
32. Rex DK, McGowan J, Cleveland Mv, et al. A randomized, controlled trial of oral sulfate solution plus polyethylene glycol as a bowel preparation for colonoscopy. Gastrointest Endosc 2014;80(3):482–91.
33. Flemming JA, Vanner SJ, Hookey LC. Split-dose picosulfate, magnesium oxide, and citric acid solution markedly enhances colon cleansing before colonoscopy: a randomized, controlled trial. Gastrointest Endosc 2012;75(3):537–44.
34. Manes G, Repici A, Hassan C, et al, Magic-P Study Group. Randomized controlled trial comparing efficacy and acceptability of split- and standard-dose sodium picosulfate plus magnesium citrate for bowel cleansing prior to colonoscopy. Endoscopy 2014;46:662–9.
35. Markowitz GS, Perazella MA. Acute phosphate nephropathy. Kidney Int 2009;76: 1027–34.
36. Brunelli SM, Lewis JD, Gupta M, et al. Risk of kidney injury following oral phosphosoda bowel preparation. J Am Soc Nephrol 2009;18:3199–205.
37. Siddique S, Lopez KT, Hinds AM, et al. Miralax with Gatorade for bowel preparation: a meta-analysis of randomized controlled trials. Am J Gastroenterol 2014; 109(10):1566–74.
38. Berkelhammer C, Ekambaram A, Silva RG. Low-volume oral colonoscopy bowel preparation: sodium phosphate and magnesium citrate. Gastrointest Endosc 2002;56(1):89–94.
39. Hassan C, Bretthauer M, Kaminski MF, et al. Bowel preparation for colonoscopy: European Society of Gastrointestinal Endoscopy (ESGE) guideline. Endoscopy 2013;45(2):142–50.
40. Park S, Lim YJ. Adjuncts to colonic cleansing before colonoscopy. World J Gastroenterol 2014;20(11):2735–40.
41. Ben-Horin S, Bar-Meir S, Avidan B. The outcome of a second preparation for colonoscopy after preparation failure in the first procedure. Gastrointest Endosc 2009;69(3 Pt 2):626–30.

42. Kim JW, Han JH, Boo SJ, et al. Rescue bowel preparation: same day 2-L polyethylene glycol addition, not superior to bisacodyl addition 7 days later. Dig Dis Sci 2014;59:2215–21.
43. Ibáñez M, Parra-Blanco A, Zaballa P, et al. Usefulness of an intensive bowel cleansing strategy for repeat colonoscopy after preparation failure. Dis Colon Rectum 2011;54(12):1578–84.
44. Wu KL, Rayner CK, Chuah SK, et al. Impact of low-residue diet on bowel preparation for colonoscopy. Dis Colon Rectum 2011;54(1):107–12.
45. Soweid AM, Kobeissy AA, Jamali FR, et al. A randomized single-blind trial of standard diet versus fiber-free diet with polyethylene glycol electrolyte solution for colonoscopy preparation. Endoscopy 2010;42(8):633–8.
46. Aoun E, Abdul-Baki H, Azar C, et al. A randomized single-blind trial of split-dose PEG-electrolyte solution without dietary restriction compared with whole dose PEG-electrolyte solution with dietary restriction for colonoscopy preparation. Gastrointest Endosc 2005;62(2):213–8.
47. Sipe BW, Fischer M, Baluyut AR, et al. A low-residue diet improved patient satisfaction with split-dose oral sulfate solution without impairing colonic preparation. Gastrointest Endosc 2013;77(6):932–6.
48. Melicharkova A, Flemming J, Vanner S, et al. A low-residue breakfast improves patient tolerance without impacting quality of low-volume colon cleansing prior to colonoscopy: a randomized trial. Am J Gastroenterol 2013;108(10):1551–5.
49. Jung YS, Seok HS, Park DI, et al. A clear liquid diet is not mandatory for polyethylene glycol-based bowel preparation for afternoon colonoscopy in healthy outpatients. Gut Liver 2013;7(6):681–7.
50. Siddiqui AA, Yang K, Spechler SJ, et al. Duration of the interval between the completion of bowel preparation and the start of colonoscopy predicts bowel-preparation quality. Gastrointest Endosc 2009;69(3 Pt 2):700–6.
51. Kilgore TW, Abdinoor AA, Szary NM, et al. Bowel preparation with split-dose polyethylene glycol before colonoscopy: a meta-analysis of randomized controlled trials. Gastrointest Endosc 2011;73(6):1240–5.
52. Bucci C, Rotondano G, Hassan C, et al. Optimal bowel cleansing for colonoscopy: split the dose! A series of meta-analyses of controlled studies. Gastrointest Endosc 2014;80(4):566–76.e2.
53. Jover R, Zapater P, Polanía E, et al. Modifiable endoscopic factors that influence the adenoma detection rate in colorectal cancer screening colonoscopies. Gastrointest Endosc 2013;77(3):381–9.
54. Gurudu SR, Ramirez FC, Harrison ME, et al. Increased adenoma detection rate with system-wide implementation of a split-dose preparation for colonoscopy. Gastrointest Endosc 2012;76(3):603–8.
55. Ton L, Lee H, Taunk P, et al. Nationwide variability of colonoscopy preparation instructions. Dig Dis Sci 2014;59(8):1726–32.
56. Matro R, Shnitser A, Spodik M, et al. Efficacy of morning-only compared with split-dose polyethylene glycol electrolyte solution for afternoon colonoscopy: a randomized controlled single-blind study. Am J Gastroenterol 2010;105(9):1954–61.
57. Longcroft-Wheaton G, Bhandari P. Same-day bowel cleansing regimen is superior to a split-dose regimen over 2 days for afternoon colonoscopy: results from a large prospective series. J Clin Gastroenterol 2012;46(1):57–61.
58. Aronchick CA, Lipshutz WH, Wright SH, et al. Validation of an instrument to assess colon cleansing [abstract]. Am J Gastroenterol 1999;4:2667.
59. Rostom A, Jolicoeur E. Validation of a new scale for the assessment of bowel preparation quality. Gastrointest Endosc 2004;59:482–6.

60. Halphen M, Heresbach D, Gruss HJ, et al. Validation of the Harefield Cleansing Scale: a tool for the evaluation of bowel cleansing quality in both research and clinical practice. Gastrointest Endosc 2013;78:121–31.
61. Lai EJ, Calderwood AH, Doros G, et al. The Boston Bowel Preparation Scale: a valid and reliable instrument for colonoscopy-oriented research. Gastrointest Endosc 2009;69:620–5.
62. Calderwood AH, Jacobson BC. Comprehensive validation of the Boston Bowel Preparation Scale. Gastrointest Endosc 2010;72:686–92.
63. Calderwood AH, Schroy PC, Lieberman DA, et al. Boston Bowel Preparation Scale scores provide a standardized definition of adequate for describing bowel cleanliness. Gastrointest Endosc 2014;80(2):269–76.
64. Kim EJ, Park YI, Kim YS, et al. A Korean experience of the use of Boston bowel preparation scale: a valid and reliable instrument for colonoscopy-oriented research. Saudi J Gastroenterol 2014;20(4):219–24.

Techniques and Technologies to Maximize Mucosal Exposure

Leon M.G. Moons, MD, PhD[a],*,
Ian M. Gralnek, MD, PhD, MSHS, FASGE[b,c],
Peter D. Siersema, MD, PhD, FASGE[a]

KEYWORDS

- Mucosal exposure • Colonoscopy • Polyp • Adenoma

KEY POINTS

- Improving withdrawal techniques supported with different maneuvers, such as positioning of the patient, a second pass in the right colon if necessary, and removal of small polyps during insertion, are likely to improve the ADR of the individual endoscopist. This can be supported with new technologies.
- More research is needed, with ADR as the primary end point, to identify the optimal and cost-effective technology that results in a lower miss rate of polyps and adenomas, is easy to implement in daily practice, and does not significantly increase health care costs.

INTRODUCTION

Removal of polyps detected during colonoscopy protects against colorectal cancer.[1] Unfortunately, although colonoscopy is the gold standard for detecting and removing polyps, colorectal carcinomas diagnosed within just a few years following a colonoscopy (interval colorectal cancer) demonstrate the fallibility of current techniques of visualization of the colon. Several factors, such as incomplete resection of polyps or different tumor biology, have been related to these interval cancers, but most are thought to develop because of missed polyps. The endoscopist adenoma detection rate (ADR) has been shown to be inversely associated with the risk of interval cancer.[2,3] Recently, a large population-based study using data from the Kaiser Permanente Northern California health service organization showed that higher ADR (above the threshold of 22%) was associated with decreasing rates of interval colorectal cancers,[3] and that for each 1% increase in ADR, the risk of an interval cancer decreased by 3%.

[a] Department Gastroenterology and Hepatology, University Medical Center Utrecht, Heidelberglaan 100, 3508CH Zeist, Utrecht, The Netherlands; [b] Department of Gastroenterology, Ha'Emek Medical Center, Afula, Israel; [c] Rappaport Faculty of Medicine, Technion-Israel Institute of Technology, Haifa, Israel
* Corresponding author.
E-mail address: l.m.g.moons@umcutrecht.nl

Gastrointest Endoscopy Clin N Am 25 (2015) 199–210
http://dx.doi.org/10.1016/j.giec.2014.11.012
1052-5157/15/$ – see front matter © 2015 Elsevier Inc. All rights reserved.

A systematic review of studies with tandem colonoscopies showed a pooled polyp miss rate of 22%.[4] The missed polyps were mainly small (5–10 mm; 13%) or diminutive (1–5 mm; 26%), but also 2.1% of the polyps greater than 1 cm were missed during colonoscopy. Virtual colonoscopy (computed tomography colography) has demonstrated that missed polyps are primarily located in the proximal colon and particularly on the proximal side of colon folds, making them more difficult to identify.[5] It is likely that an increase in ADR to a high level of detection (>40% in a symptomatic population and >50% in a Fecal immunochemical test (FIT)-based screening population) accounts for the detection of these small or diminutive polyps. Although most small or diminutive polyps will never develop into cancer, advanced histologic features are encountered in a subset of small adenomas,[6] especially in the proximal colon.[7] Risk factors for developing an interval colorectal cancer after a colonoscopy include age; location in the proximal colon; detection of an adenoma at baseline colonoscopy; advanced polyp features, such as villous histology; and a positive family history.[8,9] It therefore seems logical to assume that missing even small polyps in the proximal colon in the context of an increased risk of developing cancer (age, family history, number of polyps, and presence of advanced adenomas) is associated with an increased risk of developing an interval cancer.

Quality improvement programs should aim to train endoscopists to become high-level detectors. Several techniques and technologies are currently available to support current and future endoscopists in maximizing visualization of the mucosal surface of the colon with the objective to lower the polyp/adenoma miss rate.

TECHNIQUES TO OPTIMIZE COLONIC MUCOSAL VISUALIZATION
High-Quality Colonoscopy: Withdrawal Techniques

For complete visualization of the colon, intubation of the cecum is a necessity, and therefore proper scope and loop handling are basic skills required for a high-quality colonoscopy. Although the criterion cecum intubation rate of greater than 90% is often met in daily clinical practice, it is known that the ADR differs significantly between endoscopists.[2,3,10] This difference is partly explained by differences in the withdrawal technique. A video analysis of colonoscopy withdrawals performed by two endoscopists at opposite ends of the spectrum of ADR showed that the endoscopist with the higher ADR visualized a greater percentage of the colonic mucosa because this endoscopist (1) was more adequate in examining the proximal side of the haustral folds, flexures, and rectal valves; (2) was more thorough in removing remnant fluid or fecal material; (3) distended the colon better; and (4) spent more time viewing the mucosa. This was confirmed in another study by Lee and colleagues[11] showing that moderate-level (ADR between 21% and 42%) or high-level (ADR >42%) detectors had higher scores on their withdrawal technique after video analysis of 20 colonoscopies of each of 11 participants, all working in different facilities. The most important differences were found between low-level detectors and moderate- or high-level detectors, suggesting that proper withdrawal techniques are required for higher adenoma detection. Nonetheless, other skills, such as pattern recognition, may define even more the difference between moderate- and high-level adenoma detectors. Moreover, no difference was observed in withdrawal time between low- and high-level detectors. Increased detection of adenomas has, however, been associated with a withdrawal time of greater than or equal to 6 minutes, and this quality indicator is currently endorsed as a surrogate marker of the quality of withdrawal technique.[10,12] Nonetheless, introducing a protocol with a minimum time for withdrawal greater than or equal to 6 minutes has shown conflicting results with regard to an increase in ADR.[13,14] It is therefore likely that factors other than withdrawal time alone influence the ADR, and withdrawal skills in all aforementioned domains need to be improved.

The question of whether improving the withdrawal technique results in a higher ADR is still unanswered. Raising awareness of quality measurement by video recording has been shown to improve withdrawal techniques, but had no effect on ADR.[15] The study was, however, underpowered for this end point. Endoscopists randomized to a training program (EQUIP training) increased their ADR from an average of 36% to 47%, compared with control subjects, which remained at an ADR of 35%.[16] The EQUIP program consisted of training in the importance of good practice withdrawal techniques, but also of training in pattern recognition. This study showed that endoscopists are able to improve their ADR, but the extent to which it can be increased by only improving the level of performance in all domains of the withdrawal technique remains unknown. It seems likely that improving withdrawal techniques improves visualization of the colonic mucosa, and therefore will increase the ADR at least to some extent.

Retroflexion in the Right Colon

Retroflexion of the endoscope in the rectum to visualize the distal rectum and dentate line is a widely accepted and performed standard part of routine colonoscopy. Retroflexion can also be performed in the proximal colon. Because of the diameter of the right colon, retroflexion can be achieved in most patients, and failure to do so is mainly caused by looping of the insertion tube. It was hypothesized that retroflexion in the proximal colon could increase the detection of adenomas located on the proximal sides of haustral folds that are difficult to detect by forward viewing. A randomized study, comparing a second pass of the proximal colon in forward-viewing position in 48 patients with a second pass in retroflexed position in 50 patients, showed an adenoma miss rate of 33.3% in forward view versus 23.7% in retroflex view. Based on these findings the authors concluded that retroflex view of the proximal colon was of no additional value. This was indirectly supported by a prospective, observational study of 1000 patients that all had a second pass in the right colon in retroflex view. This study showed a polyp miss rate of 9.8%, which was much lower than the miss rate of 27% for proximal colon polyps reported in tandem colonoscopy studies. Although retroflexion in the right colon should be performed carefully to prevent mechanical damage to the bowel wall, no adverse events were reported in either study. Based on the aforementioned studies, routine retroflex view of the proximal colon is not expected to increase adenoma detection compared with a second pass of the proximal colon in forward view. Because the detection of a proximal neoplasia at first pass was an important predictor of missed polyps in the proximal colon,[17] a second pass in forward view may be useful in those patients with a proximal neoplasia detected. This strategy has, however, not been formally tested.

Use of Antispasmodic Agents on Colonic Surface Area Visualization

Besides remnant fecal material, haustral folds, and sharp bends, colonic motility can interfere with good visualization of the colonic mucosa. It has been hypothesized that inhibiting smooth muscle contractions during withdrawal may increase mucosal visualization, and thereby polyp and adenoma detection. Hyoscine-N-butylbromide has a superior safety profile and costs less than glucagon, making it the preferred agent to inhibit colonic motility. Although increased polyp detection was reported with hyoscine-N-butylbromide in retrospective and prospective cohorts, recently published randomized placebo-controlled studies did not show a significant increase in ADR with regular use of hyoscine-N-butylbromide.[18–21] Lee and colleagues[22] found a nonsignificant increase in polyp detection (1.2 vs 0.41; $P = .06$) in patients with more than grade 3 spasm of the colon during insertion. The observed difference was small, however, and the ADR was not mentioned. Two meta-analyses on the use of hyoscine-*N*-butylbromide did not show a significant increase in polyp or adenoma detection between hyoscine-*N*-butylbromide and placebo.[23,24] In a recent randomized controlled study of hyoscine-*N*-butylbromide including 402 participants, visualization of nonpolypoid lesions was higher in the placebo arm of the study (1 vs 11)[18]; however, this finding was not confirmed in another study (Ter Borg F, personal communication, 2014).[20] Based on these observations, the routine use of hyoscine-*N*-butylbromide is of no benefit for mucosal visualization, and there is concern whether this hampers the visualization of nonpolypoid lesions.

Positioning of the Patient

Adequate luminal distention is essential for full visualization of the colonic mucosa. This can be partly achieved with insufflation of room air or CO_2, but may be unsuccessful as the air travels to proximal segments of the colon leading to excessive insufflation, which is associated with abdominal symptoms during or after colonoscopy. Position changes have been shown to increase visualization at virtual colonoscopy.[25] In addition, in a video analysis of tandem colonoscopies, luminal distention of several segments of the colon was scored during different positions. Better luminal distention was achieved with the left lateral position for the cecum toward the hepatic flexure, the supine position for the transverse colon, and the right lateral position for the splenic flexure and the descending colon (**Fig. 1**).[26] This prompted the authors of this study to perform a randomized crossover trial to validate the effect of better luminal distention on the ADR in the proximal colon. Patients were randomized to withdrawal of the colonoscope in left lateral position only or in the previously summarized dynamic sequence. Each segment was examined in tandem fashion. Dynamic positioning was associated with an 11% increase in ADR from 23% to 34%, with 61 adenomas detected with dynamic positioning compared with 42 adenomas detected with

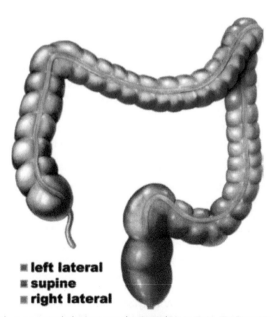

■ left lateral
■ supine
■ right lateral

Fig. 1. Position changes used during extubation. (*From* East JE, Bassett P, Arebi N, et al. Dynamic patient position changes during colonoscope withdrawal increase adenoma detection: a randomized, crossover trial. Gastrointest Endosc 2011;73(3):458; with permission.)

standard left lateral positioning.[27] The differences in polyp and adenoma detection were particularly observed in the transverse colon, splenic flexure, and descending colon, with the most apparent improvement in the transverse colon. Another study with comparable design reported an increase in ADR from 24% to 33% with dynamic positioning with an increase from 42 to 53 detected adenomas.[28] A more recent study in 776 patients comparing dynamic positioning with standard care did not confirm these results.[29] Several explanations can be provided for these conflicting data. In the study by Ou and colleagues,[29] position changes were allowed in the control arm of the study, and 32% had at least one position change during endoscope withdrawal. Furthermore, ADR was 40% in the dynamic positioning group against 39% in the control group. The authors suggested that the benefit of position changes may be of less value when appropriate withdrawal techniques are applied. Despite these contradictory results, it seems reasonable to assume that position changes can be of added value for the endoscopist as one of the options to improve distention of the colon segments when standard options, such as insufflation, are unsuccessful.

Removing Polyps During Insertion

Prevention of postcolonoscopy interval colorectal cancer is not only related to detection of adenomas, but also their removal. It is recognized that small polyps visualized during insertion may be difficult to find during withdrawal. Several explanations have been postulated, such as a different anatomic position of the colon during insertion of the endoscope, exposing other parts of the mucosal surface.[30] In a prospective study of 368 patients, 61.5% of the nonadvanced adenomas were already detected during insertion with an additional detection of 38.5% nonadvanced adenomas during withdrawal.[31] Most polyps were detected in the sigmoid during insertion. A study randomized patients between polypectomy of less than 10-mm polyps during insertion and withdrawal (N = 150) or during withdrawal only (N = 151). This study concluded that adenomas were missed in 7.3% of patients when removing polyps only during withdrawal of the endoscope.[32] These missed polyps were primarily located in the sigmoid and descending colon.[32] This considerable adenoma miss rate suggests that small polyps should be removed during insertion. However, two recent studies, randomizing patients between polypectomy during insertion and withdrawal versus during withdrawal only, showed no benefit of removing small and diminutive polyps during insertion.[30,33] There were, however, some major differences between the studies. The study by Hewitt and colleagues[30] evaluated the effect of an additional 3 minutes inspection on ADR during insertion, whereas removal of polyps during insertion was also allowed in the control arm consisting of inspection during withdrawal only. In contrast, in the study by Sanaka and colleagues[33] polyps were only removed in the withdrawal phase of the colonoscopy. In both studies, most colonoscopies were performed by high-level detectors (ADR ranging from 34% to 58%) in populations with a different case mix of colonoscopy indications. Notwithstanding these conflicting data, it seems reasonable to assume that removing all small polyps detected during insertion, especially diminutive polyps in the sigmoid or descending colon, may be beneficial.

TECHNOLOGIES TO LOOK BEHIND THE FOLDS
Third-Eye Retroscope

A device specifically designed to enhance the visualization on the proximal side of colonic folds is the Third-Eye Retroscope (Avantis Medical Systems, Inc, Sunnyvale, CA). The retroscope is advanced through the working channel of the colonoscope and after retroflexion to 180 degrees it provides a 135-degree retrograde view of the colon. The efficacy of the Third-Eye Retroscope was initially studied in three colon models with simulated polyps.[34] Standard colonoscopy detected 12% of the polyps located on the proximal side of folds, whereas 81% of these polyps were detected with the Third-Eye Retroscope. The first pilot study in 24 patients resulted in an 11.8% increase in diagnostic yield, with 34 polyps detected in the antegrade view and four additional polyps in the retrograde view.[35] In two nonrandomized studies,[36,37] the additional diagnostic yield of the Third-Eye Retroscope was investigated by evaluating whether polyps detected with the Third-Eye Retroscope could also be seen with the antegrade view of the colonoscope. In the first study, 182 polyps in 298 subjects were found with the antegrade view and 27 additional polyps were found with the Third-Eye Retroscope, resulting in a 14.8% increase in polyp detection and a 16.0% increase in adenoma detection.[36] The second study reported a similar result with a 13.2% increase in polyp detection and an 11.0% increase in adenoma detection.[37] A single randomized back-to-back study has been performed, the TERRACE study.[38] In this multicenter study including 349 patients, a net additional detection rate with the Third-Eye Retroscope of 29.8% for polyps and 23.2% for adenomas was reported. This study was criticized because the mean withdrawal time was almost 2 minutes longer with the Third-Eye Retroscope compared with standard colonoscopy. Nevertheless, studies that have investigated the Third-Eye Retroscope have shown a significant additional diagnostic yield when using this technology, but there are some limitations inherent to the device. First, thorough suctioning of colonic debris must be done during insertion of the colonoscope because of a 50% reduced suctioning capacity when the retroscope is in position. A second disadvantage is that the Third-Eye Retroscope needs to be removed from the working channel when an accessory device is required, such as a biopsy forceps or a polypectomy snare, which is cumbersome and increases procedure time.

Wide-Angle Colonoscopy

The recently developed Full Spectrum Endoscopy (FUSE; EndoChoice, Alpharetta, GA) colonoscope allows a high-resolution 330° "full spectrum" viewing of the colonic lumen while maintaining the standard colonoscope technical features and capabilities of a standard 140° and 170° colonoscope. The FUSE system consists of a main control unit and a video colonoscope with three imagers and LED groups located at the front and both sides of the flexible colonoscope tip. The video images transmitted from the three cameras on the left side, front, and right side of the colonoscope are displayed on three contiguous monitors corresponding with each individual camera. The two additional side cameras incorporated in the FUSE colonoscope provide a better and more comprehensive view of the total colonic lumen and surface area. Frequently encountered blind spots, such as the internal lining of flexures and proximal aspects of folds, should be easily visualized with this system. An international, randomized, multicenter, tandem colonoscopy crossover trial was performed, comparing standard forward-viewing colonoscopy with FUSE colonoscopy.[39] Same-day colonoscopies with FUSE and standard colonoscopes were performed in 185 randomized subjects. Eighty-eight patients (48%) were randomly assigned to receive standard forward-viewing colonoscopy first and 97 (52%) to receive full-spectrum endoscopy colonoscopy first. The adenoma miss rate was significantly lower in patients in the full-spectrum endoscopy group (7%; 5 of 67 adenomas) than in those in the standard forward-viewing procedure group (41%; 20 of 49 adenomas). The withdrawal time was shorter for standard forward-viewing colonoscopy examinations (5.6 [interquartile range, 4.1–6.8] vs 6.2 minutes [interquartile range, 5.1–8.3]). Although this cannot be excluded, it is unlikely that this time difference has a clinically significant influence on the difference in observed adenoma miss rate. Five (6%) patients in the standard forward-viewing first group had no adenomas detected at first-pass examination, but had adenomas detected by full-spectrum endoscopy. By contrast, no patients in the full-spectrum endoscopy first group had additional adenomas detected by standard forward-viewing colonoscopy. This trial was not statistically powered for per-patient analyses, and although full-spectrum colonoscopy yielded significantly fewer false-negative examinations than standard forward-viewing colonoscopy, no significant increase in ADR was observed.[39]

Cap-Assisted Colonoscopy

Transparent caps attached to the distal tip of the colonoscope have been suggested to be of help in flattening colonic folds to improve visualization of their proximal side. Randomized controlled trials that evaluated the additional diagnostic yield of cap-assisted colonoscopy were mostly performed in Asian countries and have shown mixed results.[40,41] In a study by Kondo and colleagues,[41] 684 subjects were randomized to colonoscopy with a 4-mm transparent cap, a 2-mm rubber cap, or without a cap. Polyp detection rates for colonoscopies with the transparent cap, rubber cap, or no cap were 49.3%, 44.7%, and 39.1%, respectively; only the difference between the transparent 4-mm cap and no cap was statistically significant. In a randomized controlled trial by Rastogi and colleagues[42] ADR was 13% higher with cap-assisted colonoscopy compared with standard colonoscopy, but this was only observed for diminutive ($\leq$5 mm) adenomas. In contrast, in the single largest randomized trial published thus far (1000 patients included), a lower ADR (30.5% vs 37.5%) and mean number of adenomas per subject were reported with cap-assisted colonoscopy compared with standard colonoscopy.[43] Other studies also showed no increased yield with cap-assisted colonoscopy.[44,45]

A meta-analysis of randomized controlled trials comparing cap-assisted colonoscopy with standard colonoscopy included 16 randomized controlled trials, in which 4501 subjects had cap-assisted colonoscopy and 4490 standard colonoscopy. Cap-assisted colonoscopy detected a higher proportion of subjects with polyps compared with standard colonoscopy (52.5% vs 47.5%). A subanalysis of six trials investigating ADR showed no benefit of cap-assisted colonoscopy over standard colonoscopy (46.8% vs 45.3%). Although a cap may be helpful during insertion of the endoscope and assist during polypectomy, routine use of cap-assisted colonoscopy probably does not increase ADR.

Endocuff

The Endocuff (Arc Medical Design Ltd, Leeds, UK) is a device that can be attached to the tip of the colonoscope. It is designed to provide a better view of the proximal sides of haustral folds by stretching the folds backward with the arms of the Endocuff during withdrawal. It is also hypothesized that the arms of the device aid in obtaining a stable position in the center of the colonic lumen. In a recent prospective cohort study in 50 Endocuff-assisted colonoscopies, the cecum was reached in 98%, and the terminal ileum intubated in 76%. In 15 of 50 (30%) subjects, scratch-like lesions were observed on the colonic mucosa, but no severe adverse events, such as bleeding or perforation, were reported. A randomized controlled study randomizing 498 patients to standard forward-viewing colonoscopy with or without Endocuff showed an overall 14% increase in ADR with the Endocuff (ADR, 42% vs 56%). The use of the Endocuff was associated with minimal mucosal lacerations (nine vs two patients) which was no longer observed after examination of six cases. The results of ongoing randomized controlled studies are awaited, but the existing data seem promising.

EndoRings

EndoRings (EndoAid Ltd, Caesarea, Israel) is a silicone rubber device that is fitted onto the distal end of the colonoscope. Its flexible circular rings engage and mechanically stretch colonic folds during withdrawal. In a multicenter, tandem colonoscopy, cross-over study comparing standard colonoscopy with EndoRings-assisted colonoscopy, an adenoma miss rate of 10% (7 of 69 adenomas) was found when EndoRings-assisted colonoscopy was the first procedure compared with 48% when started with standard colonoscopy (28 of 58 adenomas).[46] Insertion and withdrawal times were not different between the two groups.

Because the Endocuff and the EndoRings are easily mounted on currently available colonoscopes, they are attractive alternatives to other currently available technologies, such as the FUSE colonoscope and Third-Eye Retroscope.

G-Eye Balloon

The NaviAid G-EYE System (SMART Medical Systems, Ra'anana, Israel) includes the G-EYE balloon-colonoscope and the NaviAid SPARK2C inflation system. The NaviAid G-EYE colonoscope permanently integrates an inflatable, reusable, and reprocessable balloon onto the flexible tip of a standard colonoscope. The integrated balloon can be inflated by the endoscopist upon colonoscope withdrawal to perform balloon-assisted colonoscopy. The mechanical flattening and straightening of haustral folds with the inflated balloon allows visualization of hidden colonic areas. The balloon can also be inflated to a set pressure of 70 mbar to anchor the colonoscope and stabilize it within the colon lumen during endoscopic interventions (eg, biopsy, polypectomy), thereby minimizing movement of the colonoscope. To prevent excessive insufflation, the NaviAid SPARK2C includes pressure sensors with dedicated software. A prospective cohort study in 47 patients showed that introduction and balloon-assisted withdrawal

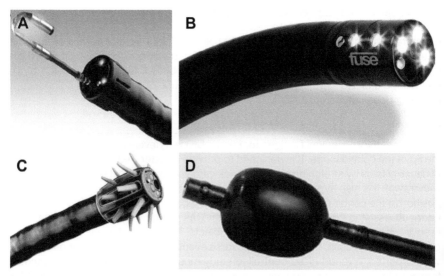

Fig. 2. Overview of several new technologies to improve mucosal visualization of the colon. (A) Third-Eye Retroscope. (B) FUSE colonoscope. (C) Endocuff. (D) G-EYE balloon colonoscope. (*Courtesy of* [A] Avantis Medical Systems, Inc, Sunnyvale, CA; [B] EndoChoice, Alpharetta, GA; [C] Arc Medical Design Ltd, Leeds, UK; and [D] SMART Medical Systems, Ra'anana, Israel; with permission.)

Table 1

Overview of tandem colonoscopy studies and randomized controlled studies of techniques and technologies to improve mucosal visualization of the colon

Author, Year	Technique	Study Design	Study Arms	End Point	N	Withdrawal Time (min)	Total Procedure Time (min)	PDR	Total Patients with Adenomas (%)	Number of Adenomas/ Patients	Adenoma Miss Rates
Rex et al,[15] 1997	Second look	Tandem colonoscopy	SFV	Adenoma miss rate	183 SFV	—	—	145/183 (79%)	104/183 (57%)	2.07	89/289 (24%)
Leufkens et al,[38] 2011	Third-Eye Retroscope	Tandem colonoscopy	SFV + TER / TER + SFV	Number of adenomas	173 SFV / 176 TER	TER 9.52 / SFV 7.58	20.87 / 16.97	— / —	— / —	0.90 / 0.80	49/156 (31%) / 26/141 (18%)
Gralnek et al,[39] 2014	FUSE	Tandem colonoscopy	SFV + FUSE / FUSE + SFV	Adenoma miss rates	88 SFV / 97 FUSE	5.6 (4.1–6.8) / 6.2 (5.1–8.3)	12.2 (9.2–16.5) / 14.5 (10.8–20.2)	—	30 (34%) / 33 (34%)	0.56 / 0.69	20/49 (41%) / 5/67 (7%)
Dik et al,[46] 2014	EndoRings	Tandem colonoscopy	EndoRings + SFV / SFV + EndoRings	Adenoma miss rates	62 EndoRings / 64 SFV	7.4 ± 1.9 / 7.2 ± 2.2	21.6 ± 8.9 / 18.5 ± 8.2	68% / 41%	29/62 (47%) / 17/64 (27%)	1.11 / 0.91	7/69 (10%) / 28/58 (48%)
Biecker,[48] 2014	Endocuff	RCT	Endocuff / SFV	Number of polyps/ colonoscopy	239 Endocuff / 247 SFV	n.m. / n.m.	23.11 ± 8.83 / 21.51 ± 8.00	56% / 42%	87 (36%) / 69 (28%)	— / —	— / —
Harrison,[49] 2004	Retroflexion	RCT	SFV + SFV / SFV + retroflexion	Adenoma miss rates	48 SFV / 50 Retroflexion	10.4 / 10.3	— / —	— / —	— / —	0.88 / 0.76	14/42 (33.3%) / 9/38 (23.7%)

Abbreviations: PDR, polyp detection rate; RCT, randomized controlled trial; SFV, standard forward viewing; TER, Third-Eye Retroscope.

were safe and feasible.[47] Prospective trials comparing G-EYE balloon colonoscopy with standard colonoscopy are underway to test the additional value of this technology compared with standard forward-viewing colonoscopy.

SUMMARY

Improving withdrawal techniques, supported with different maneuvers, such as positioning of the patient, a second pass in the right colon if necessary, and removal of small polyps during insertion, are likely to improve the ADR of the individual endoscopist. This can be supported with new technologies, as discussed previously (**Fig. 2**). Although new technologies seem promising, it should be stressed that most studies were not powered to detect a difference in ADR, and most technologies are evaluated in single studies (**Table 1**). Therefore more research is needed, with ADR as the primary end point, to identify the optimal and cost-effective technology that results in a lower miss rate of polyps and adenomas, is easy to implement in daily practice, and does not significantly increase health care costs.

REFERENCES

1. Zauber AG, Winawer S, O'Brien MJ, et al. Colonoscopic polypectomy and long-term prevention of colorectal-cancer deaths. N Engl J Med 2012;366(8):687–96.
2. Kaminski MF, Regula J, Kraszewska E, et al. Quality indicators for colonoscopy and the risk of interval cancer. N Engl J Med 2010;362(19):1795–803.
3. Corley DA, Jensen CD, Marks AR, et al. Adenoma detection rate and risk of colorectal cancer and death. N Engl J Med 2014;370(14):1298–306.
4. van Rijn JC, Reitsma JB, Stoker J, et al. Polyp miss rate determined by tandem colonoscopy: a systematic review. Am J Gastroenterol 2006;101(2):343–50.
5. Pickhardt PJ, Nugent PA, Mysliwiec PA, et al. Location of adenomas missed by optical colonoscopy. Ann Intern Med 2004;141(5):352–9.
6. Repici A, Hassan C, Vitetta E, et al. Safety of cold polypectomy for <10 mm polyps at colonoscopy: a prospective multicenter study. Endoscopy 2012;44(1):27–31.
7. Rondagh EJ, Bouwens MW, Riedl RG, et al. Endoscopic appearance of proximal colorectal neoplasms and potential implications for colonoscopy in cancer prevention. Gastrointest Endosc 2012;75(6):1218–25.
8. Samadder NJ, Curtin K, Tuohy TM, et al. Characteristics of missed or interval colorectal cancer and patient survival: a population-based study. Gastroenterology 2014;146(4):950–60.
9. Bressler B, Paszat LF, Chen Z, et al. Rates of new or missed colorectal cancers after colonoscopy and their risk factors: a population-based analysis. Gastroenterology 2007;132(1):96–102.
10. Barclay RL, Vicari JJ, Doughty AS, et al. Colonoscopic withdrawal times and adenoma detection during screening colonoscopy. N Engl J Med 2006;355(24):2533–41.
11. Lee RH, Tang RS, Muthusamy VR, et al. Quality of colonoscopy withdrawal technique and variability in adenoma detection rates (with videos). Gastrointest Endosc 2011;74(1):128–34.
12. Overholt BF, Brooks-Belli L, Grace M, et al. Withdrawal times and associated factors in colonoscopy: a quality assurance multicenter assessment. J Clin Gastroenterol 2010;44(4):e80–6.
13. Barclay RL, Vicari JJ, Greenlaw RL. Effect of a time-dependent colonoscopic withdrawal protocol on adenoma detection during screening colonoscopy. Clin Gastroenterol Hepatol 2008;6(10):1091–8.

14. Sawhney MS, Cury MS, Neeman N, et al. Effect of institution-wide policy of colonoscopy withdrawal time > or = 7 minutes on polyp detection. Gastroenterology 2008;135(6):1892–8.

15. Rex DK, Cutler CS, Lemmel GT, et al. Colonoscopic miss rates of adenomas determined by back-to-back colonoscopies. Gastroenterology 1997;112(1):24–8.

16. Coe SG, Crook JE, Diehl NN, et al. An endoscopic quality improvement program improves detection of colorectal adenomas. Am J Gastroenterol 2013;108(2): 219–26 [quiz: 227].

17. Laiyemo AO, Doubeni C, Sanderson AK, et al. Likelihood of missed and recurrent adenomas in the proximal versus the distal colon. Gastrointest Endosc 2011; 74(2):253–61.

18. Rondonotti E, Radaelli F, Paggi S, et al. Hyoscine N-butylbromide for adenoma detection during colonoscopy: a randomized, double-blind, placebo-controlled study. Dig Liver Dis 2013;45(8):663–8.

19. Mui LM, Ng EK, Chan KC, et al. Randomized, double-blinded, placebo-controlled trial of intravenously administered hyoscine N-butyl bromide in patients undergoing colonoscopy with patient-controlled sedation. Gastrointest Endosc 2004; 59(1):22–7.

20. de Brouwer EJ, Arbouw ME, van der Zwet WC, et al. Hyoscine N-butylbromide does not improve polyp detection during colonoscopy: a double-blind, randomized, placebo-controlled, clinical trial. Gastrointest Endosc 2012;75(4):835–40.

21. Corte C, Dahlenburg L, Selby W, et al. Hyoscine butylbromide administered at the cecum increases polyp detection: a randomized double-blind placebo-controlled trial. Endoscopy 2012;44(10):917–22.

22. Lee JM, Cheon JH, Park JJ, et al. Effects of Hyosine N-butyl bromide on the detection of polyps during colonoscopy. Hepatogastroenterology 2010;57(97): 90–4.

23. Cui PJ, Yao J, Han HZ, et al. Does hyoscine butylbromide really improve polyp detection during colonoscopy? A meta-analysis of randomized controlled trials. World J Gastroenterol 2014;20(22):7034–9.

24. Rondonotti E, Zolk O, Amato A, et al. The impact of hyoscine-N-butylbromide on adenoma detection during colonoscopy: meta-analysis of randomized, controlled studies. Gastrointest Endosc 2014;80(6):1103–12.e2.

25. Mulhall BP, Veerappan GR, Jackson JL. Meta-analysis: computed tomographic colonography. Ann Intern Med 2005;142(8):635–50.

26. East JE, Suzuki N, Arebi N, et al. Position changes improve visibility during colonoscope withdrawal: a randomized, blinded, crossover trial. Gastrointest Endosc 2007;65(2):263–9.

27. East JE, Bassett P, Arebi N, et al. Dynamic patient position changes during colonoscope withdrawal increase adenoma detection: a randomized, crossover trial. Gastrointest Endosc 2011;73(3):456–63.

28. Koksal AS, Kalkan IH, Torun S, et al. A simple method to improve adenoma detection rate during colonoscopy: altering patient position. Can J Gastroenterol 2013; 27(9):509–12.

29. Ou G, Kim E, Lakzadeh P, et al. A randomized controlled trial assessing the effect of prescribed patient position changes during colonoscope withdrawal on adenoma detection. Gastrointest Endosc 2014;80(2):277–83.

30. Hewett DG, Rex DK. Inspection on instrument insertion during colonoscopy: a randomized controlled trial. Gastrointest Endosc 2012;76(2):381–7.

31. Morini S, Hassan C, Zullo A, et al. Detection of colonic polyps according to insertion/withdrawal phases of colonoscopy. Int J Colorectal Dis 2009;24(5):527–30.

32. Wildi SM, Schoepfer AM, Vavricka SR, et al. Colorectal polypectomy during insertion and withdrawal or only during withdrawal? A randomized controlled trial. Endoscopy 2012;44(11):1019–23.
33. Sanaka MR, Parsi MA, Burke CA, et al. Adenoma detection at colonoscopy by polypectomy in withdrawal only versus both insertion and withdrawal: a randomized controlled trial. Surg Endosc 2015;29(3):692–9.
34. Triadafilopoulos G, Watts HD, Higgins J, et al. A novel retrograde-viewing auxiliary imaging device (Third Eye Retroscope) improves the detection of simulated polyps in anatomic models of the colon. Gastrointest Endosc 2007;65(1):139–44.
35. Triadafilopoulos G, Li J. A pilot study to assess the safety and efficacy of the Third Eye retrograde auxiliary imaging system during colonoscopy. Endoscopy 2008; 40(6):478–82.
36. DeMarco DC, Odstrcil E, Lara LF, et al. Impact of experience with a retrograde-viewing device on adenoma detection rates and withdrawal times during colonoscopy: the Third Eye Retroscope study group. Gastrointest Endosc 2010;71(3):542–50.
37. Waye JD, Heigh RI, Fleischer DE, et al. A retrograde-viewing device improves detection of adenomas in the colon: a prospective efficacy evaluation (with videos). Gastrointest Endosc 2010;71(3):551–6.
38. Leufkens AM, DeMarco DC, Rastogi A, et al. Effect of a retrograde-viewing device on adenoma detection rate during colonoscopy: the TERRACE study. Gastrointest Endosc 2011;73(3):480–9.
39. Gralnek IM, Siersema PD, Halpern Z, et al. Standard forward-viewing colonoscopy versus full-spectrum endoscopy: an international, multicentre, randomised, tandem colonoscopy trial. Lancet Oncol 2014;15(3):353–60.
40. Ng SC, Tsoi KK, Hirai HW, et al. The efficacy of cap-assisted colonoscopy in polyp detection and cecal intubation: a meta-analysis of randomized controlled trials. Am J Gastroenterol 2012;107(8):1165–73.
41. Kondo S, Yamaji Y, Watabe H, et al. A randomized controlled trial evaluating the usefulness of a transparent hood attached to the tip of the colonoscope. Am J Gastroenterol 2007;102(1):75–81.
42. Rastogi A, Bansal A, Rao DS, et al. Higher adenoma detection rates with cap-assisted colonoscopy: a randomised controlled trial. Gut 2012;61(3):402–8.
43. Lee YT, Lai LH, Hui AJ, et al. Efficacy of cap-assisted colonoscopy in comparison with regular colonoscopy: a randomized controlled trial. Am J Gastroenterol 2009;104(1):41–6.
44. de Wijkerslooth TR, Stoop EM, Bossuyt PM, et al. Adenoma detection with cap-assisted colonoscopy versus regular colonoscopy: a randomised controlled trial. Gut 2012;61(10):1426–34.
45. Tee HP, Corte C, Al-Ghamdi H, et al. Prospective randomized controlled trial evaluating cap-assisted colonoscopy vs standard colonoscopy. World J Gastroenterol 2010;16(31):3905–10.
46. Dik VK, Gralnek IM, Segol O, et al. Comparing standard colonoscopy with EndoRings colonoscopy: a randomized, multicenter tandem colonoscopy study: interim results of the CLEVER study. Gastroenterology 2014;146(5 Suppl 1):S160.
47. Gralnek IM, Suissa A, Domanov S. Safety and efficacy of a novel balloon colonoscope: a prospective cohort study. Endoscopy 2014;46(10):883–7.
48. Biecker E, Floer M, Heinecke A, et al. Novel endocuff-assisted colonoscopy significantly increases the polyp detection rate: a randomized controlled trial. J Clin Gastroenterol 2014;11.
49. Harrison M, Singh N, Rex DK. Impact of proximal colon retroflexion on adenoma miss rates. Am J Gastroenterol 2004;99(3):519–22.

Water-Aided Colonoscopy

Joseph C. Anderson, MD[a,b],*

KEYWORDS

- Colonoscopy • Water immersion • Water infusion • Adenoma detection • Sedation

KEY POINTS

- Water-assisted colonoscopy involves the infusion of water without air and subsequent suctioning during insertion (exchange) or withdrawal (immersion or infusion).
- Water-assisted colonoscopy can be used to decrease sedation requirements in patients undergoing colonoscopy.
- Water-assisted colonoscopy can increase completion rate in examinations not using sedation.
- Water-assisted colonoscopy can be used to complete difficult examinations owing to redundancy or severe angulation in the distal colon.
- Water-assisted colonoscopy may yield more proximal adenomas than air insufflation for some operators, perhaps due to longer withdrawal/examination time and bowel preparation salvaging.
- Water exchange may be superior to water immersion with regards to pain experience by patients.
- Water infusion has been shown to not deleteriously alter serum electrolyte levels or vital signs.

INTRODUCTION

Colorectal cancer prevention with colonoscopy depends on the successful insertion of the colonoscope to the cecum with subsequent careful mucosal inspection on withdrawal. The recommended target for an endoscopist's cecal intubation rate is 90% for all examinations and 95% for healthy screening patients.[1,2] Thus, a significant number of colonoscopies may still be incomplete. In addition, colonoscope insertion, even in those examinations with ultimately successful cecal intubation, can still be associated with many challenges. Previous investigators have observed that

The contents of this work do not represent the views of the Department of Veterans Affairs or the United States Government.
J.C. Anderson is the guarantor of the article and has no conflicts of interest to disclose.
[a] Department of Veterans Affairs Medical Center, Department of Medicine, 215 North Main Street, White River Junction, VT 05009, USA; [b] The Geisel School of Medicine at Dartmouth Medical, Department of Medicine, Hanover, NH 03755, USA
* Department of Veterans Affairs Medical Center, 215 North Main Street, White River Junction, VT 05009.
E-mail address: joseph.anderson@dartmouth.edu

Gastrointest Endoscopy Clin N Am 25 (2015) 211–226
http://dx.doi.org/10.1016/j.giec.2014.11.002
1052-5157/15/$ – see front matter Published by Elsevier Inc.

predictors such as female gender and thin body habitus may be associated with difficult or incomplete examinations.[3,4] There have been attempts to produce new scopes that may aid in the completion of colonoscopies.[5] In addition, new techniques such as water-aided colonoscopy have been developed.

The infusion of water during colonoscopy has been used in an attempt to allow easier insertion of the scope. One of the initial studies involved the use of 100 to 200 mL of sterile water to facilitate the passage of the colonoscope through the left colon.[6] The investigators observed that water infusion in the left colon reduced insertion time by nearly one-third as compared with the traditional insertion method. Since that publication, several studies have examined the utility of water infusion as well as water exchange. This review provides insight into the rationale and utility of water-assisted colonoscopy and highlights important clinical studies.

DIFFICULT COLONOSCOPIES

When assessing the efficacy of any modality designed to assist the endoscopist during colonoscope insertion, the clinically important outcomes and benchmarks need to be identified. Thus, it is important to examine how difficulty in colonoscopy insertion can be defined, measured, and characterized. The most important outcome for colonoscopy is completion of the examination as defined by successful cecal intubation. Because this rate is often greater than 95%, other important measures may be considered. Despite the potential for gaming, time to the cecum or insertion time has been used to determine the difficulty of colonoscopy.[3] Other measures may include the ability to retroflex in the cecum, which can often be a manifestation of redundancy or looping of the scope,[5] and the need for maneuvers such as abdominal pressure, stiffening of the colonoscope, and changing the position of the patient. These measures likely reflect the degree to which the colonoscope is looping in the patient. The ability to perform endoscopy without sedation or the amount of sedation medication required may also be considered relevant measures. Finally, the patient's experience, often reported as pain during or after the examination, is also an important outcome. Except for cecal intubation, these measures are subjective, and thus the results of studies based exclusively on them may be difficult to interpret.

Adequate discussion of difficult insertion requires understanding the underlying mechanisms. Difficult insertion is often related to the anatomic location of the colonoscope tip when the challenge is encountered and can be categorized into challenges that are distal or in the sigmoid and those that are related to redundancy or persistent looping.[7] Sigmoid challenges might be observed in patients with severe angulation, such as thin women or patients with diverticular disease.[3,4] Issues related to redundancy or excessive looping may be seen in patients with central obesity or severe constipation.[3]

RATIONALE FOR USE OF WATER-ASSISTED COLONOSCOPY

There are several proposed mechanisms through which water may facilitate the passage of a colonoscope through the colon. When filled with water, the sigmoid colon may be weighted down into the left lower quadrant if the patient is in the left lateral decubitus position. This can straighten the sigmoid and make tight angles less acute. Another mechanism may be related to the shortening of the colon through the use of water as opposed to air, which may elongate the colon.[8] In addition, the use of water may help to lubricate the scope, allowing for easier passage. Other proposed mechanisms include decreased colonic spasm.

TECHNIQUE OF WATER-ASSISTED COLONOSCOPIES: IMMERSION VERSUS EXCHANGE

During water immersion, water is infused during insertion and the air pump is turned off. Infused water is then aspirated during scope withdrawal. Water exchange involves the infusion of clean water with suction and removal of the fecal suspension during insertion. Water exchange also involves turning off of the air pump. A hybrid of these methods is often used in practice and in trials. In this technique, water is used as an adjunct to air insufflation during the passage through tight strictures or angles often observed in the sigmoid colon.[9]

With regards to water exchange, one expert has offered helpful maneuvers in a recent editorial.[9] These maneuvers include the infusion of a minimal amount of water that is sufficient to open the lumen or spasm. The investigator suggests that to minimize inadvertent mucosal suction, the endoscopist should decrease the level of suction and point the suction port toward the center of the lumen. In addition, if bowel preparation is not optimal, the endoscopist should infuse clean water and suction the debris simultaneously. In the author's opinion, cleaning of the bowel is easier in a water-filled colon than in an air-filled lumen because the simultaneous infusion and suctioning of water creates a turbulent environment that suspends the fecal debris, allowing for efficient suctioning of fecal debris. Finally, although maneuvers such as abdominal compression and change of patient position may be required less often in water techniques, these adjunctive techniques should still be considered an integral part of the examination.

LEARNING THE WATER TECHNIQUE

It has been suggested that the water technique may seem too cumbersome for endoscopists who are accustomed to air insufflation.[10] One report examined the cecal intubation rate for an experienced endoscopist during the learning phase of the water technique. The investigators examined 4 groups or quartiles of 25 water-aided colonoscopies and compared these examinations to 100 historical colonoscopies performed by the same endoscopist in which air insertion was used. The cecal intubation for the water technique increased from 76% in the first quartile to 96% in the fourth quartile. The cecal intubation rate for the final quartile was comparable to the 98% observed in the air cohort. Other trends observed included a faster cecal intubation time, higher adenoma detection rate (ADR), and a lower rate of change in patient position when compared with the air cohort. These data suggest that an experienced endoscopist might require only 100 examinations to become proficient at the water technique. The most common reason for failure to intubate the cecum was misidentification of the cecum. The identification of the usual landmarks was initially more difficult in the water-filled colon. The hepatic flexure was the most common anatomic location that was mistaken for the cecum. The investigators observed that suction marks on the cecum were good indicators of cecal intubation. They speculated that these marks were the result of the attempts by the endoscopist to open the appendix, believing that this was the lumen. Another reliable indicator of cecal intubation was the insertion of 90 cm of colonoscope.

WATER-ASSISTED COLONOSCOPY AND COMPLETION RATE

Cecal intubation has been assessed by several trials, which are shown in **Table 1**.[11–18] One meta-analysis observed no difference between water infusion and air insufflation in 6 randomized controlled studies (odds ratio [OR] = 1.0; 95% confidence interval [CI], 0.96–1.03).[19] Another meta-analysis also observed that there was no difference in cecal

Table 1
Review of salient studies examining the use of water during colonoscopy

Author, Year, Country	Subjects	Design	Comparison	Outcome	Results	Limitations	Conclusions
Brocchi et al,[11] 2008, Italy	Colonoscopy patients	RCT (170 patients in each arm)	Standard jelly for lubricating vs corn seed oil vs warm water	CI rate; Time to cecum and for examination; Pain; Difficulty of examination for endoscopist	1. CI rate higher in oil/water than standard 2. Less intubation time in oil 3. Less pain in oil/water 4. Oil/water examinations less difficult 5. No difference between oil and water groups	Unblinded single center	Warm water– and oil-assisted examinations may allow for easier cecal intubation and less pain for patient
Leung J, et al,[17] 2009, USA	Minimally sedated Veterans Affairs patients	RCT (28 patients in each arm)	WI vs AI	Sedation; Pain; CI rate; Willingness to repeat examination	1. Pain reduced in WI 2. Less medications in WI 3. CI rate and willingness to repeat examination were similar	Older male population	WI may be superior to AI in minimally sedated patients
Leung F, et al,[22] 2009, USA	Two consecutive groups of unsedated Veterans Affairs patients	Observational (62 AI & 63 WI)	WI vs AI	CI rate; Willingness to repeat examination	1. CI rate higher in WI a compared to air (97% vs 76%) 2. WI had more patients willing to repeat (90% vs 69%)	Nonrandomized older men	RCT required to examine WI vs AI

Study	Population	Design	Outcomes	Results	Limitations	Comments
Radaelli et al,[18] 2010, Italy	Consecutive outpatients initially having no sedation	RCT (116 WI & 114 AI)	Warm WI vs AI	Patients requesting sedation; CI rate	1. % requesting sedation less in WI (P = .07) 2. CI rate similar in WI/air 3. Less pain WI (P = .05) 4. ADR higher in WI	Single center physicians not blinded	Borderline significant results suggest more data needed to support the decreased need for sedation in WI examinations
Leung F, et al,[15] 2010, USA	Unsedated Veterans Affairs patients	RCT (40 AI & 42 WI)	WI vs AI (some WE occurred in poor preparations)	Pain; CI rate; Willingness to repeat examination	1. CI rate higher in WI (78% vs 98%) 2. WI associated with higher willingness for repeat examination 3. Less pain in WI	Older male population	Water infusion may increase CI rate and decrease patient pain in unsedated male patients
Pohl et al,[21] 2011, Germany	Consecutive outpatients initially having no sedation	RCT (58 patients in each arm)	WI vs AI	Patients requesting sedation	1. % requesting sedation less in WI 2. Less pain in WI 3. CI rate for unsedated examinations higher in WI but lower than AI overall 4. Similar ADR in AI/WI	Single center physicians not blinded	Suboptimal bowel preparation may limit benefit of using water method

(continued on next page)

Table 1
(continued)

Author, Year, Country	Subjects	Design	Comparison	Outcome	Results	Limitations	Conclusions
Ramirez & Leung,[31] 2011, USA	368 consecutive screening patients	RCT	WI vs AI	ADR CI rate WT Sedation required Abdominal pressure used	1. ADR higher in WI 2. Similar CI rates 3. WI had longer insertion time but similar WT 4. Less abdominal pressure needed in WI	Male population	WI may increase yield of proximal adenomas perhaps due to longer insertion time
Hsieh et al,[12] 2011, China	Consecutive minimally sedated patients	RCT (AI 89 & 90 WI)	WI in left colon vs AI	CI rate Time for insertion Need for maneuvers during examination such as abdominal pressure Pain	1. CI rate and need for maneuvers similar in both groups 2. Less pain in WI 3. Longer insertion time in WI	Single center	Limited water infusion may lower pain but lengthen insertion time
Leung J, et al,[16] 2011, USA	Veterans Affairs patients accepting on demand sedation	RCT (50 patients in each arm)	WI vs AI (some WE occurred in poor preparations)	proportion of patients completing examination with no sedation CI rate Sedation medications Pain	1. More patients in WI had complete examination with no sedation 2. Overall CI rates similar 3. Lower medication need in WI 4. Lower pain in WI	Older male population	Benefit of WI in reducing sedation requirement is confirmed in this study

Leung F, et al,[23] 2011, USA	Combination of 2 RCTs (see earlier text) from Veterans Affairs health centers[5,9]	WI (92) and AI (90) WI vs air	CI rate ADR	1. Higher CI rate in water-assisted examinations 2. Higher ADR for water for small proximal adenomas 3. Longer WT in WI 4. Better bowel preparation score in WI	Older male population	Water had modest increase in yield of small proximal adenomas but with higher WT
Vemulapalli & Rex,[8] 2012, USA	Patients referred for incomplete colonoscopy	Observational: 345 patients	WI vs AI	CI rate Equipment required	1. CI rates similar in AI and WI 2. Fewer external straightening device in WI	Single endoscopist	Water immersion may aid in completing examinations of patients with previously incomplete colonoscopies using standard equipment
Leung F, et al,[28] 2012, USA	Various published studies	Systematic review WI vs WE vs AI	Pain ADR	1. ADR higher in WE vs AI especially in proximal colon 2. Pain is reduced in WE more than WI as compared with AI	Differences in study design	WE may be superior to WI and a study examining 3 approaches is needed

(continued on next page)

Table 1
(continued)

Author, Year, Country	Subjects	Design	Comparison	Outcome	Results	Limitations	Conclusions
Jun & Bing,[19] 2013, China	Various published studies	Meta-analysis	WI vs air	CI rate Total examination time Abdominal compression or position change ADR Pain On demand sedation	1. No difference in CI rates, adenoma detection rate 2. Less abdominal compression or position change required in WI 3. Less pain in WI 4. Less on demand sedation for WI	Few studies and differences in study design	WI may be associated with less patient discomfort
Lee et al,[38] 2012, USA	175 Patients having colonoscopy with sedation	RCT	Warm vs cold water-assisted colonoscopy	Sedation medication used Pain score CI rate Time Satisfaction Willingness to repeat examination	No differences between warm and cold water groups	Results may be limited to sedated patients with good to excellent bowel preparations	Temperature may not matter in water-assisted colonoscopies
Leung F, et al,[39] 2013, USA	Various published studies	Meta-analysis	WI or WE vs AI	Insertion pain ADR	1. Less pain in WE and WI than AI 2. No difference in ADR for WI and AI 3. Higher ADR in WE than WI	Differences in study design	Pain may be reduced in water technique. ADR may be higher in WE

Luo et al,[26] 2013, China	Patients with previous abdominal surgery having colonoscopy without sedation	RCT (55 patients in WE vs AI each arm)	CI rate	1. Higher CI rate in WE vs AI (92.7% vs 76.4%) 2. Pain lower in WE	Single center unblinded physicians	WE may help in patient with previous surgery having examination with no sedation
Lin et al,[20] 2013, China	Various published studies	Meta-analysis	Pain, CI rate, Sedation required	1. Less sedation in WI 2. Lower pain scores in WI 3. Higher CI rate in WI 4. No difference in ADR	Differences in study design	Water can reduce sedation requirement and lower pain with higher CI rates
Hsieh et al,[24] 2014, China	Patients having minimally sedated colonoscopy	RCT (90 patients in WE vs WI vs AI each arm)	Painless insertion, Pain scores, ADR, CI rate	1. Highest proportion of painless insertion in WE 2. Lowest pain in WE and WI 3. Overall ADR the same but proximal ADR highest in WE 4. Lowest CI rate in AI 5. Longer insertion time in WE (16.4 minutes) as compared to WI (5.7) or AI (6.3)	Single center and single unblinded endoscopist	WE may be better than AI or WI in achieving painless colonoscopy

Abbreviations: ADR, adenoma detection rate; AI, air insufflation; CI, cecal intubation; RCT, randomized controlled trial; WE, water exchange; WI, water immersion/infusion.

intubation rate between the standard air and water methods (OR = 0.67; 95% CI, 0.24–1.89).[20] However, the investigators of this meta-analysis highlighted that 4 trials used the assistance of air insufflation in their water method groups; this might also explain the moderate heterogeneity observed in the previous meta-analysis (I^2 = 61%), which examined a similar group of trials. The examinations that used adjunctive air were considered as incomplete in these 4 trials.[12,13,18,21] When the cecal intubation rates were recalculated after reclassifying the examinations with air as complete, the cecal intubation rates were higher for water infusion as compared with air insufflation. Thus, the published data regarding cecal intubation and the use of water infusion seem to be inconsistent. As stated earlier, the completion rates in average patients, with no risk factors that predict difficult colonoscopy, may be close to 100%. Therefore, even large studies or meta-analyses may not detect significant differences.

One scenario in which water-assisted colonoscopy may be advantageous over air insufflation for cecal intubation is in the performance of colonoscopies without use of sedation. One of the earliest trials examined 125 male veterans who had colonoscopies without sedation.[22] The percentage of complete examinations as well as the number of patients willing to have another colonoscopy without sedation was significantly higher in the water immersion group than in the air insufflation group.[22] One small study of 82 veterans showed a higher cecal intubation rate for patients undergoing colonoscopy without sedation in water-assisted examinations as opposed to air insufflation.[15] Another study combined the results of 2 smaller studies of Veterans Affairs (VA) patients undergoing colonoscopy without sedation and observed a higher rate for cecal intubation in the water group.[23] One of the common limitations in the water-assisted examination studies has been the performance of these trials in predominantly older male populations. One recent trial, which enrolled men and women, compared 3 insertion methods, air, water immersion, and exchange.[24] These investigators observed a higher cecal intubation rate in the water groups than in the air method.

WATER-ASSISTED COLONOSCOPY AND PATIENT PAIN AND SEDATION REQUIREMENT

One important outcome is the proportion of patients requesting sedation during an examination without sedation. One study from Italy showed that there was a trend toward fewer patients in the water-assisted colonoscopy requesting sedation as compared with the standard air method.[18] Another trial from Germany observed that fewer patients in the water group requested sedation.[21] However, the percentage of patients who had a complete examination with no sedation was not significantly different in colonoscopies with water as compared with air. A trial of 100 male veterans having a colonoscopy with on-demand sedation reported that more patients in the water-assisted group could have a complete colonoscopy with no sedation as compared with the air insertion group.[16] Another study of 82 male veterans demonstrated similar results.[15] In this study, a larger proportion of patients in the water group were willing to have a repeat colonoscopy with no sedation. A meta-analysis of 5 studies demonstrated that water infusion colonoscopy was associated with a lower rate of patients receiving sedation than examinations with air insufflation.[20] However, many of the studies that showed a benefit from water were performed in largely male cohorts.

One of the proposed benefits of water-assisted colonoscopy is the reduction of pain and an attendant reduction in medication used for sedation.[25] Many of the studies examining water-assisted colonoscopy have been performed in patients undergoing examinations without sedation.[15,16,18,21,22,26] In addition, several studies were performed in older male populations, potentially limiting the generalizability of their findings.[15,16,22] With regards to reduction in pain, one meta-analysis demonstrated a lower maximum pain as well as total pain score for patients having water infusion as compared with the traditional air method.[19] Another meta-analysis of 8 trials confirmed the observation that water infusion was associated with lower pain scores than air infusion.[11–18,21,27] In this meta-analysis, the finding of a lower pain score for water-assisted examinations was observed regardless of trial quality. A systematic review[28] that included only 3 water exchange studies[15–17] concluded that the pain reduction might be greater for water exchange than for water infusion. Thus, the results of these meta-analyses suggest that water infusion and water exchange reduce pain experienced during colonoscopy. However, the results of the analysis of a small number of studies suggest that more data are needed to compare the 2 water techniques.

A published trial was designed to compare both water techniques with air in colonoscopies with minimal sedation. The goal of the study was to identify the method that could produce the highest proportion of patients reporting painless insertion. The study randomized 270 patients into 1 of 3 arms, air insufflation, water immersion, and water exchange. All patients received minimal sedation in the form of 25 mg of intramuscular meperidine. During insertion and withdrawal, a nurse recorded the patient's level of pain every 2 to 3 minutes. The results showed that the water exchange group had the highest proportion of patients reporting painless insertion (61.1%) as compared with water immersion (43.3%) or air (30.0%) ($P<.001$). Pain scores during insertion were lower for water exchange than for water immersion or the air group. These data suggest that water exchange may be superior to water immersion with regards to pain reported by patients during colonoscopies with minimal sedation. However, there were limitations that apply to many of these studies, including the use of a single center, 1 unblinded endoscopist, and unblinded assistants. In addition, the method for recording the patient's pain may be a potential source of bias and the long insertion time observed in the water exchange group (about 16 minutes) may have contributed to less painful insertion, rather than an independent effect of water immersion itself.[25]

IMPACT ON ADENOMA DETECTION RATE

A low ADR is associated with increased risk of interval colorectal cancers.[29,30] Thus, the potential for water techniques to improve endoscopists' ADR may aid in reducing the risk of interval cancer. Water infusion or exchange may improve adenoma detection through one of a few proposed mechanisms.[25] The introduction of water may aid in clearing the bowel of any residual stool. In addition, the distention of the lumen with water is different from that with air. In the water technique, the lumen is not fully distended and thus polyps are not flattened and may be visualized better than with the air method. Finally, water has a magnifying effect, which may increase polyp detection.

One small study of 82 male patients showed a trend toward an increase in detection of adenomas, especially proximal polyps, in patients who had water infusion as compared with air insufflation.[15] Although the overall detection rate was 27.5% (11 of 40) in the air group and 40% (17 of 42) in the water group, this difference was not statistically significant. One study combined the results of the previous study with another small trial of VA patients.[15,16,23] Although there was increased detection of small proximal adenomas in the water-assisted colonoscopy, this method was associated with a longer procedure time. Thus, the increase in adenoma detection in water may be due to longer examination times. Another small trial of 100 male veterans also showed a smaller and not statistically significant difference between water and air methods (40% vs 36%, respectively).[16] A study of 368 male patients demonstrated a higher ADR for water-assisted colonoscopy than for the standard air method (57.1% vs 46.1%; $P = .04$).[31] The difference was more pronounced in the right side of the colon. The procedure time in the water group was longer than in the air group and was due to a longer insertion time in the water group. The withdrawal times were similar in both arms. Thus, the increased detection may be due to increased time for mucosal inspection during the insertion of the colonoscope in the water group. All the aforementioned studies were performed in a VA setting, and the patients were predominantly male, potentially affecting generalizability.

One retrospective study of nonveterans compared 50 patients who underwent air insufflation colonoscopy with 50 patients who had the water technique.[32] Although there was no difference in overall adenoma detection, there was a higher proximal ADR for patients who had water-assisted examinations. One study of 230 Italian patients observed that the ADR for warm water infusion was lower than that for air (25% vs 40.1%; $P = .013$).[18] The investigators speculated that air might distend the ascending colon more than water, allowing for increased mucosal inspection. There was no difference in the detection of advanced adenomas. One study from Germany of 116 patients observed a higher ADR for examinations with water than for those with air, but the difference was not statistically significant.[21] One study from China randomized patients to air- or water-assisted colonoscopy in the left side of the colon and observed no difference in ADRs.[12]

Given the inconsistent literature regarding water-assisted colonoscopy and ADRs, aggregate studies in the form of systematic reviews and meta-analyses have been performed. One systematic review suggested that, although there was inconsistency in trials examining water-assisted colonoscopy, water exchange might increase proximal adenoma detection.[28] One meta-analysis observed no overall difference in adenoma detection for water-assisted examinations as compared to air (OR, 1.01; 95% CI, 0.79–1.29).[19] Another meta-analysis also observed no difference between water and air methods (OR, 0.91; 95% CI, 0.68–1.22).[20] Finally, a recent meta-analysis showed no overall difference in ADR between water-assisted techniques and air method. However, a subgroup analysis demonstrated that water exchange might be associated with a higher ADR than water immersion.[33]

One trial,[14] described previously, compared the 3 insertion techniques and examined ADR as one outcome. The overall ADR for the water exchange (56.7%) was higher than that for water immersion (45.6%) or air (43.3%), but this was not statistically significant ($P = .16$). An interesting finding was that the ADR for insertion was the highest for the water exchange method, although this did not reach statistical significance. However, the ADR for right-sided adenomas was statistically higher for water exchange than for the other 2 methods. These data suggest that water exchange may be superior in adenoma detection, especially those that are proximal. However, one confounding factor might be the longer insertion time in the water exchange group, which may have allowed for higher adenoma detection. The largest difference between the 3 groups was observed in the number of patients with adenomas detected during insertion. In addition, water exchange may allow for bowel preparation salvaging,[25] as suggested by the superior bowel preparation score in the water exchange groups as compared with the other 2 methods. As pointed out in an accompanying editorial, the lack of blinding of the endoscopist or the assistant, differences in insertion time, as well as the method for assigning polyps to colon segments may be potential sources of bias.[25] Thus, more data from controlled studies are needed to clarify the impact of water-aided colonoscopy on adenoma detection.

COMPLETION OF DIFFICULT OR INCOMPLETE EXAMINATIONS

The use of water may aid in facilitating the passage of the colonoscope from the anus to the cecum. Obstacles to easy passage of the scope may be due to an angulated or strictured distal colon or due to a redundant colon. With regards to the former, one study randomized 110 patients with prior abdominal or pelvic surgery who were undergoing colonoscopies without sedation to either air or water exchange colonoscopy.[26] The sample included mostly women with a low body mass index and almost half who had had pelvic surgery, thus expected to have difficult or challenging distal colons owing to severe angulation.[3,4] The examinations performed in the water group had a higher cecal intubation rate than those in the air group (92.7% vs 76.4%; $P = .033$). In addition, the water group had lower pain scores and required fewer changes in patients' positions, and more patients were willing to have a repeat examination. This study demonstrated the possible benefit of water exchange in achieving less painful cecal intubation in patients with difficult distal colons.

Another study demonstrated the potential benefit of water-assisted techniques in achieving cecal intubation in examinations that were previously incomplete.[8] This study was a retrospective analysis of repeat colonoscopies in 345 patients using water (178) and air techniques (167). There was no significant difference in cecal intubation between the air (162/167; 97%) and water groups (170/178; 96%). Among the 148 patients with redundant colons, there was a slight trend toward a higher cecal intubation rate for the water group (79/80; 99%) as compared with the air examinations (64/68; 94%) ($P = .18$). One interesting finding was that the examinations in the water group were more likely to be completed with a standard adult colonoscope than the examinations using air, whereas the latter were more likely to require enteroscopes and/or straighteners. These data underscore the benefit of water immersion for redundant colons, as water distends the colon to a lesser degree than air. In addition, when the patient is in the left lateral decubitus position, the sigmoid colon is weighted down. The result of these 2 actions is the straightening of the colon, especially in the sigmoid. Thus, the water method seems to be a potential asset for the endoscopist when challenged by a patient with a redundant colon, including tall or obese patients,[34] especially men[4] or those who have constipation.[3]

One interesting application of water-assisted colonoscopy is the treatment of sigmoid volvulus.[35] One case series reported 21 patients with sigmoid volvulus who were all successfully treated using water immersion. Ten patients had a recurrence within a 6-month follow-up period. The method included the introduction of water with the aspiration of residual air. The colonoscope was inserted with a torque in the direction of the twist until the point of the obstruction. If no necrosis was present, the scope was passed through the twist in an effort to straighten the bowel. Air from the proximal colon was removed to decompress the bowel, and no decompression tube was placed. Although this method is similar to the standard approach, one potential benefit of the water method in patients with obstruction may be the introduction of less air into the colon.

COMPLICATIONS AND SAFETY OF WATER TECHNIQUE

As with any technique, there may be concerns regarding the possible complications that may arise with water-assisted colonoscopy. One meta-analysis pointed out that few studies have reported their complications.[20] Two of these trials reported a total of 2 unexpected cardiopulmonary events.[16,17] Another study from Italy reported 2 vagal-associated events, 9 patients with oxygen desaturation in the air group, 4 cases of desaturation in the water group, and 1 polypectomy bleed in each arm.[18]

Thus, complications that occur in standard colonoscopies also apply to water-assisted colonoscopies. The fact that up to 2 L of water may be infused into the patient's colon raises concerns regarding the safety of water-assisted colonoscopy. One study examined the effect of water method on the vital signs, cardiac rhythm, and serum electrolyte levels in patients having water-assisted examinations.[36] The investigators examined the results from 2 separate studies. In the first study, patients' vital signs and cardiac rhythm were monitored before and after the colonoscopies. There were no differences observed between the preexamination and postexamination mean blood pressures, pulse measurements, and oxygen saturation for the patients enrolled in the water group. In addition, there were no observed differences between these values in the air versus the water groups. In the second study, electrolyte levels for sodium and potassium were measured preexamination and postexamination. There were also no observed differences in these levels precolonoscopy and postcolonoscopy in patients in the water-assisted examinations.

Another study prospectively examined the effect of water exchange on serum electrolyte levels.[37] These investigators collected clinical data as well as blood before and 10 minutes postcolonoscopy from 140 patients. In this study, 1.8 L was infused and a similar volume was subsequently suctioned out of the colon. As observed in the previous study, there was no difference between serum potassium and sodium levels before and after water-assisted colonoscopy. In addition, there were no differences in the serum chloride and bicarbonate levels. These data suggest that water infusion and exchange may not pose additional risks for patients who undergo colonoscopies with these techniques.

SUMMARY

In summary, water-assisted colonoscopy offers the endoscopist a unique method for addressing challenges in navigating the colonoscope through difficult colons. It seems to be a safe and cheap method. One benefit of the water technique is the reduction of the requirement for medications used for sedation. Another application may be the use of water-aided colonoscopy in the performance of examinations without sedation. When comparing water exchange with water immersion, the former may be superior with regards to insertion. However, there is a trade-off in the form of a longer procedure time, mostly due to insertion. The possible benefit of higher proximal adenoma detection requires additional studies that include colonoscopies performed by several endoscopists to minimize potential bias present in previous studies that use only a few examiners. Finally, as pointed out by one expert,[25] the choice to use the water techniques is ultimately up to the endoscopist and there is still much contention among endoscopists regarding the true benefit of the water-assisted methods.

REFERENCES

1. Rex DK, Bond JH, Winawer S, et al. Quality in the technical performance of colonoscopy and the continuous quality improvement process for colonoscopy: recommendations of the U.S. Multi-Society Task Force on Colorectal Cancer. Am J Gastroenterol 2002;97:1296–308.
2. Rex DK, Petrini JL, Baron TH, et al. Quality indicators for colonoscopy. Am J Gastroenterol 2006;101:873–85.
3. Anderson JC, Messina CR, Cohn W, et al. Factors predictive of difficult colonoscopy. Gastrointest Endosc 2001;54:558–62.
4. Anderson JC, Gonzalez JD, Messina CR, et al. Factors that predict incomplete colonoscopy: thinner is not always better. Am J Gastroenterol 2000;95:2784–7.

5. Anderson JC, Walker G, Birk JW, et al. Tapered colonoscope performs better than the pediatric colonoscope in female patients: a direct comparison through tandem colonoscopy. Gastrointest Endosc 2007;65:1042–7.
6. Baumann UA. Water intubation of the sigmoid colon: water instillation speeds up left-sided colonoscopy. Endoscopy 1999;31:314–7.
7. Rex DK, Chen SC, Overhiser AJ. Colonoscopy technique in consecutive patients referred for prior incomplete colonoscopy. Clin Gastroenterol Hepatol 2007;5: 879–83.
8. Vemulapalli KC, Rex DK. Water immersion simplifies cecal intubation in patients with redundant colons and previous incomplete colonoscopies. Gastrointest Endosc 2012;76:812–7.
9. Leung FW. Water exchange may be superior to water immersion for colonoscopy. Clin Gastroenterol Hepatol 2011;9:1012–4.
10. Ramirez FC, Leung FW. The water method for aiding colonoscope insertion: the learning curve of an experienced colonoscopist. J Interv Gastroenterol 2011;1: 97–101.
11. Brocchi E, Pezzilli R, Tomassetti P, et al. Warm water or oil-assisted colonoscopy: toward simpler examinations? Am J Gastroenterol 2008;103:581–7.
12. Hsieh YH, Lin HJ, Tseng KC. Limited water infusion decreases pain during minimally sedated colonoscopy. World J Gastroenterol 2011;17:2236–40.
13. Hsieh YH, Tseng KC, Hsieh JJ, et al. Feasibility of colonoscopy with water infusion in minimally sedated patients in an Asian Community Setting. J Interv Gastroenterol 2011;1:185–90.
14. Leung CW, Kaltenbach T, Soetikno R, et al. Water immersion versus standard colonoscopy insertion technique: randomized trial shows promise for minimal sedation. Endoscopy 2010;42:557–63.
15. Leung FW, Harker JO, Jackson G, et al. A proof-of-principle, prospective, randomized, controlled trial demonstrating improved outcomes in scheduled unsedated colonoscopy by the water method. Gastrointest Endosc 2010;72: 693–700.
16. Leung J, Mann S, Siao-Salera R, et al. A randomized, controlled trial to confirm the beneficial effects of the water method on U.S. veterans undergoing colonoscopy with the option of on-demand sedation. Gastrointest Endosc 2011;73: 103–10.
17. Leung JW, Mann SK, Siao-Salera R, et al. A randomized, controlled comparison of warm water infusion in lieu of air insufflation versus air insufflation for aiding colonoscopy insertion in sedated patients undergoing colorectal cancer screening and surveillance. Gastrointest Endosc 2009;70:505–10.
18. Radaelli F, Paggi S, Amato A, et al. Warm water infusion versus air insufflation for unsedated colonoscopy: a randomized, controlled trial. Gastrointest Endosc 2010;72:701–9.
19. Jun WU, Bing HU. Comparative effectiveness of water infusion vs air insufflation in colonoscopy: a meta-analysis. Colorectal Dis 2013;15:404–9.
20. Lin S, Zhu W, Xiao K, et al. Water intubation method can reduce patients' pain and sedation rate in colonoscopy: a meta-analysis. Dig Endosc 2013;25:231–40.
21. Pohl J, Messer I, Behrens A, et al. Water infusion for cecal intubation increases patient tolerance, but does not improve intubation of unsedated colonoscopies. Clin Gastroenterol Hepatol 2011;9:1039–43.e1.
22. Leung FW, Aharonian HS, Leung JW, et al. Impact of a novel water method on scheduled unsedated colonoscopy in U.S. veterans. Gastrointest Endosc 2009; 69:546–50.

23. Leung FW, Leung JW, Siao-Salera RM, et al. The water method significantly enhances proximal diminutive adenoma detection rate in unsedated patients. J Interv Gastroenterol 2011;1:8–13.
24. Hsieh YH, Koo M, Leung FW. A patient-blinded randomized, controlled trial comparing air insufflation, water immersion, and water exchange during minimally sedated colonoscopy. Am J Gastroenterol 2014;109:1390–400.
25. Rex DK. Water exchange vs. water immersion during colonoscope insertion [editorial]. Am J Gastroenterol 2014;109:1401–3.
26. Luo H, Zhang L, Liu X, et al. Water exchange enhanced cecal intubation in potentially difficult colonoscopy. Unsedated patients with prior abdominal or pelvic surgery: a prospective, randomized, controlled trial. Gastrointest Endosc 2013;77: 767–73.
27. Church JM. Warm water irrigation for dealing with spasm during colonoscopy: simple, inexpensive, and effective. Gastrointest Endosc 2002;56:672–4.
28. Leung FW, Amato A, Ell C, et al. Water-aided colonoscopy: a systematic review. Gastrointest Endosc 2012;76:657–66.
29. Corley DA, Jensen CD, Marks AR, et al. Adenoma detection rate and risk of colorectal cancer and death. N Engl J Med 2014;370:1298–306.
30. Kaminski MF, Regula J, Kraszewska E, et al. Quality indicators for colonoscopy and the risk of interval cancer. N Engl J Med 2010;362:1795–803.
31. Ramirez FC, Leung FW. A head-to-head comparison of the water vs. air method in patients undergoing screening colonoscopy. J Interv Gastroenterol 2011;1: 130–5.
32. Tejaswi S, Stondell J, Ngo C, et al. Increase in proximal adenoma detection rate after transition from air to water method for screening colonoscopy in a community-based setting in the United States. J Interv Gastroenterol 2013;3: 53–6.
33. Bayupurnama P, Ratnasari N, Indrarti F, et al. The water method colonoscopy in routine unsedated colonoscopy examinations: a randomized controlled trial in diagnostic cases in Indonesian patients. J Interv Gastroenterol 2013;3:12–7.
34. Waye JD. Completing colonoscopy. Am J Gastroenterol 2000;95:2681–2.
35. Sugimoto S, Hosoe N, Mizukami T, et al. Effectiveness and clinical results of endoscopic management of sigmoid volvulus using unsedated water-immersion colonoscopy. Dig Endosc 2014;26:564–8.
36. Leung FW, Leung JW, Siao-Salera RM, et al. Vital signs and serum electrolyte levels are well preserved after large volume water exchange in the colonic lumen used with the water exchange method. J Interv Gastroenterol 2013;3:89–92.
37. Leung JW, Siao-Salera R, Abramyan O, et al. Impact of water exchange colonoscopy on serum sodium and potassium levels: an observational study. Dig Dis Sci 2014;59:653–7.
38. Lee BY, Katon R, Herzig D, et al. Warm water infusion during sedated colonoscopy does not decrease amount of sedation medication used. Gastrointest Endosc 2012;76:1182–7.
39. Leung FW, Hu B, Wu J. Comparative effectiveness of water immersion and water exchange versus air insufflation for colonoscopy. J Interv Gastroenterol 2013;3: 100–3.

Electronic Imaging to Enhance Lesion Detection at Colonoscopy

Shara Nguyen Ket, MBBS, FRACP,
Elizabeth Bird-Lieberman, MRCP, PhD, James E. East, MD(res), FRCP*

KEYWORDS

- Colonoscopy • Colorectal cancer • Colonic polyps • Surveillance • Adenoma
- Lynch syndrome • Inflammatory bowel disease • Molecular imaging • Lectins

KEY POINTS

- Electronic imaging has shown no utility in enhancing adenoma detection in average risk patients.
- Patients with Lynch syndrome or serrated polyposis syndrome may benefit from electronic imaging.
- Electronic imaging seems to offer limited benefit for patients undergoing surveillance for longstanding inflammatory bowel disease.
- The addition of molecular imaging probes may be needed to fully realize the benefits of electronic imaging for polyp detection in the colon.

INTRODUCTION

Colorectal cancer (CRC) can be considered a heterogenous disease appearing in various clinical contexts, such as sporadically, in those with an inherited predisposition, or in chronic inflammatory processes of the colon such as inflammatory bowel disease (IBD).

There are multiple molecular pathways that can lead to CRC,[1–3] reviewed in the article Colorectal Neoplasia Pathways: State-of-the-Art by Ijspeert and colleagues elsewhere in this issue. Adenomatous polyps undergo sporadic accumulation of genetic mutations in multiple molecular pathways, including the adenomatous polyposis coli tumor suppressor gene and DNA mismatch repair genes,[4] which can lead to mutations in the KRAS oncogene and p53 suppressor gene. Sessile serrated adenomas/

Translational Gastroenterology Unit, John Radcliffe Hospital, Headley Way, Headington, Oxford OX3 9DU, UK
* Corresponding author. Translational Gastroenterology Unit, Experimental Medicine Division, Nuffield Department of Clinical Medicine, University of Oxford, John Radcliffe Hospital, Headley Way, Headington, Oxford OX3 9DU, UK.
E-mail address: jameseast6@yahoo.com

Gastrointest Endoscopy Clin N Am 25 (2015) 227–242
http://dx.doi.org/10.1016/j.giec.2014.11.011
1052-5157/15/$ – see front matter © 2015 Elsevier Inc. All rights reserved.
giendo.theclinics.com

polyps develop into CRC via a separate molecular pathway involving BRAF mutations and DNA methylation.[5,6] Recent data suggest that traditional serrated adenomas develop through a pathway driven by epithelial over expression of the bone morphogenic protein antagonist GREM1.[7]

Hereditary or familial syndromes give rise to approximately 3% of cases of CRC. The most common is hereditary nonpolypsis CRC or the Lynch syndrome, where a germline mutation in DNA mismatch repair genes occurs leading to microsatellite instability. The less well-recognized serrated polyposis syndrome is characterized by multiple serrated polyps, defined as patients with more than 20 serrated polyps throughout the colon or 5 or more serrated polyps proximal to the sigmoid with 2 or more that are at least 10 mm in size.[8] Other genetic syndromes are either less common or produce so many polyps that advanced endoscopic imaging is not needed, for example, in familial adenomatous polyposis.

IBD has long been recognized to be associated with CRC, related to the carcinogenic effect of chronic inflammation combined with a genetic predisposition. A meta-analysis has estimated the cumulative probability of developing CRC in any patient, 30 years after a diagnosis of ulcerative colitis, at 18%[9]; however, population-based studies suggest that for patients with IBD overall, the risk may in fact be minimally elevated.[10,11] There are no large studies confirming that surveillance reduces the mortality of ulcerative colitis–associated CRC. However, the benefit of continued surveillance has been described[12] and it remains recommended practice in all international guidelines,[13–17] with increasing focus on risk stratification to target efforts on higher risk patients.

Recognition of lesions with malignant potential is crucial, because detection and early removal of polyps reduces CRC mortality compared with population risk estimates.[18] No randomised studies for colonoscopy for CRC prevention are available; however, a meta-analysis looking at 4 randomised, controlled trials and 10 observational studies found that flexible sigmoidoscopy for population screening showed a reduction in CRC rates in the distal colon.[19] Variation in adenoma detection correlates with the incidence of postcolonoscopy CRC and death from CRC.[20] Current white light techniques for colonoscopic detection of polyps and neoplasia yield a high miss rate of up to 22% of all adenomas[21] and 2% to 6% of advanced colorectal adenomas and cancers.[22]

It is, therefore, imperative to maximize polyp detection rates and to avoid missing polyps to maximize cancer prevention and minimize the risk of postcolonoscopy CRCs. Missed polyps and subsequent cancers can arise through suboptimal mucosal visualization,[23] failure of complete polyp resection,[24] or failed polyp detection.[25]

In this review, we assess the potential benefits of additional electronic imaging above and beyond standard white light to improve polyp detection at colonoscopy.

HISTORY OF COLONIC POLYP DETECTION

The ability to reliably detect subcentimeter polyps is a relatively new phenomenon that has come with the advent of increasingly sophisticated endoscopic equipment. Before the 1950s, barium radiographic studies and rigid sigmoidoscopy were used for investigation of the colon. Flexible endoscopic visualization of the mucosa of the gastrointestinal tract was made possible by the development of a coherent optical fiber bundle by Hopkins and Kapany.[26] This led to the development of the first flexible gastroscope "fiberscope" reported in 1958, which was developed commercially by 1960.[27] Combined with the use of fluoroscopy, endoscope location could be confirmed and correlated with the endoscopic findings.[28] The next major development in endoscopy came when Sivak and Fleischer[29] published findings of a new endoscope where the optical fiber bundle was replaced with an image sensor or charge-coupled device at the tip of the endoscope. This allowed the conversion of the light into electrical charges and reconstruction on a television monitor. By the 1990s, videocolonoscopy had largely replaced fiberoptic colonoscopy and as technology advanced, high-resolution endoscopy (HRE), and most recently high-definition endoscopy with 1080 lines of pixels was introduced in 2005 (see **Fig 1**A and **2**A). Nevertheless, polyp miss rates continued to be significant for both adenomas and polyps.[30]

Colonoscopic chromoendoscopy was introduced in the 1970s and involves enhancement of the mucosa by segmentally applying stains, such as methylene blue or indigo carmine.[31] This not only improves localization and characterization of lesions during endoscopy (see **Fig. 2**B), but also allows targeted biopsies of enhanced mucosal abnormality improving dysplasia detection in long-standing IBD,[32] as well as increasing detection of neoplastic lesions in average risk subjects.[33] Despite evidence supporting the use of chromoendoscopy, it has not become a widely adopted practice. This low use may be owing to a number of factors, including increased time required, cost, inadequate training, and interobserver variability.

Narrowed Spectrum Endoscopy (Virtual Chromoendoscopy)

Virtual chromoendoscopy may provide an alternative to conventional chromoendoscopy, because it does not require dye spray catheters and the use of dye. Rather, it relies on built-in technologies within the endoscope and processor that uses the innate properties of light to generate a tissue enhanced pseudoimage.

Conventional white light endoscopy (WLE) generates endoscopic images by shining white light (400–700 nm) onto tissue and uses a charge-coupled device to capture reflected light. Specific components of the mucosa and submucosa can be enhanced by manipulating the light reflected and the generated endoscopic images. This maneuver allows for detailed endoscopic examination of the mucosa and any abnormalities, without the need for dye.

Currently there are 3 different systems that enhance the mucosal appearance that are available commercially: (1) narrow band imaging (NBI) by Olympus (Tokyo, Japan), (2) Fuji intelligent color enhancement (FICE) by Fujinon (Tokyo, Japan), and (3) i-scan (Pentax, Tokyo, Japan).

NBI utilizes the principle that light wavelength determines depth of tissue penetration. Special filters are placed in front of the xenon lamp that narrows the spectrum to blue light of 400 to 430 nm and green light of 525 to 555 nm. The blue short wavelength (centered at 415 nm) not only has penetration limited to the mucosa, but has been shown to correspond with the peak absorption spectrum of hemoglobin[34]; thus, mucosal structures containing high hemoglobin content, such that vessels seem to be brown. The longer wavelength light (centered at 540 nm) penetrates deeper into the submucosa and corresponds with a secondary absorption peak of hemoglobin, highlighting submucosal vasculature as cyan (**Figs. 1** and **2**C).

FICE uses an algorithm that takes an ordinary endoscope image and decomposes the light according to wavelengths. Selective wavelength images are then combined to reconstruct a real-time image. There are 10 channels with each channel corresponding with 3 specific virtual, electronic filters resulting in images with various tissue depth penetrations, and hence tissue enhancements.[35]

I-scan uses 3 algorithms for image enhancement. (1) Surface enhancement allows minor changes in structure to be seen by enhancing the edge. This is achieved by analyzing the difference in luminance intensity of the pixels in this area with the edge components being enhanced. (2) Contrast enhancement identifies pixels of lower luminance intensity and subsequently enhancing the blue component of these

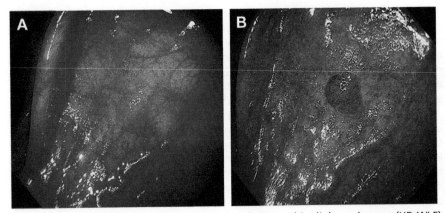

Fig. 1. A sporadic adenoma viewed using high-definition white light endoscopy (HD-WLE) and narrow band imaging (NBI). (*A*) A 7-mm adenoma seen with HD-WLE in the ascending colon (Lucera Elite, Olympus Keymed, UK). (*B*) The same adenoma seen with NBI. Note the lesion stands out browner owing to highlighting of increased microvessel density compared with the background mucosa; however, this has not translated into higher detection rates in meta-analysis.

pixels. This gives areas of low luminance such as depressed areas a bluish color. (3) Tone enhancement decomposes the ordinary color image into light wavelength components of red, green, and blue. These components are then adjusted along a tone curve and reconstructed to produce an image with increased contrast of color tone.[36]

AUTOFLUORESCENCE IMAGING

Autofluorescence imaging (AFI) is another modality of mucosal enhancement manufactured by Olympus (Tokyo, Japan). Autofluorescence is the natural emission of light from biological molecules, endogenous fluorophores, when light of a suitable wavelength is absorbed. When cellular components and tissue state changes during pathologic processes, this alters the amount and distribution of endogenous fluorophores; hence, the autofluorescence generated. In neoplastic epithelial cells, there is increased fluorescence from mitochondrial cofactors nicotinamide adenine dinucleotide (plus hydrogen) and flavin adenine dinucleotide (FAD), but reduced fluorescence from collagen in the stroma.[37] Thickening of the mucosa and increased blood flow in adenomatous lesions also attenuate excitation light and block the autofluorescence signal.

The autofluorescence endoscope generates blue light (390–470 nm) and green light (540–560 nm) via rotating color filters in front of the xenon light. After excitation by the shorter wavelength blue light, fluorophores emit autofluorescence of longer wavelengths (500–630 nm). A filter in front of the separate AFI charge-coupled device blocks the reflected blue excitation light, but enables the tissue autofluorescence as well as the reflected green light to filter through. These images are then integrated by the processor to generate a pseudocolor image where normal tissue and vessels appear green and dysplastic tissue as magenta (see **Fig. 2**D).

CLINICAL APPLICATION OF ELECTRONIC IMAGING AT COLONOSCOPY
Average-Risk Populations

In average-risk populations, the use of NBI has been compared with WLE for detection of colonic lesions in 5 meta-analyses (**Table 1**). Overall, the evidence that NBI is better than WLE for adenoma detection is not convincing. Similarly, polyp detection was not

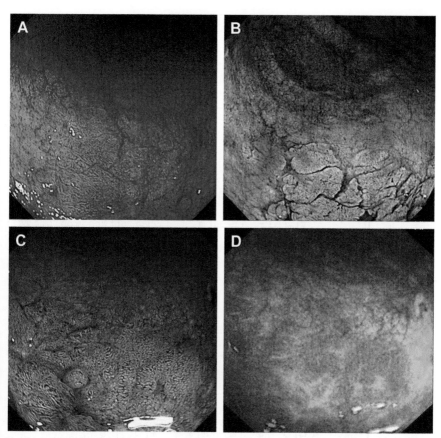

Fig. 2. A nonpolypoid colorectal neoplasm in quiescent ulcerative colitis. (*A*) An area of abnormal pit pattern with a "velvety" appearance was seen during high definition white light colonoscopy for surveillance of longstanding ulcerative colitis. (*B*) Use of chromoendoscopy (*dye spray*) with indigocarmine 0.2% revealed a flat (Paris 0-IIb) lesion with a circumscribed boarder with a diameter of approximately 30 mm. (*C*) Assessment with narrow band imaging (NBI; Olympus, Tokyo, Japan) is also shown to clarify the pit pattern, but the border is not as distinct as with chromoendoscopy. (*D*) Assessment with autofluorescence imaging (AFI; Olympus) also helps to differentiate the neoplastic tissue (*pink/purple*) from the surrounding normal mucosa (*green*). Biopsy confirmed low-grade dysplasia.

improved with NBI and only 1 meta-analysis found that NBI increased detection of flat adenomas (95% CI, 1.09–3.52, $P = .02$).[38]

Other virtual chromoendoscopy modalities have limited data. A randomized, tandem trial in patients undergoing surveillance colonoscopy compared NBI, FICE, and WLE on first withdrawal. The authors recruited 550 patients into each group and neither NBI nor FICE improved adenoma detection or miss rates, with no benefit over WLE demonstrated.[39] Two prospective, randomized, controlled trials, which enrolled a total of 1230 patients combined, compared WLE with FICE.[40,41] These trials did not demonstrate an improvement in adenoma miss rate of FICE over WLE. A third prospective trial of 1318 patients (68% undergoing screening colonoscopies, the remaining diagnostic) also did not demonstrate significant benefit of FICE over white light for adenoma detection.[42] Similarly, when assessing i-scan, 1 study has not

Table 1
Summary of meta-analyses comparing advanced electronic imaging modalities and white light

Author, Year of Publication	No. of Studies Included	Method	Study Design	No. of Patients	Adenoma Detection Rate	Polyps per Patient	Flat Adenoma Detection
Pasha et al,[75] 2012	9	NBI vs WLE	Meta-analysis	3059	OR, 1.01; 95% CI, 0.74-1.37	OR, 1.17; 95% CI, 0.8-1.71	OR, 1.26; 95% CI, 0.62-2.57
Dinesen et al,[76] 2012	7	NBI vs WLE	Meta-analysis	2936	RR, 1.06; 95% CI, 0.97-1.16	RR, 1.22[a]; 95% CI, 0.85-1.76	WMD 0.06; 95% CI, -0.01-0.13
Nagorni et al,[77] 2012	8	NBI vs WLE	Meta-analysis	3673	RR, 1.03; 95% CI, 0.92-1.16	RR, 1.01; 95% CI, 0.96-1.06	RR, 0.87; 95% CI, 0.72-1.04
Jin et al,[38] 2011	8	NBI vs WLE	Meta-analysis	3049	RR, 1.09; 95% CI, 1.00-1.19	—	RR, 1.96; 95% CI, 1.09-3.52
Omata et al,[44] 2014	5	AFI vs WLE	Meta-analysis	758	RR, 1.04; 95% CI, 0.87-1.24	—	—
	5	FICE/i-scan vs WLE		3032	RR, 1.09; 95% CI, 0.97-1.23	—	—
	14	NBI vs WLE		5074	RR, 1.03; 95% CI, 0.96-1.11	—	—
Zhao et al,[50] 2014	6	AFI vs WLE	Meta-analysis	1199	OR, 1.01; 95% CI, 0.74-1.37	OR, 0.86; 95% CI, 0.57-1.30	—

Abbreviations: AFI, autofluorescence imaging; FICE, Fujinon intelligent color enhancement; NBI, narrow band imaging; OR, Odds ratio; RR, relative risk; WLE, white light endoscopy; WMD, weighted mean difference.
[a] Polyp detection rate.

demonstrated improvement in adenoma detection during screening colonoscopy.[43] A meta-analysis that combined FICE and i-scan also showed no benefit of these modalities.[44] Regarding AFI versus high-definition (HD)-WLE in average risk populations, the results are inconsistent, with 2 Japanese studies finding improved outcome with AFI. One study found that the miss rate for all polyps with AFI (30%) was significantly less than with WLE (49%; $P = .01$)[45] and a second study detected significantly more colorectal neoplasms with AFI, although a transparent hood was also used in this study.[46] Interestingly, 3 European trials have not demonstrated a significant adenoma miss rate difference.[47–49] Two meta-analyses of AFI did not find that it improved adenoma detection.[44,50]

In summary, there is insufficient evidence to support the routine use of electronic imaging enhancement in average-risk populations to increase adenoma yield during colonoscopy, irrespective of the system used.

Hereditary Syndromes

Screening of patients with hereditary nonpolyposis syndromes reduces the risk of CRC by one half.[51,52] A prospective cohort study of patients with the Lynch syndrome found that an additional pass with NBI compared with a single pass with HD-WLE significantly increased adenoma detection (absolute difference, 15%; 95% CI, 4%–25%).[53]

Pancolonic chromoendoscopy seems to have benefit in screening colonoscopies in this patient population. Chromoendoscopy compared with conventional colonoscopy significantly improved detection of significant neoplastic lesions (24 lesions in 13 patients compared with 52 lesions in 16 patients; $P = .004$).[54] In another cohort study, an additional pass with conventional chromoendoscopy after a first pass with HD-NBI significantly increased the number of adenomas detected.[55] A further study found that chromoendoscopy is superior to white light, AFI, and NBI for the detection of diminutive polyps in adenomatous polyposis.[56] However, some studies have found that chromoendoscopy did not perform better for missed adenomas than intensive inspection.[57] Data using other virtual chromoendoscpy modalities are very limited.

AFI was found to improve adenoma detection in a prospective single-center study that enrolled 75 asymptomatic patients with the Lynch syndrome or familial CRC families ($P = .01$).[58] In the context of serrated polyposis syndrome, a randomized crossover study of consecutive patients who underwent tandem colonoscopy with HRE and NBI found the polyp miss rates was 36% (95% CI, 28%–45%) for HRE compared with a significantly lower 10% (95% CI, 5.5%–19%) for NBI ($P<.001$).[59] Similarly, a pilot study comparing HRE, AFI, and NBI showed significantly lower polyp miss rates with HD-NBI compared with HD WLE. Endoscopic differentiation between hyperplastic polyps and sessile serrated adenomas/polyps using endoscopic trimodal imaging did not demonstrate a significant difference; however, hyperplastic polyps and adenomas could be differentiated with NBI but not AFI.[60]

The use of electronic imaging in the high-risk populations of hereditary syndromes may have some benefit, but has not been shown to be superior to conventional chromoendoscopy.

Inflammatory Bowel Disease

Patients with long-standing and extensive ulcerative colitis benefit from colonoscopic surveillance[12] given their increased risk of CRC compared with the average-risk population. In 3 randomized, controlled trials comparing NBI with WLE for the detection of neoplasia in long-standing IBD, it was found that NBI did not increase significantly the detection rate of neoplastic lesions compared with WLE.[61–63] Random biopsies taken with both NBI as well as WLE (n = 1348 and 1359, respectively) yielded only 1 biopsy demonstrating histologic evidence of low-grade dysplasia, suggesting that this practice should be abandoned.[61]

Two randomized, controlled trials have compared the detection of neoplasia in long-standing IBD using HD-NBI with HD conventional chromoendoscopy. One study found that NBI had a significantly inferior false-positive biopsy rate ($P = .001$) but a higher percentage of missed neoplastic lesions (31.8% with NBI compared with 13.6% using chromoendoscopy).[64] Similarly, a second study found that chromoendoscopy identified more lesions than NBI (131 vs 102; $P<.001$), but histology revealed most of these lesions to be nondysplastic. In the same study, chromoendoscopy identified more neoplastic lesions (23 lesions in 11 patients vs 20 lesions in 10 patients), but this difference was not statistically significant ($P = .180$).[65]

There are 2 studies comparing HD-WLE with AFI for the detection of colorectal neoplasia in IBD. A pilot study showed that protruding lesions with a low autofluorescence signal were more likely to be neoplastic than lesions with a high autofluorescence signal,[66] and in a randomized, controlled trial, the miss rate for neoplastic lesions was statistically significantly lower with AFI compared with HD-WLE.[67]

Overall, advanced electronic imaging has demonstrated limited utility compared with conventional chromoendoscopy in the detection of neoplastic lesions in patients with long-standing IBD.

MOLECULAR IMAGING ENHANCED ELECTRONIC IMAGING: AN EMERGING TECHNOLOGY

Given the overall lack of evidence supporting the routine use of electronic imaging modalities in surveillance colonoscopy to enhance polyp detection, further technological advancements are needed. Molecular imaging has the potential to facilitate this step forward in our endoscopic diagnostic and perhaps even prognostic ability. This technique takes advantage of molecular changes that occur early in the pathogenesis of disease and allows these molecular changes to be detected at endoscopy to highlight areas of concern. The key to success in this technique will be the ability to detect these molecular changes using an endoscope with a wide field of view (ie, not needing confocal endomicroscopy), without the need for specialist interpretation or expensive equipment, and to identify imaging probes for the molecular changes that are sufficiently sensitive and specific in their binding to a defined target. Ultimately, such a technique may even allow a degree of quantification of biomarker expression.

Ideally, probes would have a high binding affinity to a specific target relative to background; they would remain structurally stable until imaging is complete, and be rapidly cleared in a nontoxic manner. It must also be possible to combine the probe with a fluorescent tag to allow its endoscopic detection, without alteration in the binding properties of the probe. The ideal endoscopic detector for such a system would be able to excite at a specific wavelength to excite the fluorochrome labeling the probe to emit light, which can then be identified by the endoscope. To avoid confounding signal from autofluorescence, it is expected that it will be optimal to undertake this endoscopic imaging in the near infrared spectrum. Optical imaging is the most sensitive way of detecting molecular changes and this is perfectly suited to endoscopic imaging of the epithelium where we have the ability to get close to the epithelium with our endoscopes.

Molecular imaging for the endoscopic detection of dysplasia that is not macroscopically evident has been shown, in proof-of-principle work, to allow identification of dysplasia within the esophagus using lectin probes.[68] Molecular imaging has also been used within the colon for endoscopic detection of the tumor necrosis factor in

Crohn's disease, using a fluorescently labeled antibody to predict clinical response to anti-tumor necrosis factor therapy, although these molecular changes were detected using confocal endoscopy and therefore subject to the same sampling error encountered with random biopsies.[69]

Studies of molecular imaging for the detection of dysplasia within the human colon are few and are listed in **Table 2**. Part of the problem has been getting probes through the necessary regulatory steps before in vivo use. This process is costly and regulatory bodies have not yet defined pathways for approval of these imaging agents, which are currently subject to the same standards as new, intravenously administered drugs. The possibility of topical application of these probes at microdosing quantities is not likely to be associated with significant toxicity, particularly within the colon. These regulatory issues have led investigators to pragmatically choose probes that are already used as therapeutic agents and have therefore already gone through the regulatory processes, such as the anti-tumor necrosis factor antibodies.[69]

Antibodies as probes have the advantage of excellent specificity; however, their cost would prohibit their use in the routine clinical setting. They are also associated with a degree of immunogenicity and therefore risk toxicity, and their binding specificity can be altered when labeled with a fluorescent probe. Keller and colleagues[70] used antibodies to carcinoembryonic antigen; however, the limitations associated with antibody probes, as well as lack of early abnormal expression of carcinoembryonic antigen in the majority of patients, limit the clinical usefulness of this probe. Peptide probes have been considered as an alternative to antibodies, because their smaller size means that they are associated with a lower degree of antigenicity and they are cheap to produce from phage libraries; however, their smaller size is associated with decreased binding specificity and an increased risk that their binding will be altered when labeled. Another problem, as seen with Hsiung and colleagues,[71] is that the molecular target of the probe may be unknown. This issue of unclear target was overcome by Hardwick and colleagues[72] when they looked for a peptide probe against a specific molecular change, known to occur early in colon cancer carcinogenesis (c-MET); however, the need for intravenous application makes such a probe more problematic to use in the routine clinical setting.

Lectin probes are an alternative to antibodies and peptides. They are naturally occurring and can therefore be obtained at low cost. They are large and relatively stable and their specificity is therefore less likely to be altered when labeled. A great deal is known about their binding specificities, but their binding to glycans is not as specific as the antibody–antigen interaction.[68] Lectin probes have been used topically in colon resection specimens to highlight dysplasia in IBD, flat polyps, and cancers using standard wide-field of view endoscopes[73] and are now being taken forward to in vivo use (**Fig. 3**). It is interesting that lectin molecular imaging probes have thus far been used as negative markers, in that they bind to normal tissue, but not to precancerous tissue,[68,73] whereas most other molecular imaging techniques have looked at increases in probe binding as disease develops. This is not a problem for endoscopic molecular imaging, because it still creates a clear color difference owing to the alteration of lectin binding that can be seen endoscopically, with a good signal:background ratio and signal:noise ratio of 5.2 (SD, 1.2–9.1) and 30.3 (SD, 15.2–45.5), respectively, in the esophagus.[68] The key to these imaging modalities is that lesions are not missed, whereas the level of false positives does not need to be controlled tightly.

This exciting progress in molecular probe development, combined with endoscopic detection, offers the potential for a giant leap forward in our endoscopic diagnostic ability and may simultaneously facilitate the guidance of endoscopic and surgical therapy, assist in risk prognostication for individual patients, and even allow more

Table 2
Molecular imaging trials reported in human colon

Author, Year of Publication	Molecular Target	Probe	Route of Administration	Detector System	Tissue Used	Key Statistics	Limitations
Hsiung et al,[71] 2008	Unknown	Fluorescein conjugated heptapeptide	Topical	Confocal laser endoscopy	During colonoscopy	81% sensitivity and 82% specificity for dysplastic colonocytes	Polyps identified were visible with white light. Field of view. Unclear molecular target.
Keller et al,[70] 2002	CEA	Fluorescein-labelled antibody against CEA	Topical	Conventional endoscope with 2 narrow-band filters	During colonoscopy	Fluorescence was present in 19/25 CRCs and 3/8 adenomas. If cases with bleeding or ulceration were excluded specificity 100%, sensitivity 78.6%, accuracy 89.3%.	Rate of CEA expression in early lesions
Yeung et al,[73] 2013	Terminal β1-4-linked GalNAc residues	Fluorescently labeled lectin (WFA)	Topical	Conventional endoscope or IVIS camera	Colectomy specimens	WFA binds more strongly to normal colonic epithelium than to cancer tissue from the same patient. Mean fluorescence 27.6 vs 4.80 arbitrary units, $P<.0001$	In vivo trials pending
Hardwick et al,[72] 2014	c-Met	Fluorescent cyanine-labelled 26-amino acid cyclic peptide	Intravenous	Dual white-light and near infrared fluorescent light endoscopic imaging system	During colonoscopy	All neoplastic lesions had increased fluorescence. 9 nonpolypoid adenomas were visible with fluorescent light but not white light	Need for IV administration means high dose and cost and increased risk of toxicity c-MET expression was reported as higher in adenomas and hyperplastic polyps

Abbreviations: CEA, carcinoembryonic antigen; IVIS, in vivo imaging system; WFA, Wisteria floribunda.

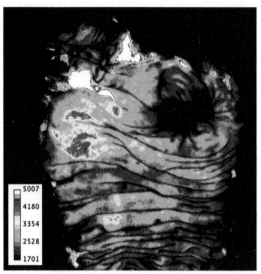

Fig. 3. Molecular imaging of a right hemicolectomy specimen after application of fluorescently labeled lectin. Cecal cancer is clearly demarcated (the *red* showing low lectin binding) from the surrounding normal mucosa with high lectin binding (*blue*). (*Courtesy of* Mr Trevor Yeung, MA, MBBChir, MRCS, DPhil, Nuffield Department of Surgical Sciences, University of Oxford, Oxford, United Kingdom.)

personalized drug therapies based on the individual molecular abnormalities that we may be able to detect in real time at endoscopy.

SUMMARY

The current generation of electronic imaging either via virtual chromoendoscopy or AFI has not delivered the hoped for benefits in terms of polyp and specifically adenoma detection. Their use is not supported in average-risk patients in recent guidelines, and is only recommended for certain specific indications (the Lynch syndrome and serrated polyposis syndrome surveillance).[74] The reasons for this may include a darker image, insufficient contrast versus background mucosa, and loss of resolution and image quality. The current reference standard, now HD-WLE, has improved. There has been a focus on quality in endoscopy and on the detection of subtle and flat lesions, which may have improved endoscopist performance, obviating the need for additional enhancements beyond high-quality white light examinations. Nevertheless, adenomas and sessile serrated adenomas/polyps are still missed at an alarming rate and seem likely to be significant factors in postcolonoscopy CRC.[20,30] Molecular imaging is an alternate modality that may offer specific highlighting of lesions to allow adequate contrast in the detection of CRC precursor lesions.

REFERENCES

1. De Sousa EM, Wang X, Jansen M, et al. Poor-prognosis colon cancer is defined by a molecularly distinct subtype and develops from serrated precursor lesions. Nat Med 2013;19(5):614–8.

2. Sadanandam A, Lyssiotis CA, Homicsko K, et al. A colorectal cancer classification system that associates cellular phenotype and responses to therapy. Nat Med 2013;19(5):619–25.

3. Marisa L, de Reynies A, Duval A, et al. Gene expression classification of colon cancer into molecular subtypes: characterization, validation, and prognostic value. PLoS Med 2013;10(5):e1001453.

4. Bond JH. Clinical evidence for the adenoma-carcinoma sequence, and the management of patients with colorectal adenomas. Semin Gastrointest Dis 2000;11: 176–84.

5. East JE, Saunders BP, Jass JR. Sporadic and syndromic hyperplastic polyps and serrated adenomas of the colon: classification, molecular genetics, natural history, and clinical management. Gastroenterol Clin North Am 2008;37(1):25–46, v.

6. Leggett B, Whitehall V. Role of the serrated pathway in colorectal cancer pathogenesis. Gastroenterology 2010;138(6):2088–100.

7. Davis HL, Irshad S, Rafferty H, et al. 399 aberrant epithelial grem1 expression promotes stem-cell plasticity and ectopic crypt formation in the pathogenesis of familial and sporadic human polyps. Gastroenterology 2014;146:S-86.

8. Snover D, Ahnen DJ, Burt RW, et al. Serrated polyps of the colon and rectum and serrated polyposis. In: Bosman FT, Carneiro F, Hruban RH, et al, editors. WHO Classification of Tumours of the Digestive System. LYON: IARC; 2010. p. 160–5.

9. Eaden JA, Abrams KR, Mayberry JF. The risk of colorectal cancer in ulcerative colitis: a meta-analysis. Gut 2001;48:526–35.

10. Jess T, Simonsen J, Jorgensen KT, et al. Decreasing risk of colorectal cancer in patients with inflammatory bowel disease over 30 years. Gastroenterology 2012; 143(2):375–81.e1 [quiz: e13–4].

11. Herrinton LJ, Liu L, Levin TR, et al. Incidence and mortality of colorectal adenocarcinoma in persons with inflammatory bowel disease from 1998 to 2010. Gastroenterology 2012;143(2):382–9.

12. Rutter MD, Saunders BP, Wilkinson KH, et al. Thirty-year analysis of a colonoscopic surveillance program for neoplasia in ulcerative colitis. Gastroenterology 2006;130(4):1030–8.

13. Annese V, Daperno M, Rutter MD, et al. European evidence based consensus for endoscopy in inflammatory bowel disease. J Crohns Colitis 2013;7(12): 982–1018.

14. Cairns SR, Scholefield JH, Steele RJ, et al. Guidelines for colorectal cancer screening and surveillance in moderate and high risk groups (update from 2002). Gut 2010;59(5):666–89.

15. Farraye FA, Odze RD, Eaden J, et al. Aga technical review on the diagnosis and management of colorectal neoplasia in inflammatory bowel disease. Gastroenterology 2010;138(2):746–74, 774e1–4; [quiz: e12–3].

16. Laine L, Kaltenbach T, Barkun A, et al. SCENIC International Consensus Statement on Surveillance and Management of Dysplasia in Inflammatory Bowel Disease. Gastroenterology 2015;148:639–51.

17. Colonoscopic surveillance for prevention of colorectal cancer in people with ulcerative colitis, Crohn's disease or adenomas: NICE guideline. http://www.nice.org.uk/nicemedia/live/13415/57930/57930.pdf. Accessed November 7, 2014.

18. Zauber AG, Winawer SJ, O'Brien MJ, et al. Colonoscopic polypectomy and long-term prevention of colorectal-cancer deaths. N Engl J Med 2012;366(8): 687–96.

19. Brenner H, Stock C, Hoffmeister M. Effect of screening sigmoidoscopy and screening colonoscopy on colorectal cancer incidence and mortality: systematic

review and meta-analysis of randomised controlled trials and observational studies. BMJ 2014;348:g2467.

20. Corley DA, Jensen CD, Marks AR, et al. Adenoma detection rate and risk of colorectal cancer and death. N Engl J Med 2014;370:1298–306.

21. van Rijn JC, Reitsma JB, Stoker J, et al. Polyp miss rate determined by tandem colonoscopy: a systematic review. Am J Gastroenterol 2006;101(2): 343–50.

22. Bressler B, Paszat LF, Chen Z, et al. Rates of new or missed colorectal cancers after colonoscopy and their risk factors: a population-based analysis. Gastroenterology 2007;132(1):96–102.

23. East JE, Saunders BP, Burling D, et al. Surface visualization at ct colonography simulated colonoscopy: effect of varying field of view and retrograde view. Am J Gastroenterol 2007;102(11):2529–35.

24. Pohl H, Srivastava A, Bensen SP, et al. Incomplete polyp resection during colonoscopy-results of the complete adenoma resection (care) study. Gastroenterology 2013;144(1):74–80.e1.

25. Rex DK, Cutler CS, Lemmel GT, et al. Colonoscopic miss rates of adenomas determined by back-to-back colonoscopies. Gastroenterology 1997;112(1):24–8.

26. Hopkins. A flexible fibrescope, using static scanning. Nature 1954;173(4392): 39–41.

27. Hirschowitz BI, Curtiss LE, Peters CW, et al. Demonstration of a new gastroscope, the fiberscope. Gastroenterology 1958;35(1):50 [discussion: 51–3].

28. Gaisford WD. Fiberoptic colonoscopy total colonoscopy–an office procedure. Dis Colon Rectum 1976;19(5):388–94.

29. Sivak MV Jr, Fleischer DE. Colonoscopy with a videoendoscope: preliminary experience. Gastrointest Endosc 1984;30(1):1–5.

30. Heresbach D, Barrioz T, Lapalus MG, et al. Miss rate for colorectal neoplastic polyps: a prospective multicenter study of back-to-back video colonoscopies. Endoscopy 2008;40(4):284–90.

31. Tada M, Katoh S, Kohli Y, et al. On the dye spraying method in colonofiberscopy. Endoscopy 1977;8(2):70–4.

32. Kiesslich R, Fritsch J, Holtmann M, et al. Methylene blue-aided chromoendoscopy for the detection of intraepithelial neoplasia and colon cancer in ulcerative colitis. Gastroenterology 2003;124(4):880–8.

33. Brown SR, Baraza W. Chromoscopy versus conventional endoscopy for the detection of polyps in the colon and rectum. Cochrane Database Syst Rev 2010;(10):CD006439.

34. Du Le VN, Wang Q, Gould T, et al. Vascular contrast in narrow-band and white light imaging. Appl Opt 2014;53(18):4061–71.

35. Coriat R, Chryssostalis A, Zeitoun JD, et al. Computed virtual chromoendoscopy system (fice): a new tool for upper endoscopy? Gastroenterol Clin Biol 2008; 32(4):363–9.

36. Kodashima S, Fujishiro M. Novel image-enhanced endoscopy with i-scan technology. World J Gastroenterol 2010;16(9):1043–9.

37. Monici M. Cell and tissue autofluorescence research and diagnostic applications. Biotechnol Annu Rev 2005;11:227–56.

38. Jin XF, Chai TH, Shi JW, et al. Meta-analysis for evaluating the accuracy of endoscopy with narrow band imaging in detecting colorectal adenomas. J Gastroenterol Hepatol 2012;27(5):882–7.

39. Chung SJ, Kim D, Song JH, et al. Comparison of detection and miss rates of narrow band imaging, flexible spectral imaging chromoendoscopy and white light at

screening colonoscopy: a randomised controlled back-to-back study. Gut 2014; 63(5):785–91.

40. Pohl J, Lotterer E, Balzer C, et al. Computed virtual chromoendoscopy versus standard colonoscopy with targeted indigocarmine chromoscopy: a randomised multicentre trial. Gut 2009;58(1):73–8.

41. Chung SJ, Kim D, Song JH, et al. Efficacy of computed virtual chromoendoscopy on colorectal cancer screening: a prospective, randomized, back-to-back trial of Fuji intelligent color enhancement versus conventional colonoscopy to compare adenoma miss rates. Gastrointest Endosc 2010;72(1):136–42.

42. Aminalai A, Rosch T, Aschenbeck J, et al. Live image processing does not increase adenoma detection rate during colonoscopy: a randomized comparison between fice and conventional imaging (berlin colonoscopy project 5, becop-5). Am J Gastroenterol 2010;105(11):2383–8.

43. Hong SN, Choe WH, Lee JH, et al. Prospective, randomized, back-to-back trial evaluating the usefulness of i-scan in screening colonoscopy. Gastrointest Endosc 2012;75(5):1011–21.e2.

44. Omata F, Ohde S, Deshpande GA, et al. Image-enhanced, chromo, and cap-assisted colonoscopy for improving adenoma/neoplasia detection rate: a systematic review and meta-analysis. Scand J Gastroenterol 2014;49(2):222–37.

45. Matsuda T, Saito Y, Fu KI, et al. Does autofluorescence imaging videoendoscopy system improve the colonoscopic polyp detection rate?–a pilot study. Am J Gastroenterol 2008;103(8):1926–32.

46. Takeuchi Y, Inoue T, Hanaoka N, et al. Autofluorescence imaging with a transparent hood for detection of colorectal neoplasms: a prospective, randomized trial. Gastrointest Endosc 2010;72(5):1006–13.

47. Kuiper T, van den Broek FJ, Naber AH, et al. Endoscopic trimodal imaging detects colonic neoplasia as well as standard video endoscopy. Gastroenterology 2011;140(7):1887–94.

48. van den Broek FJ, Fockens P, Van Eeden S, et al. Clinical evaluation of endoscopic trimodal imaging for the detection and differentiation of colonic polyps. Clin Gastroenterol Hepatol 2009;7(3):288–95.

49. Rotondano G, Bianco MA, Sansone S, et al. Trimodal endoscopic imaging for the detection and differentiation of colorectal adenomas: a prospective single-centre clinical evaluation. Int J Colorectal Dis 2012;27(3):331–6.

50. Zhao Z, Guan Y, Li B, et al. Autofluorescence imaging for the detection and miss rate of adenomatous and polypoid lesions by colonoscopy: a systematic review and meta-analysis. Endoscopy International Open 2014, in press.

51. Jarvinen HJ, Aarnio M, Mustonen H, et al. Controlled 15-year trial on screening for colorectal cancer in families with hereditary nonpolyposis colorectal cancer. Gastroenterology 2000;118(5):829–34.

52. Vasen HF, Abdirahman M, Brohet R, et al. One to 2-year surveillance intervals reduce risk of colorectal cancer in families with lynch syndrome. Gastroenterology 2010;138(7):2300–6.

53. East JE, Suzuki N, Stavrinidis M, et al. Narrow band imaging for colonoscopic surveillance in hereditary non-polyposis colorectal cancer. Gut 2008;57(1):65–70.

54. Hurlstone DP, Karajeh M, Cross SS, et al. The role of high-magnification-chromoscopic colonoscopy in hereditary nonpolyposis colorectal cancer screening: a prospective "Back-to-back" Endoscopic study. Am J Gastroenterol 2005; 100(10):2167–73.

55. Huneburg R, Lammert F, Rabe C, et al. Chromocolonoscopy detects more adenomas than white light colonoscopy or narrow band imaging colonoscopy in

hereditary nonpolyposis colorectal cancer screening. Endoscopy 2009;41(4): 316–22.

56. Matsumoto T, Esaki M, Fujisawa R, et al. Chromoendoscopy, narrow-band imaging colonoscopy, and autofluorescence colonoscopy for detection of diminutive colorectal neoplasia in familial adenomatous polyposis. Dis Colon Rectum 2009;52(6):1160–5.

57. Stoffel EM, Turgeon DK, Stockwell DH, et al. Missed adenomas during colonoscopic surveillance in individuals with lynch syndrome (hereditary nonpolyposis colorectal cancer). Cancer Prev Res (Phila) 2008;1(6):470–5.

58. Ramsoekh D, Haringsma J, Poley JW, et al. A back-to-back comparison of white light video endoscopy with autofluorescence endoscopy for adenoma detection in high-risk subjects. Gut 2010;59(6):785–93.

59. Boparai KS, van den Broek FJ, van Eeden S, et al. Increased polyp detection using narrow band imaging compared with high resolution endoscopy in patients with hyperplastic polyposis syndrome. Endoscopy 2011;43(8):676–82.

60. Boparai KS, van den Broek FJ, van Eeden S, et al. Hyperplastic polyposis syndrome: a pilot study for the differentiation of polyps by using high-resolution endoscopy, autofluorescence imaging, and narrow-band imaging. Gastrointest Endosc 2009;70(5):947–55.

61. Ignjatovic A, East JE, Subramanian V, et al. Narrow band imaging for detection of dysplasia in colitis: a randomized controlled trial. Am J Gastroenterol 2012; 107(6):885–90.

62. Dekker E, van den Broek FJ, Reitsma JB, et al. Narrow-band imaging compared with conventional colonoscopy for the detection of dysplasia in patients with long-standing ulcerative colitis. Endoscopy 2007;39(3):216–21.

63. van den Broek FJ, Fockens P, van Eeden S, et al. Narrow-band imaging versus high-definition endoscopy for the diagnosis of neoplasia in ulcerative colitis. Endoscopy 2011;43(2):108–15.

64. Pellise M, Lopez-Ceron M, Rodriguez de Miguel C, et al. Narrow-band imaging as an alternative to chromoendoscopy for the detection of dysplasia in long-standing inflammatory bowel disease: a prospective, randomized, crossover study. Gastrointest Endosc 2011;74(4):840–8.

65. Efthymiou M, Allen PB, Taylor AC, et al. Chromoendoscopy versus narrow band imaging for colonic surveillance in inflammatory bowel disease. Inflamm Bowel Dis 2013;19(10):2132–8.

66. Matsumoto T, Nakamura S, Moriyama T, et al. Autofluorescence imaging colonoscopy for the detection of dysplastic lesions in ulcerative colitis: a pilot study. Colorectal Dis 2010;12(10 Online):e291–7.

67. van den Broek FJ, Fockens P, van Eeden S, et al. Endoscopic tri-modal imaging for surveillance in ulcerative colitis: Randomised comparison of high-resolution endoscopy and autofluorescence imaging for neoplasia detection; and evaluation of narrow-band imaging for classification of lesions. Gut 2008;57(8):1083–9.

68. Bird-Lieberman EL, Neves AA, Lao-Sirieix P, et al. Molecular imaging using fluorescent lectins permits rapid endoscopic identification of dysplasia in Barrett's esophagus. Nat Med 2012;18:315–21.

69. Atreya R, Neumann H, Neufert C, et al. In vivo imaging using fluorescent antibodies to tumor necrosis factor predicts therapeutic response in Crohn's disease. Nat Med 2014;20:313–8.

70. Keller R, Winde G, Terpe HJ, et al. Fluorescence endoscopy using a fluorescein-labeled monoclonal antibody against carcinoembryonic antigen in patients with colorectal carcinoma and adenoma. Endoscopy 2002;34:801–7.

71. Hsiung PL, Hardy J, Friedland S, et al. Detection of colonic dysplasia in vivo using a targeted heptapeptide and confocal microendoscopy. Nat Med 2008;14:454–8.
72. Hardwick J, Burggraaf J, Kemerling I, et al. Detection of colorectal polyps using an intravenously administered fluorescent peptide targeted against c-met. European Molecular Imaging Meeting. June 4–6, 2014. Antwerp (Belgium), 2014. p. FS VI - 2.
73. Yeung T, East J, Wang LM, et al. Molecular imaging of dysplasia and cancer using fluorescent lectins. Dis Colon Rectum 2013;56:E104–5.
74. Kaminski MF, Hassan C, Bisschops R, et al. Advanced imaging for detection and differentiation of colorectal neoplasia: European society of gastrointestinal endoscopy (ESGE) guideline. Endoscopy 2014;46(5):435–49.
75. Pasha SF, Leighton JA, Das A, et al. Comparison of the yield and miss rate of narrow band imaging and white light endoscopy in patients undergoing screening or surveillance colonoscopy: a meta-analysis. Am J Gastroenterol 2012;107(3):363–70 [quiz: 371].
76. Dinesen L, Chua TJ, Kaffes AJ. Meta-analysis of narrow-band imaging versus conventional colonoscopy for adenoma detection. Gastrointest Endosc 2012; 75(3):604–11.
77. Nagorni A, Bjelakovic G, Petrovic B. Narrow band imaging versus conventional white light colonoscopy for the detection of colorectal polyps. Cochrane Database Syst Rev 2012;(1):CD008361.

Chromocolonoscopy

Michael J. Bartel, MD, Michael F. Picco, MD, PhD,
Michael B. Wallace, MD, MPH*

KEYWORDS

- Chromocolonoscopy • Chromoendoscopy • Advanced imaging
- Screening colonoscopy • Inflammatory bowel disease • Society guidelines

KEY POINTS

- Chromoendoscopy techniques improve the visualization of mucosal structures.
- Chromoendoscopy differentiates neoplastic from non-neoplastic polyps in the average-risk population with high accuracy but does not distinguish both reliably in inflammatory bowel disease (IBD).
- Dye-based chromoendoscopy improves neoplasia detection in colonic IBD surveillance, with the potential to replace random colonic biopsies as the preferred surveillance option.

CHROMOENDOSCOPY

Chromoendoscopy refers to image-enhanced endoscopy through the use of dye spraying or optical techniques. Although initially limited to dye spraying, over the last decade, equipment-based imaging-enhanced optical colonoscopy techniques have been developed that are commonly referred to as *dyeless* or *digital chromoendoscopy*. Chromoendoscopy techniques improve the visualization of mucosal structures and, thus, improve recognition of borders and surface topography of pathologic lesions compared with standard white light colonoscopy. This review focuses on the role of these imaging techniques in the detection of colonic neoplasia.

Why Do We Need Chromoendoscopy?

Polypectomy of colonic neoplasms is the backbone of colorectal cancer (CRC) screening and health prevention measures, as it is associated with a 53% reduction of mortality.[1,2] However, colonoscopy does not fully protect against CRC, with interval CRCs representing between 2% and 6% of all CRCs.[3] There is evidence that most interval cancers arise from missed, rather than new, colorectal neoplastic lesions.[4]

Disclosures: M.J. Bartel and M.F. Picco have no disclosure; M. Wallace receives research grants from Cosmo Pharmaceutical, Olympus, Boston Scientific, and NinePoint Medical.
Gastroenterology and Hepatology, Mayo Clinic, 4500 San Pablo Road, Jacksonville, FL 32224, USA
* Corresponding author.
E-mail address: wallace.michael@mayo.edu

Gastrointest Endoscopy Clin N Am 25 (2015) 243–260
http://dx.doi.org/10.1016/j.giec.2014.11.010
1052-5157/15/$ – see front matter © 2015 Elsevier Inc. All rights reserved.

Adenoma miss rates average 24% and are highest for diminutive adenomas (26%) compared with adenomas greater than 10 mm (2%).[5,6] The reasons for missing colorectal neoplasms during colonoscopy include inadequate bowel preparation; presence of flat polyps, which often resemble normal mucosa at first glance; and technical challenges of colonoscopy limiting mucosal visualization behind folds and in the right colon.[7–9] Fortunately, flat neoplasms, which have a prevalence of 5% to 10%, appear preferentially in the right colon allowing endoscopists to focus their attention in this region when looking for such polyps.[10–12] Sessile serrate adenoma/polyps account for an important subtype of mostly flat and right colonic neoplastic lesions, of which 9.5% contain high-grade dysplasia.[13]

Since Kaminski and colleagues[14] and Corley and colleagues[15] found that a low adenoma detection rate (ADR) is an independent predictor for interval CRC, significant attention has been directed at increasing the ADR.[14,15] Unfortunately, the introduction of high-definition (HD) colonoscopy has resulted in a diagnostic average gain of only 3.8% compared with standard white light colonoscopy.[16] The marginal increase of ADR is mainly limited to diminutive polyps.[17]

Chromoendoscopy has emerged as a method to improve ADR for both average and high-risk CRC screening populations, including those with inflammatory bowel disease (IBD). Chromoendoscopy may also have a role in distinguishing between neoplastic and non-neoplastic colonic lesions allowing for a resect-and-discard strategy for diminutive colonic lesions bypassing formal pathologic assessment.[18]

Application of Dye for Dye-Based Chromoendoscopy

Dye-based chromoendoscopy uses color dyes that are either absorbed by the mucosa (vital dye) or remain on the mucosal surface (nonvital dye). The dye can be applied in a nontargeted fashion to the entire colonic mucosa (pan-chromoendoscopy) or to target certain colonic sections to define borders and predict histology of an area of interest. The two most common dyes used for staining are indigo carmine and methylene blue. Both dyes seem to be equally effective in enhancing dysplasia detection (**Table 1**).

Indigo Carmine

Indigo carmine is not absorbed by cells (nonvital dye). It coats the mucosa highlighting mucosal pits, grooves, erosions, depressions, and subtle colonic contour irregularities. Its deep-blue color enhances the visualization of mucosal structures and allows better distinguishing of borders, depth, and surface topography of lesions.[19]

Methylene Blue

Methylene blue is actively absorbed by small intestine and colonic epithelium (vital dye). This absorption requires waiting about 60 seconds before adequate staining is achieved. Colonic dysplastic and inflamed tissue absorb less or no dye resulting in different staining characteristics compared with normal mucosa. The different staining characteristics provides better resolution to distinguish borders and surface topography of lesions, similar to the application of indigo carmine.[19]

Crystal Violet

Crystal violet is also a vital dye that stains colonic crypts by being preferentially absorbed by the crypts of Lieberkühn. Similar to methylene blue, crystal violet is absorbed by noninflamed mucosa better than by neoplasia and inflamed tissue. Crystal violet was shown to be useful in characterizing pit patterns, particularly in conjunction with indigo carmine.[19,20] This dye is not used commonly in practice.

Table 1
Baseline information of commonly used chromoendoscopy dyes for colonoscopy

	Methylene Blue	Indigo Carmine	Crystal Violet
Dye category	Vital	Nonvital	Vital
Staining mechanism	Active absorption into intestine epithelial cells Less or no absorption by inflamed mucosa and neoplasia	Not absorbed by cells but coats intestinal lining	Active absorption by Lieberkühn crypts[100]
Staining pattern	Highlights pit pattern Increases contrast between mucosal structures Inflamed mucosa or neoplasia appears brighter than normal mucosa	Highlights pit pattern Increases contrast between mucosal structures	Highlights pit pattern
Dye application	Spray catheter or standard water pump	Spray catheter or standard water pump	Spray catheter
Concentration	0.1%	0.03%–0.5%	0.05%–0.2%
Color	Blue	Blue	Blue
Staining time	1 min to allow staining of normal mucosa	No waiting time following dye application	Typically sprayed after indigo carmine application
Duration of staining	Lasts for up to 20 min	Lasts for few minutes, disappears because of dilution throughout colon	n/a

Abbreviation: n/a, not applicable.

Safety of Dye Application

Generally, mucosal dyes used by gastroenterologists are safe; no significant adverse drug reactions are reported with the exception of methylene blue, which was shown to damage DNA when used in the evaluation of Barrett esophagus. The clinical importance of this finding is not known, and methylene blue is generally considered to be safe.[21] Recent unpublished studies (Alessandro Repici, MD, verbal communication including data submitted to the US Food and Drug Administration, 2014) suggest that there is no clinically relevant DNA damage caused by methylene blue for colonic dye spraying.

Method of Dye Application

Adequate colonic preparation is paramount to achieve good mucosal visualization during chromoendoscopy. The endoscopist should lavage the colon on insertion to remove any remaining material. Once the cecum is reached, the dye is applied to the colonic mucosa. In this context, decompression of the colon allows better mucosal dye coverage.

The concentration of the indigo carmine and methylene blue has varied in studies from 0.03% to 0.5% mixed in water (indigo carmine 0.03%–0.5%[22,23]; methylene blue 0.1%[24]). The dye may be sprayed directly through the accessory channel of the colonoscope using a 60-mL syringe and a spray catheter. The spray catheter does, however, increase the cost of the procedure.[22] Picco and colleagues[25] outlined a more practical approach of dye application. The dye mixed in 1 L of sterile water was administered by a standard water pump device attached to the colonoscope, enabling the endoscopist to spray the dye by pressing the foot pedal with results similar to catheter-based applications (video example http://www.youtube.com/watch?v=6PJ91qYUPcE).

Most recently, Repici and colleagues[26] reported a coated methylene blue capsule allowing dye delivery limited to the colon by using a specific capsule formulation. However, it is not yet clear whether this method is an acceptable alternative to conventional chromoendoscopy.

For pancolonic chromoendoscopy, colon segments of 20 to 30 cm are sprayed with dye. Immediate evaluation can be performed following indigo carmine application after the excess dye is suctioned. Methylene blue, however, requires 60 seconds after application to achieve adequate mucosal staining. The steps are repeated during colonoscope withdrawal until the entire mucosa is visualized.

Kiesslich and Neurath[27] proposed several technical guidelines (SURFACE) for the use of chromoendoscopy in ulcerative colitis that included assurance of optimal visualization with excellent bowel prep and targeted chromoendoscopy with indigo carmine or methylene blue. The use of a spasmolytic was also included, but it is typically not necessary. Classification of polyp pit pattern was also recommended but does require significant expertise.

EQUIPMENT-BASED IMAGING-ENHANCED COLONOSCOPY (DIGITAL OR DYELESS CHROMOENDOSCOPY)

Since the introduction of HD colonoscopy, several equipment-based imaging-enhanced colonoscopy techniques have become available. The techniques have improved mucosal visualization of surface and vascular structures through the use of optical filters or utilization of software-based technologies. These technologies are reviewed in detail elsewhere in this issue.

Narrow-Band Imaging

Narrow-band imaging (NBI) is an optic filter-based method that allows blue and green wavelengths from the white light spectrum to pass through but blocks red wavelengths. Green and especially blue light wavelengths fall into the peak absorption of hemoglobin. As a consequence, blue and green light are absorbed by superficial and deep mucosal vessels, respectively, but are reflected by the remaining mucosa. This reflection improves visualization of mucosal vessels, which are frequently altered in form, density, and size in neoplastic colorectal lesions.[28]

Fujinon Intelligent Color Enhancement

Fujinon Intelligent Color Enhancement (FICE) (Fujinon Inc, Japan) emits and captures the entire white light spectrum without the use of any optical filters. Following light capture, digital software-based computer algorithms modify the captured images. Thus, certain combinations of wavelengths are selectively enhanced, which results in improved visualization of subtle mucosal surface changes, especially of mucosal vessels and pit patterns.

iScan

Similar to FICE, iScan (Pentax, Japan) is a postprocessing, software-based technology functioning as a digital filter. The digital filter alters certain wavelengths of reflected white light, which results in enhancement of different elements of the mucosa. Three different filter algorithms allow for surface enhancement, contrast enhancement, and tone enhancement.

CHROMOENDOSCOPY FOR AVERAGE-RISK PATIENTS
Adenoma Detection Rate in Dye-Based Chromoendoscopy

Early randomized controlled trials failed to demonstrate a significant increase in ADR with dye-based chromoendoscopy compared with standard white light colonoscopy. In these studies, ADR with white light and chromoendoscopy ranged from 25% to 31% and 33% to 39%, respectively.[29,30] The largest benefit of chromoendoscopy was an increase of the total number of detected diminutive adenomas from 37 in 135 patients to 89 in 124 patients.[29] Two additional studies found significantly more patients with 3 or more adenomas in the chromoendoscopy group compared with the standard white light colonoscopy group (12% [15 of 124] vs 2% [3 of 135] and 10% [13 of 128] vs 3% [4 of 132], respectively).[29,31] Also, more proximal colonic adenomas were detected by chromoendoscopy, although the results were only significant for diminutive adenomas (80% [71 of 89] vs 73% [27 of 37]). The prevalence of flat colorectal neoplasia in chromoendoscopy was up to 3 times greater than in regular screening colonoscopies.[12,30] This finding was confirmed by a Cochrane meta-analysis of 5 randomized controlled studies that found that chromoendoscopy detected significantly more patients with at least one lesion neoplastic (odds ratio [OR] 1.67) and significantly more patients with 3 or more neoplastic lesions (OR 2.55).[32]

Results were mixed comparing HD colonoscopy with chromoendoscopy. One study demonstrated similar ADRs (48.4% and 55.5%, no significant difference), whereas another showed a significant increase in ADR from 36.3% to 46.2%.[10,33] Once again, the differences were mostly limited to a higher detection rate of diminutive lesions (30.4% vs 23.2%), serrated lesions (46.2% vs 29.5%), and flat adenomas.[10,33] However, no significant difference was found for adenomas larger than 1 cm (12.9% vs 9.4%).[10]

These data indicate that chromoendoscopy achieves marginally higher ADR than standard or HD colonoscopy, with an advantage limited to the detection of diminutive, flat neoplastic and serrated lesions. A disadvantage of chromoendoscopy is a significantly longer procedure duration. Studies addressing the rate of interval colon cancer following screening colonoscopy with chromoendoscopy do not exist but are of interest as chromoendoscopy seems to target lesions that are frequently missed in standard colonoscopy (**Table 2**).[4]

ADENOMA DETECTION RATE IN DIGITAL CHROMOENDOSCOPY

NBI is the most thoroughly studied digital chromoendoscopy in average-risk patients undergoing screening colonoscopy. Multiple studies, including tandem colonoscopy studies and randomized controlled trials, failed to detect a significantly different ADR when comparing standard white light colonoscopy with NBI.[34,35] A subsequent meta-analysis of 2936 patients showed no significant difference in the overall ADR (36% vs 34%) with NBI. The average number of adenomas per patient also did not differ significantly (0.645 vs 0.59).[36] The only significant advantage of NBI over standard white light colonoscopy was the higher number of detected diminutive adenomas, flat adenomas, and hyperplastic polyps, especially in the distal colon. Moreover, no difference for right- versus left-sided colonic polyps was found.[37–39] Analogously, a meta-analysis comparing HD colonoscopy with or without NBI also

Table 2
Main outcomes (ADR, dysplasia detection rate) in average and high-risk patients with IBD undergoing white light colonoscopy, dye-based chromoendoscopy, and digital chromoendoscopy

	White Light Colonoscopy (%)	Methylene Blue Chromoendoscopy (%)	Indigo Carmine Chromoendoscopy (%)	NBI/FICE/ iScan (%)
Average-risk screening colonoscopy				
ADR	25.0–48.4	Not reported	33.0–55.5	28–64
Differentiating neoplastic from non-neoplastic lesions				
Sensitivity	33.0–95.5	Not reported	82–98	78–98
Specificity	74–97	Not reported	72.7–95.0	61.2–93.0
PPV	87.9–93.4	Not reported	98.1	89–93
NPV	63–100	Not reported	88	76–100
Accuracy	61.0–93.3	Not reported	75–94	79.0–98.6
IBD surveillance colonoscopy				
Dysplasia detection rate per patient	2.0–8.8	13.8–16.7	7.0–19.7	9–19
Differentiating neoplastic from non-neoplastic lesions				
Sensitivity	38–88	72–97	89–100	75–76
Specificity	65.6–93.8	92–93	91.0–96.8	66–81
PPV	93.4	Not reported	16.5–62.5	Not reported
NPV	63.3	Not reported	99.6–100	Not reported
Accuracy	72–84	Not reported	Not reported	67–80

Abbreviations: NPV, negative predictive value; PPV, positive predictive value.

found no significant difference in ADR or detection of flat adenomas and adenomas less than 10 mm of size.[40]

In summary, NBI technology did not show any significant advantage over HD white light colonoscopy in terms of ADR. Therefore, it is not recommended as an ADR-improving strategy.

The data for iScan are less consistent. Hoffman and colleagues[41] demonstrated a higher ADR and rate of flat adenoma detection in screening colonoscopies with iScan in relation to standard colonoscopy (38% vs 13% and 58% vs 23%). These differences were caused by improved detection of diminutive and flat adenomas with mean polyp sizes of 5.6 mm and 6.7 mm, respectively. It is important to note that the ADR in the control group was low, which may have exaggerated the effect of iScan. The same investigators also reported a lower adenoma miss in a tandem study with iScan compared with standard colonoscopy (30.0% vs 62.5%) but again most significantly in nonpolypoid lesions less than 5 mm of size.[42] Others have reported no significant differences in ADR and adenoma miss rate comparing HD colonoscopy and iScan in tandem fashion (31.9% vs 36.5% and 22.9% vs 19.3%).[43] Lastly, following an iScan, a tandem dye-based chromoendoscopy increased the number of detected polyps less than 5 mm in size by 92% in an evaluation limited to the distal colon. Most of the polyps were, however, non-neoplastic polyps.[44]

The least amount of evidence is available for FICE, which did not demonstrate a significant advantage over standard white light colonoscopy in terms of ADR (64% vs 55%).[45] A randomized trial showed similar results with no significant difference in

ADR when compared with HD colonoscopy: 28% versus 28%.[46] The only prospective randomized trial comparing FICE with chromoendoscopy for screening colonoscopy also demonstrated no significant difference in ADR (64% vs 68%).[47]

In summary, NBI and iScan primarily improved the detection of diminutive and hyperplastic polyps; however, the overall ADR was not improved. FICE was also unable to improve ADR. Therefore, the routine use of digital chromoendoscopy is not recommended as a tool to improve ADR.

CHROMOENDOSCOPY IN INFLAMMATORY BOWEL DISEASE

IBD involving the colon is a well-recognized risk factor for the development of CRC. The cancer risk increases with both the extent and duration of colitis as well as the presence of primary sclerosing cholangitis.[48] A population surveillance study estimated the CRC risk for left-sided and pancolitis to be 2.5% at 20 years, 7.6% at 30 years, and 10.8% at 40 years following the development of ulcerative colitis; however, higher incidences have been reported.[49] Similar risks have been reported for Crohn colitis.[50] A Cochrane analysis found no evidence that survival is prolonged in patients with IBD who underwent surveillance colonoscopy. Although CRCs were detected at an early stage, which was linked with a better prognosis, a lead-time bias could not be excluded.[51]

Historically, colonoscopy for IBD surveillance consists of 4 quadrant biopsies obtained every 10 cm during colonoscopy withdrawal as well as targeted biopsies as indicated for visible mucosal abnormalities. This recommendation was based on the assumption that dysplastic lesions in IBD are flat and endoscopically invisible. In this context, a minimum of 33 biopsies is required to detect dysplasia with a probability of 90%.[52] This theory has been challenged by several investigators who reported that dysplasia is visible with white light colonoscopy in 58.5% to 87.9% of dysplastic lesions and 80% of cancers.[53,54] Further, it was shown that the yield of nontargeted, random surveillance biopsies is very low, with a neoplasia detection rate per specimen of less than 0.5%.[55,56] In contrast, targeted biopsies of the lesions present on white light colonoscopy resulted in neoplasia detection rates per specimen of 23% in a trial with 466 surveillance colonoscopies (166 patients) over 10 years.[57]

Dye-Based Chromoendoscopy in Inflammatory Bowel Disease

Several investigators addressed whether targeted biopsies during chromoendoscopy can further improve the neoplasia detection rate in IBD surveillance. In a cohort study, Hurlstone and colleagues[58] analyzed the yield of targeted biopsies in chromoendoscopy and standard colonoscopy. Chromoendoscopy detected dysplasia in 8% of specimens (49 of 644 specimens), whereas standard colonoscopy yielded dysplasia in only 1.6% (6 of 369 specimens). Consistent with previous reports, yield of random biopsies for dysplasia detection ranged between 0.14% (18 of 12,482 specimens) and 0.16% (20 of 12,850 specimens).

A tandem colonoscopy study by Rutter and colleagues[55] documented a dysplasia detection rate per patient of 7% following targeted biopsies in chromoendoscopy (9 dysplastic lesions in 7 of 100 patients) and 2% in standard colonoscopy (2 dysplastic lesions in 2 of 100 patients). Another prospective tandem study by Marion and colleagues[56] showed comparable results, with dysplasia detection rates per patient of 16.6% in chromoendoscopy (17 of 102 patients) and 8.8% in standard colonoscopy (9 of 102 patients). Of note, none of the 2904 random biopsies in the first study and only 16 of 3245 random biopsies (0.4%) in the second tandem study harbored dysplasia.

Lastly, a randomized, controlled trial reported a dysplasia detection rate per patient of 15.5% (13 of 84 patients, total of 32 dysplastic lesions) following chromoendoscopy and 7.4% (6 of 81 patients, total of 10 dysplastic lesions) in the standard colonoscopy group, although the findings were not significantly different.[59]

In summary, these studies indicate a 2 to 3 times higher yield per patient of dysplasia detection with chromoendoscopy compared with regular white light colonoscopy. A meta-analysis that included most of the aforementioned studies measured an increased detection of 44% for all dysplastic lesions and 27% for flat dysplastic lesions favoring chromoendoscopy over white light colonoscopy. This finding corresponded with an OR of 8.9 and 5.2, respectively. In addition, chromoendoscopy had a 40% lower miss rate for dysplastic lesions.[60,61] Another meta-analysis of 6 randomized controlled trials calculated the pooled sensitivity, specificity, and diagnostic OR of 83.0%, 91.3%, and 17.5, respectively, to detect dysplasia in long-standing ulcerative colitis with chromoendoscopy.[62]

The advantages of chromoendoscopy are limited by a significantly longer withdrawal time (pooled difference 11 minutes).[60,61] However, the time-consuming 32 random biopsies are often not taken into account. In this context, Rutter and colleagues[55] measured an average withdrawal time of 10 minutes for standard surveillance colonoscopy and 11 minutes for chromoendoscopy. Picco and colleagues[25] established a learning curve for chromoendoscopy in non-IBD endoscopists. The curve plateaued following 15 procedures at an average withdrawal time of 19 minutes that included both visualization with white light and chromoendoscopy.

Digital Chromoendoscopy in Inflammatory Bowel Disease

With the development of digital chromoendoscopy, gastroenterologists expected detection yield of dysplasia in colonic IBD comparable with dye-based chromoendoscopy, with the advantage of shortened withdrawal time as dye application became obsolete. Unfortunately, multiple studies have proven otherwise and have not demonstrated NBI to be superior to white light colonoscopy.

NBI does not detect more dysplastic lesions than standard and HD colonoscopy based on targeted biopsies (9% vs 9% and 19% vs 17%).[63,64] Similarly, the proportion of patients with at least one dysplastic lesion was not significantly different between NBI and HD colonoscopy (73% vs 64%).[63] Pellise and colleagues[65] randomized patients with longstanding IBD into surveillance with HD colonoscopy with NBI or chromoendoscopy. The investigators found no significant difference in the detection rate of dysplastic lesions. However, NBI had a higher miss rate of neoplastic lesions compared with chromoendoscopy (miss rate per lesion 13.6% vs 31.8%; miss rate per patient 15.4% vs 46.1%), although not reaching a statistical significance.

In summary, NBI has not been shown to improve the detection rate of dysplasia in IBD. Moreover, it was associated with a higher dysplasia miss rate compared with chromoendoscopy. Studies addressing FICE and iScan for IBD surveillance are not available.

Dysplasia-Associated Lesion or Mass

Special attention needs to be drawn for neoplasms arising within an area of inflammation, which is termed *dysplasia-associated lesion or mass* (DALM). It can be difficult to distinguish these lesions from sporadic polyps that would otherwise develop among patients without colitis because of age or family history.[66] Sessile lesions resemble a sporadic adenoma, termed *adenomalike DALM* or *adenomalike mass* (ALM) (Fig. 1). Endoscopic and pathologic features favoring sporadic adenoma include polyps in an area without colitis, short disease duration, the absence of primary

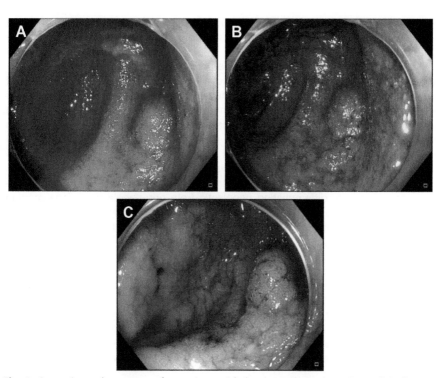

Fig. 1. Screening colonoscopy of a patient with long-standing ulcerative colitis demonstrating a flat lesion in the ascending colon consistent with an ALM. (*A*) ALM in standard white light. (*B*) ALM in NBI. (*C*) ALM in chromoendoscopy with 0.1% indigo carmine.

sclerosing cholangitis, a well-circumscribed lesion, and typical histologic characteristics.[67] In contrast, non-adenomalike DALM are highly irregular neoplastic lesions that do not resemble a sporadic adenoma located in an area of chronic inflammation.[68] Current guidelines recommend proctocolectomy for patients with IBD with invasive carcinoma, flat high-grade dysplasia, and non-adenomalike DALM.[67,69] This guideline is based on the fact that DALM harbors a high risk for synchronous CRC.[70]

Several trials showed that polyps with characteristics of ALM in areas of inflammation can be resected successfully.[71,72] More importantly, the frequency of cancer in patients following endoscopic resection of neoplasia did not differ from that of the IBD surveillance population. In this context, targeted chromoendoscopy can play a role by defining the borders of ALM and assuring complete removal.[72,73] Based on these data, a subset of patients with dysplastic polyps can be managed conservatively with close colonoscopy surveillance and, by doing so, avoid colectomy.[74]

REAL-TIME OPTICAL PREDICTION OF POLYP HISTOLOGY
Dye-Based Chromoendoscopy

High-quality and real-time imaging is paramount to adopt a resect-and-discard strategy for diminutive colorectal polyps.[18] The American Society for Gastrointestinal Endoscopy (ASGE) has defined basic requirements for endoscopic methods, which are named "*preservation and incorporation of valuable endoscopic innovations*"

(PIVI). PIVI requires greater than 90% agreement in determining postpolypectomy surveillance intervals and a greater than 90% negative predictive value (NPV) for adenomatous histology.[75]

The concept that histopathology can be predicted by endoscopic polyp appearance was initially studied by Kudo and colleagues.[20] Characteristic pit patterns of colonic mucosa following cresyl violet staining (Kudo classification) distinguished non-neoplastic from neoplastic colonic mucosal lesions. Pit pattern 1 (round pits) and 2 (stellar or papillary pits) were associated with non-neoplastic lesions, whereas 3 (tubular pits), 4 (branchlike or gyruslike pits), and 5 (nonstructural pits) predicted neoplastic lesions, including intramucosal cancer. Dye-based chromoendoscopy is known to improve visualization of superficial colonic mucosa.

Early studies measuring the effect of chromoendoscopy showed accuracy, sensitivity, and specificity differentiating neoplastic from non-neoplastic lesions ranging 95% to 99%, 94% to 98%, and 65.0% to 99.8%, respectively.[31,76–79] This finding has been confirmed by 2 separate meta-analyses with sensitivities of 92% and 94% and specificities of 82% and 86% using chromoendoscopy to differentiate neoplastic and non-neoplastic lesions based on the Kudo pit pattern.[34,80]

In a direct comparison, the highest accuracy in distinguishing neoplastic from non-neoplastic colorectal lesions was found in HD chromoendoscopy (96%), followed by chromoendoscopy (89%) and conventional colonoscopy (84%).[81]

In terms of polyp size, chromoendoscopy predicted large polyps (mean 14 mm) as neoplastic with a higher sensitivity and specificity than diminutive (<5 mm) polyps (92% vs 82% and 93% vs 82%).[77,82] Neoplastic and non-neoplastic polyps of the right colon can be distinguished with a high sensitivity (91%) but low specificity (62%).[77]

Digital Chromoendoscopy

Digital chromoendoscopy has the advantage over dye-based chromoendoscopy in that the optical enhancement mode can be simply switched on or off with a button and no procedure-prolonging dye application is required. NBI was shown to be superior over HD colonoscopy in differentiating non-neoplastic and neoplastic lesions.[83] Differences in the microvascular capillary pattern were shown to be particularly helpful for predicting polyp histology.[84] This finding was further elaborated in the NBI International Colorectal Endoscopic classification. Both surface color and vessel surface structure of diminutive colorectal polyps predicted polyp histology with a high sensitivity (98%), NPV (95%), and accuracy (89%).[85] Focusing on diminutive polyps, Rastogi and colleagues[86] predicted neoplastic polyps with a sensitivity, specificity, and accuracy of 95%, 88%, and 92% with NBI and only 33%, 97%, and 61% with HD colonoscopy. Correct surveillance guidelines for polyps less than 10 mm were given in 95% to 98% only based on NBI, meeting the PIVI criteria.[18] In the most recent meta-analysis of 28 studies, NBI differentiated between neoplastic and non-neoplastic lesions with a sensitivity, specificity, and NPV of 91.0%, 82.6%, and 90.0%, again meeting the PIVI criteria.[87]

Similarly, iScan was shown to predict histology with an accuracy, sensitivity, and specificity of 86.3% to 98.6%, 78.0%, and 93.0% respectively.[41,42] Two prospective studies compared HD colonoscopy with iScan. Hong and colleagues[43] showed significantly improved accuracy, sensitivity, and specificity distinguishing neoplastic from non-neoplastic colorectal lesions with iScan (79.3% vs 75.0%, 86.5% vs 72.6%, and 91.4% vs 80.6%). In contrast, no significant difference was reported by Basford and colleagues[88] for neoplastic and non-neoplastic polyps less than 10 mm (accuracy 93.3% vs 94.7%, sensitivity 95.5% vs 97.0%, specificity 89.3% vs 90.7%, NPV for adenoma 100% and 100%). Similarly, no significant differences between NBI and iScan were reported (sensitivity 88.8% vs 94.6%; specificity 86.8% vs 86.4%; accuracy 87.8% vs 90.7%).[89]

FICE also showed high sensitivity of 93%, positive predictive value (PPV) of 89%, and NPV of 85% in distinguishing neoplastic from non-neoplastic colorectal lesions.[90] Compared with white light colonoscopy, FICE had higher sensitivity, specificity, and accuracy in distinguishing neoplastic and non-neoplastic colorectal polyps (90% vs 97%, 74% vs 80%, and 83% vs 90%).[91] However, no significant differences were found between FICE and dye-based chromoendoscopy, yielding accuracy, sensitivity, specificity, PPV, and NPV of 87.0% to 92.7%, 93%, 61.2% to 70.0%, 90%, and 76%, respectively.[47,92] Focusing on diminutive polyps, Longcroft-Wheaton and colleagues[93] also showed no significant difference between FICE and dye-based chromoendoscopy in distinguishing neoplastic from non-neoplastic lesions.

In summary, most studies that addressed the in vivo prediction of polyp histology with digital chromoendoscopy showed consistently high accuracy, sensitivity, specificity, PPV, and NPV, which met the PIVI criteria. However, none of these techniques are endorsed at this point by the Gastroenterology Societies guidelines as alternatives for histopathology. A substantial limitation of all advanced imaging studies is that they originate from experts in endoscopy. It remains unanswered whether the data can be generalized to community practices, which represent the largest proportion of screening and surveillance colonoscopies in the United States.

Real-Time Optical Prediction of Polyp Histology in Inflammatory Bowel Disease

Digital chromoendoscopy was evaluated to predict neoplastic lesions in IBD. In contrast to chromoendoscopy in average-risk patients, multiple studies proved that NBI, which was the main studied digital chromoendoscopy technique, insufficiently distinguished neoplastic from non-neoplastic lesions in patients with IBD, with sensitivity, specificity, and accuracy ranging only between 75% and 76%, 66% and 81%, and 67% and 80%, respectively.[94,95] Therefore, NBI is not recommended to predict polyp histology in vivo in IBD; histopathology remains the standard of care.

GASTROENTEROLOGY SOCIETY'S GUIDELINES AND ENDORSEMENT OF CHROMOENDOSCOPY

Chromoendoscopy has no relevance in the current guidelines from the Gastroenterology Societies for screening colonoscopy of average-risk patients. However, it is conceivable that, in the future, advanced imaging will play a role in distinguishing neoplastic from non-neoplastic polyps, once the resect-and-discard strategy of diminutive colorectal polyps gains acceptance.

As of now, chromoendoscopy is an accepted and often preferred screening and surveillance tool in patients with IBD. All major society guidelines (American Gastroenterological Association [AGA], American College of Gastroenterology [ACG], ASGE, European Crohn's and Colitis Organization [ECCO], British Society of Gastroenterology [BSG], Crohn's and Colitis Foundation of America [CCFA]) agree that surveillance is indicated during clinical remission of IBD, although differences exist in terms of timing for the first screening colonoscopy as well as surveillance intervals.

European guidelines (ECCO, BSG) endorse chromoendoscopy with targeted biopsies in IBD surveillance as the procedure of choice.[74,96,97] However, the experts acknowledge that chromoendoscopy requires sufficient expertise, which, when not available, makes random biopsies inevitable.

The North American society guidelines are less clear-cut. Both the ASGE and AGA refer to chromoendoscopy as only a reasonable alternative to standard colonoscopy with random biopsies in IBD surveillance.[67,98] The CCFA still endorses random 4-quadrant biopsies; however, chromoendoscopy is accepted as an alternative surveillance protocol for appropriately trained endoscopists. Of note, the CCFA's recommendations have not been updated since 2005.[99] Only the ACG states that generalized guidelines for chromoendoscopy in IBD are premature. They stated that chromoendoscopy might be of value for follow-up of high-risk patients with known or indefinite dysplasia who do not undergo colectomy; however, they cited the lack of data regarding benefit, especially in low-risk patients with IBD.[69]

Recommendations on digital chromoendoscopy are only incorporated in European guidelines. Neither the ECCO nor the BSG recommend NBI, FICE, and iScan as alternatives for chromoendoscopy.

SUMMARY RECOMMENDATION

Chromoendoscopy techniques are useful in the detection of colonic neoplasia in both average- and high-risk populations, including those with colonic IBD. Several studies demonstrated that dye-based chromoendoscopy, in contrast to HD colonoscopy and digital chromoendoscopy, increases not only the ADR but also the total number of adenomas per patient; however, the significance in terms of decreased interval CRC rate remains unclear.

There are convincing data to support that, in experienced hands, differentiation of neoplastic from non-neoplastic polyps, especially diminutive polyps, is possible with both dye-based and digital chromoendoscopy, meeting the ASGE's PIVI criteria. Because it is not clear whether this expertise can be translated into general practice, endoscopic determination of polyp histology is not endorsed by the current Gastroenterology Societies guidelines.

The strongest evidence exists for dye-based chromoendoscopy in IBD surveillance, replacing random biopsies as the preferred option. Digital chromoendoscopy was not shown to be of benefit for IBD surveillance. Lastly, neither dye-based nor digital chromoendoscopy can be reliably used to distinguish neoplastic from non-neoplastic lesions in IBD.

REFERENCES

1. Winawer SJ, Zauber AG, Ho MN, et al. Prevention of colorectal cancer by colonoscopic polypectomy. The National Polyp Study Workgroup. N Engl J Med 1993;329(27):1977–81.
2. Zauber AG, Winawer SJ, O'Brien MJ, et al. Colonoscopic polypectomy and long-term prevention of colorectal-cancer deaths. N Engl J Med 2012;366(8):687–96.
3. Bressler B, Paszat LF, Chen Z, et al. Rates of new or missed colorectal cancers after colonoscopy and their risk factors: a population-based analysis. Gastroenterology 2007;132(1):96–102.
4. Pohl H, Robertson DJ. Colorectal cancers detected after colonoscopy frequently result from missed lesions. Clin Gastroenterol Hepatol 2010;8(10): 858–64.
5. Rex DK, Cutler CS, Lemmel GT, et al. Colonoscopic miss rates of adenomas determined by back-to-back colonoscopies. Gastroenterology 1997;112(1):24–8.
6. van Rijn JC, Reitsma JB, Stoker J, et al. Polyp miss rate determined by tandem colonoscopy: a systematic review. Am J Gastroenterol 2006;101(2):343–50.
7. Harewood GC, Sharma VK, de Garmo P. Impact of colonoscopy preparation quality on detection of suspected colonic neoplasia. Gastrointest Endosc 2003;58(1):76–9.

8. Heresbach D, Barrioz T, Lapalus MG, et al. Miss rate for colorectal neoplastic polyps: a prospective multicenter study of back-to-back video colonoscopies. Endoscopy 2008;40(4):284–90.

9. Pickhardt PJ, Nugent PA, Mysliwiec PA, et al. Location of adenomas missed by optical colonoscopy. Ann Intern Med 2004;141(5):352–9.

10. Pohl J, Schneider A, Vogell H, et al. Pancolonic chromoendoscopy with indigo carmine versus standard colonoscopy for detection of neoplastic lesions: a randomised two-centre trial. Gut 2011;60(4):485–90.

11. Bianco MA, Cipolletta L, Rotondano G, et al. Prevalence of nonpolypoid colorectal neoplasia: an Italian multicenter observational study. Endoscopy 2010; 42(4):279–85.

12. Soetikno RM, Kaltenbach T, Rouse RV, et al. Prevalence of nonpolypoid (flat and depressed) colorectal neoplasms in asymptomatic and symptomatic adults. JAMA 2008;299(9):1027–35.

13. Bouwens MW, van Herwaarden YJ, Winkens B, et al. Endoscopic characterization of sessile serrated adenomas/polyps with and without dysplasia. Endoscopy 2014;46(3):225–35.

14. Kaminski MF, Regula J, Kraszewska E, et al. Quality indicators for colonoscopy and the risk of interval cancer. N Engl J Med 2010;362(19):1795–803.

15. Corley DA, Jensen CD, Marks AR, et al. Adenoma detection rate and risk of colorectal cancer and death. N Engl J Med 2014;370(14):1298–306.

16. Subramanian V, Mannath J, Hawkey CJ, et al. High definition colonoscopy vs. standard video endoscopy for the detection of colonic polyps: a meta-analysis. Endoscopy 2011;43(6):499–505.

17. East JE, Stavrindis M, Thomas-Gibson S, et al. A comparative study of standard vs. high definition colonoscopy for adenoma and hyperplastic polyp detection with optimized withdrawal technique. Aliment Pharmacol Ther 2008;28(6): 768–76.

18. Ignjatovic A, East JE, Suzuki N, et al. Optical diagnosis of small colorectal polyps at routine colonoscopy (Detect InSpect ChAracterise Resect and Discard; DISCARD trial): a prospective cohort study. Lancet Oncol 2009; 10(12):1171–8.

19. Canto MI. Staining in gastrointestinal endoscopy: the basics. Endoscopy 1999; 31(6):479–86.

20. Kudo S, Tamura S, Nakajima T, et al. Diagnosis of colorectal tumorous lesions by magnifying endoscopy. Gastrointest Endosc 1996;44(1):8–14.

21. Olliver JR, Wild CP, Sahay P, et al. Chromoendoscopy with methylene blue and associated DNA damage in Barrett's oesophagus. Lancet 2003;362(9381): 373–4.

22. Leong RW, Butcher RO, Picco MF. Implementation of image-enhanced endoscopy into solo and group practices for dysplasia detection in Crohn's disease and ulcerative colitis. Gastrointest Endosc Clin N Am 2014;24(3):419–25.

23. Subramanian V, Bisschops R. Image-enhanced endoscopy is critical in the surveillance of patients with colonic IBD. Gastrointest Endosc Clin N Am 2014;24(3):393–403.

24. Kiesslich R, Neurath MF. Chromoendoscopy in inflammatory bowel disease. Gastroenterol Clin North Am 2012;41(2):291–302.

25. Picco MF, Pasha S, Leighton JA, et al. Procedure time and the determination of polypoid abnormalities with experience: implementation of a chromoendoscopy program for surveillance colonoscopy for ulcerative colitis. Inflamm Bowel Dis 2013;19(9):1913–20.

26. Repici A, Di Stefano AF, Radicioni MM, et al. Methylene blue MMX tablets for chromoendoscopy. Safety tolerability and bioavailability in healthy volunteers. Contemp Clin Trials 2012;33(2):260–7.
27. Kiesslich R, Neurath MF. Surveillance colonoscopy in ulcerative colitis: magnifying chromoendoscopy in the spotlight. Gut 2004;53(2):165–7.
28. Emura F, Saito Y, Ikematsu H. Narrow-band imaging optical chromocolonoscopy: advantages and limitations. World J Gastroenterol 2008;14(31): 4867–72.
29. Brooker JC, Saunders BP, Shah SG, et al. Total colonic dye-spray increases the detection of diminutive adenomas during routine colonoscopy: a randomized controlled trial. Gastrointest Endosc 2002;56(3):333–8.
30. Le Rhun M, Coron E, Parlier D, et al. High resolution colonoscopy with chromoscopy versus standard colonoscopy for the detection of colonic neoplasia: a randomized study. Clin Gastroenterol Hepatol 2006;4(3):349–54.
31. Hurlstone DP, Cross SS, Slater R, et al. Detecting diminutive colorectal lesions at colonoscopy: a randomised controlled trial of pan-colonic versus targeted chromoscopy. Gut 2004;53(3):376–80.
32. Brown SR, Baraza W. Chromoscopy versus conventional endoscopy for the detection of polyps in the colon and rectum. Cochrane Database Syst Rev 2010;(10):CD006439.
33. Kahi CJ, Anderson JC, Waxman I, et al. High-definition chromocolonoscopy vs. high-definition white light colonoscopy for average-risk colorectal cancer screening. Am J Gastroenterol 2010;105(6):1301–7.
34. van den Broek FJ, Reitsma JB, Curvers WL, et al. Systematic review of narrow-band imaging for the detection and differentiation of neoplastic and nonneoplastic lesions in the colon (with videos). Gastrointest Endosc 2009; 69(1):124–35.
35. Rex DK, Helbig CC. High yields of small and flat adenomas with high-definition colonoscopes using either white light or narrow band imaging. Gastroenterology 2007;133(1):42–7.
36. Dinesen L, Chua TJ, Kaffes AJ. Meta-analysis of narrow-band imaging versus conventional colonoscopy for adenoma detection. Gastrointest Endosc 2012; 75(3):604–11.
37. Inoue T, Murano M, Murano N, et al. Comparative study of conventional colonoscopy and pan-colonic narrow-band imaging system in the detection of neoplastic colonic polyps: a randomized, controlled trial. J Gastroenterol 2008;43(1):45–50.
38. Adler A, Pohl H, Papanikolaou IS, et al. A prospective randomised study on narrow-band imaging versus conventional colonoscopy for adenoma detection: does narrow-band imaging induce a learning effect? Gut 2008;57(1):59–64.
39. Paggi S, Radaelli F, Amato A, et al. The impact of narrow band imaging in screening colonoscopy: a randomized controlled trial. Clin Gastroenterol Hepatol 2009;7(10):1049–54.
40. Pasha SF, Leighton JA, Das A, et al. Comparison of the yield and miss rate of narrow band imaging and white light endoscopy in patients undergoing screening or surveillance colonoscopy: a meta-analysis. Am J Gastroenterol 2012;107(3):363–70 [quiz: 371].
41. Hoffman A, Sar F, Goetz M, et al. High definition colonoscopy combined with i-Scan is superior in the detection of colorectal neoplasias compared with standard video colonoscopy: a prospective randomized controlled trial. Endoscopy 2010;42(10):827–33.

42. Hoffman A, Loth L, Rey JW, et al. High definition plus colonoscopy combined with i-scan tone enhancement vs. high definition colonoscopy for colorectal neoplasia: a randomized trial. Dig Liver Dis 2014;46(11):991–6.

43. Hong SN, Choe WH, Lee JH, et al. Prospective, randomized, back-to-back trial evaluating the usefulness of i-SCAN in screening colonoscopy. Gastrointest Endosc 2012;75(5):1011–21.e2.

44. Hoffman A, Kagel C, Goetz M, et al. Recognition and characterization of small colonic neoplasia with high-definition colonoscopy using i-Scan is as precise as chromoendoscopy. Dig Liver Dis 2010;42(1):45–50.

45. Chung SJ, Kim D, Song JH, et al. Efficacy of computed virtual chromoendoscopy on colorectal cancer screening: a prospective, randomized, back-to-back trial of Fuji Intelligent Color Enhancement versus conventional colonoscopy to compare adenoma miss rates. Gastrointest Endosc 2010;72(1):136–42.

46. Aminalai A, Rosch T, Aschenbeck J, et al. Live image processing does not increase adenoma detection rate during colonoscopy: a randomized comparison between FICE and conventional imaging (Berlin Colonoscopy Project 5, BECOP-5). Am J Gastroenterol 2010;105(11):2383–8.

47. Pohl J, Lotterer E, Balzer C, et al. Computed virtual chromoendoscopy versus standard colonoscopy with targeted indigo carmine chromoscopy: a randomised multicentre trial. Gut 2009;58(1):73–8.

48. Ekbom A, Helmick C, Zack M, et al. Ulcerative colitis and colorectal cancer. A population-based study. N Engl J Med 1990;323(18):1228–33.

49. Rutter MD, Saunders BP, Wilkinson KH, et al. Thirty-year analysis of a colonoscopic surveillance program for neoplasia in ulcerative colitis. Gastroenterology 2006;130(4):1030–8.

50. Canavan C, Abrams KR, Mayberry J. Meta-analysis: colorectal and small bowel cancer risk in patients with Crohn's disease. Aliment Pharmacol Ther 2006; 23(8):1097–104.

51. Collins PD, Mpofu C, Watson AJ, et al. Strategies for detecting colon cancer and/or dysplasia in patients with inflammatory bowel disease. Cochrane Database Syst Rev 2006;(2):CD000279.

52. Rubin CE, Haggitt RC, Burmer GC, et al. DNA aneuploidy in colonic biopsies predicts future development of dysplasia in ulcerative colitis. Gastroenterology 1992;103(5):1611–20.

53. Blonski W, Kundu R, Lewis J, et al. Is dysplasia visible during surveillance colonoscopy in patients with ulcerative colitis? Scand J Gastroenterol 2008;43(6): 698–703.

54. Rubin DT, Rothe JA, Hetzel JT, et al. Are dysplasia and colorectal cancer endoscopically visible in patients with ulcerative colitis? Gastrointest Endosc 2007; 65(7):998–1004.

55. Rutter MD, Saunders BP, Schofield G, et al. Pancolonic indigo carmine dye spraying for the detection of dysplasia in ulcerative colitis. Gut 2004;53(2): 256–60.

56. Marion JF, Waye JD, Present DH, et al. Chromoendoscopy-targeted biopsies are superior to standard colonoscopic surveillance for detecting dysplasia in inflammatory bowel disease patients: a prospective endoscopic trial. Am J Gastroenterol 2008;103(9):2342–9.

57. van den Broek FJ, Stokkers PC, Reitsma JB, et al. Random biopsies taken during colonoscopic surveillance of patients with longstanding ulcerative colitis: low yield and absence of clinical consequences. Am J Gastroenterol 2014; 109(5):715–22.

58. Hurlstone DP, Sanders DS, Lobo AJ, et al. Indigo carmine-assisted high-magnification chromoscopic colonoscopy for the detection and characterisation of intraepithelial neoplasia in ulcerative colitis: a prospective evaluation. Endoscopy 2005;37(12):1186–92.

59. Kiesslich R, Fritsch J, Holtmann M, et al. Methylene blue-aided chromoendoscopy for the detection of intraepithelial neoplasia and colon cancer in ulcerative colitis. Gastroenterology 2003;124(4):880–8.

60. Subramanian V, Mannath J, Ragunath K, et al. Meta-analysis: the diagnostic yield of chromoendoscopy for detecting dysplasia in patients with colonic inflammatory bowel disease. Aliment Pharmacol Ther 2011;33(3):304–12.

61. Soetikno R, Subramanian V, Kaltenbach T, et al. The detection of nonpolypoid (flat and depressed) colorectal neoplasms in patients with inflammatory bowel disease. Gastroenterology 2013;144(7):1349–52, 1352.e1–6.

62. Wu L, Li P, Wu J, et al. The diagnostic accuracy of chromoendoscopy for dysplasia in ulcerative colitis: meta-analysis of six randomized controlled trials. Colorectal Dis 2012;14(4):416–20.

63. Ignjatovic A, East JE, Subramanian V, et al. Narrow band imaging for detection of dysplasia in colitis: a randomized controlled trial. Am J Gastroenterol 2012; 107(6):885–90.

64. Dekker E, van den Broek FJ, Reitsma JB, et al. Narrow-band imaging compared with conventional colonoscopy for the detection of dysplasia in patients with longstanding ulcerative colitis. Endoscopy 2007;39(3):216–21.

65. Pellise M, Lopez-Ceron M, Rodriguez de Miguel C, et al. Narrow-band imaging as an alternative to chromoendoscopy for the detection of dysplasia in long-standing inflammatory bowel disease: a prospective, randomized, crossover study. Gastrointest Endosc 2011;74(4):840–8.

66. Ullman T, Odze R, Farraye FA. Diagnosis and management of dysplasia in patients with ulcerative colitis and Crohn's disease of the colon. Inflamm Bowel Dis 2009;15(4):630–8.

67. Farraye FA, Odze RD, Eaden J, et al. AGA technical review on the diagnosis and management of colorectal neoplasia in inflammatory bowel disease. Gastroenterology 2010;138(2):746–74, 774.e1–4; [quiz: e12–3].

68. Bernstein CN. ALMs versus DALMs in ulcerative colitis: polypectomy or colectomy? Gastroenterology 1999;117(6):1488–92.

69. Kornbluth A, Sachar DB. Ulcerative colitis practice guidelines in adults: American College Of Gastroenterology, Practice Parameters Committee. Am J Gastroenterol 2010;105(3):501–23 [quiz: 524].

70. Murthy SK, Kiesslich R. Evolving endoscopic strategies for detection and treatment of neoplastic lesions in inflammatory bowel disease. Gastrointest Endosc 2013;77(3):351–9.

71. Engelsgjerd M, Farraye FA, Odze RD. Polypectomy may be adequate treatment for adenoma-like dysplastic lesions in chronic ulcerative colitis. Gastroenterology 1999;117(6):1288–94 [discussion: 1488–91].

72. Rubin PH, Friedman S, Harpaz N, et al. Colonoscopic polypectomy in chronic colitis: conservative management after endoscopic resection of dysplastic polyps. Gastroenterology 1999;117(6):1295–300.

73. Rutter MD, Saunders BP, Wilkinson KH, et al. Most dysplasia in ulcerative colitis is visible at colonoscopy. Gastrointest Endosc 2004;60(3):334–9.

74. Cairns SR, Scholefield JH, Steele RJ, et al. Guidelines for colorectal cancer screening and surveillance in moderate and high risk groups (update from 2002). Gut 2010;59(5):666–89.

75. Rex DK, Kahi C, O'Brien M, et al. The American Society for Gastrointestinal Endoscopy PIVI (Preservation and Incorporation of Valuable Endoscopic Innovations) on real-time endoscopic assessment of the histology of diminutive colorectal polyps. Gastrointest Endosc 2011;73(3):419–22.

76. Kato S, Fujii T, Koba I, et al. Assessment of colorectal lesions using magnifying colonoscopy and mucosal dye spraying: can significant lesions be distinguished? Endoscopy 2001;33(4):306–10.

77. Eisen GM, Kim CY, Fleischer DE, et al. High-resolution chromoendoscopy for classifying colonic polyps: a multicenter study. Gastrointest Endosc 2002; 55(6):687–94.

78. Kato S, Fu KI, Sano Y, et al. Magnifying colonoscopy as a non-biopsy technique for differential diagnosis of non-neoplastic and neoplastic lesions. World J Gastroenterol 2006;12(9):1416–20.

79. De Palma GD, Rega M, Masone S, et al. Conventional colonoscopy and magnified chromoendoscopy for the endoscopic histological prediction of diminutive colorectal polyps: a single operator study. World J Gastroenterol 2006;12(15):2402–5.

80. Brown SR, Baraza W, Hurlstone P. Chromoscopy versus conventional endoscopy for the detection of polyps in the colon and rectum. Cochrane Database Syst Rev 2007;(4):CD006439.

81. Fu KI, Sano Y, Kato S, et al. Chromoendoscopy using indigo carmine dye spraying with magnifying observation is the most reliable method for differential diagnosis between non-neoplastic and neoplastic colorectal lesions: a prospective study. Endoscopy 2004;36(12):1089–93.

82. Kiesslich R, von Bergh M, Hahn M, et al. Chromoendoscopy with indigo carmine improves the detection of adenomatous and nonadenomatous lesions in the colon. Endoscopy 2001;33(12):1001–6.

83. Rex DK. Narrow-band imaging without optical magnification for histologic analysis of colorectal polyps. Gastroenterology 2009;136(4):1174–81.

84. Katagiri A, Fu KI, Sano Y, et al. Narrow band imaging with magnifying colonoscopy as diagnostic tool for predicting histology of early colorectal neoplasia. Aliment Pharmacol Ther 2008;27(12):1269–74.

85. Hewett DG, Kaltenbach T, Sano Y, et al. Validation of a simple classification system for endoscopic diagnosis of small colorectal polyps using narrow-band imaging. Gastroenterology 2012;143(3):599–607.e1.

86. Rastogi A, Keighley J, Singh V, et al. High accuracy of narrow band imaging without magnification for the real-time characterization of polyp histology and its comparison with high-definition white light colonoscopy: a prospective study. Am J Gastroenterol 2009;104(10):2422–30.

87. McGill SK, Evangelou E, Ioannidis JP, et al. Narrow band imaging to differentiate neoplastic and non-neoplastic colorectal polyps in real time: a meta-analysis of diagnostic operating characteristics. Gut 2013;62(12):1704–13.

88. Basford PJ, Longcroft-Wheaton G, Higgins B, et al. High-definition endoscopy with i-Scan for evaluation of small colon polyps: the HiSCOPE study. Gastrointest Endosc 2014;79(1):111–8.

89. Lee CK, Lee SH, Hwangbo Y. Narrow-band imaging versus I-Scan for the real-time histological prediction of diminutive colonic polyps: a prospective comparative study by using the simple unified endoscopic classification. Gastrointest Endosc 2011;74(3):603–9.

90. Longcroft-Wheaton G, Brown J, Cowlishaw D, et al. High-definition vs. standard-definition colonoscopy in the characterization of small colonic polyps: results from a randomized trial. Endoscopy 2012;44(10):905–10.

91. Pohl J, Nguyen-Tat M, Pech O, et al. Computed virtual chromoendoscopy for classification of small colorectal lesions: a prospective comparative study. Am J Gastroenterol 2008;103(3):562–9.

92. Togashi K, Osawa H, Koinuma K, et al. A comparison of conventional endoscopy, chromoendoscopy, and the optimal-band imaging system for the differentiation of neoplastic and non-neoplastic colonic polyps. Gastrointest Endosc 2009;69(3 Pt 2):734–41.

93. Longcroft-Wheaton GR, Higgins B, Bhandari P. Flexible spectral imaging color enhancement and indigo carmine in neoplasia diagnosis during colonoscopy: a large prospective UK series. Eur J Gastroenterol Hepatol 2011;23(10): 903–11.

94. van den Broek FJ, Fockens P, van Eeden S, et al. Endoscopic tri-modal imaging for surveillance in ulcerative colitis: randomised comparison of high-resolution endoscopy and autofluorescence imaging for neoplasia detection; and evaluation of narrow-band imaging for classification of lesions. Gut 2008;57(8): 1083–9.

95. van den Broek FJ, Fockens P, van Eeden S, et al. Narrow-band imaging versus high-definition endoscopy for the diagnosis of neoplasia in ulcerative colitis. Endoscopy 2011;43(2):108–15.

96. Annese V, Daperno M, Rutter MD, et al. European evidence based consensus for endoscopy in inflammatory bowel disease. J Crohns Colitis 2013;7(12): 982–1018.

97. Van Assche G, Dignass A, Bokemeyer B, et al. Second European evidence-based consensus on the diagnosis and management of ulcerative colitis part 3: special situations. J Crohns Colitis 2013;7(1):1–33.

98. Sharaf RN, Shergill AK, Odze RD, et al. Endoscopic mucosal tissue sampling. Gastrointest Endosc 2013;78(2):216–24.

99. Itzkowitz SH, Present DH. Consensus conference: colorectal cancer screening and surveillance in inflammatory bowel disease. Inflamm Bowel Dis 2005;11(3): 314–21.

100. Thorlacius H, Toth E. Role of chromoendoscopy in colon cancer surveillance in inflammatory bowel disease. Inflamm Bowel Dis 2007;13(7):911–7.

Tools for Polyp Histology Prediction

Shreyas Saligram, MD, MRCP[a,b], Amit Rastogi, MD[a,b],*

KEYWORDS

- Colonoscopy • Advanced imaging • Polyp histology prediction • Adenoma
- Hyperplastic polyps • Electronic chromoendoscopy

KEY POINTS

- Real-time polyp histology prediction during colonoscopy is feasible and can result in significant cost savings.
- Several imaging technologies have been studied and most have shown good accuracy in polyp histology prediction.
- Electronic chromoendoscopy is a practical and easy to use technology that is accurate for real-time histology prediction of polyps.

INTRODUCTION

Colonoscopy is the favored modality for screening and prevention of colorectal cancer in the United States. Removal of adenomatous polyps during colonoscopy can prevent the development of colorectal cancer, because most cancers arise from adenomatous polyps following the adenoma-carcinoma pathway.[1,2] Another type of colon polyp are hyperplastic polyps,[3,4] which are in general not considered to be premalignant, especially those present in the distal colon and 5 mm or less in size.[5] Most polyps (>80%) detected during colonoscopy are diminutive (ie, ≤5 mm). Current practice is to remove all polyps detected during colonoscopy, irrespective of their size, and send them to pathology for evaluation. Because diminutive polyps rarely harbor any advanced histology, such as high-grade dysplasia or cancer,[6] histopathologic evaluation of these lesions determines whether they are adenomatous, which then dictates the postpolypectomy surveillance intervals. This practice entails a huge cost burden to the health care system, with limited clinical benefits in return. If the histology of diminutive polyps can be predicted real-time during colonoscopy by the endoscopist, then the cost of histology can potentially be avoided ("resect and discard").

Conflicts of Interest: Research grant support and Consultant from Olympus America (A. Rastogi). No conflict of Interest (S. Saligram).

[a] University of Kansas School of Medicine, University of Kansas, Department of Gastroenterology, 3901 Rainbow Blvd, Kansas City, KS 66160, USA; [b] Veterans Affairs Medical Center, Department of Gastroenterology, 4801 Linwood Blvd, Kansas City, MO 64128, USA
* Corresponding author. University of Kansas, Kansas City, KS 66160.
E-mail address: arastogi@kumc.edu

Gastrointest Endoscopy Clin N Am 25 (2015) 261–286
http://dx.doi.org/10.1016/j.giec.2014.11.009
1052-5157/15/$ – see front matter Published by Elsevier Inc.

giendo.theclinics.com

Moreover, although histopathologic diagnosis is considered the gold standard, another advantage of predicting polyp histology relates to diminutive hyperplastic polyps. Because these are not considered to have malignant potential, their removal and routine pathologic evaluation are seemingly wasteful and time-consuming endeavors. If these can be accurately characterized during colonoscopy, then they can potentially be left behind ("do not resect"), thereby saving further costs and also decreasing the risks associated with polypectomy. Cost-savings estimates of the "predict, resect, and discard" strategy have ranged from $33 million to $1 billion annually in the United States.[7,8]

Several novel imaging modalities have been developed during the past decade that have expanded the scope of colonoscopy and enabled the endoscopist to predict polyp histology. These imaging systems can be broadly divided into large-field and small-field technologies depending on the area of mucosa that is imaged. Large-field technologies include high-definition white light, chromoendoscopy, electronic chromoendoscopy, and autofluorescence. Small-field technologies include confocal endomicroscopy and endocytoscopy. This article reviews each technology as it relates to predicting polyp histology.

HIGH-DEFINITION WHITE LIGHT ENDOSCOPY
Technology

The older-generation white light endoscopy used a charge-coupled device (CCD) chip with an average of 300,000 pixels. Over the past decade, technology has evolved, with advancements in miniaturization and a specialized design of the CCD chip. CCD chips now have a 3-fold higher pixel density than standard-definition white light endoscopy (ie, >1 million pixels). This resolution, along with a high-definition video processor and a high-definition monitor, produces a high-definition image with 1080 effective scan lines.[9,10] Although some data suggest that high-definition white light (HD-WL) endoscopy may improve the adenoma detection rate, this improvement in technology has not had a significant impact on the ability to characterize the histology of polyps.

Performance

A randomized controlled study reported no difference in the performance between standard-definition and HD-WL endoscopy in characterizing the histology of 293 consecutive polyps smaller than 10 mm, as measured by sensitivity (76% vs 76%; $P = .96$), specificity (59% vs 67%; $P = .44$), and accuracy (70% vs 73%; $P = .6$).[10] Another prospective, randomized controlled trial showed slightly superior accuracy of HD-WL compared with standard-definition endoscopy in predicting adenomatous polyps (73.2% versus 68.5%, $P<.0001$).[11] A third prospective study compared HD-WL endoscopy and narrow band imaging (NBI) in the prediction of histology of 236 polyps in 100 patients. HD-WL endoscopy had a significantly lower sensitivity (38% vs 96%; $P<.0001$) and lower accuracy (61% vs 93%; $P<.0001$) than NBI in distinguishing adenomas from hyperplastic polyps.[12]

CHROMOENDOSCOPY
Technique

Chromoendoscopy involves the spraying of dyes, such as methylene blue, cresyl violet, and indigo carmine, using a spray catheter.[13,14] Methylene blue and cresyl violet stain the surface of a lesion by being actively absorbed and interacting with cell constituents. Contrast dyes such as indigo carmine are not absorbed by the mucosa and pool in the pits and mucosal crevices on the surface of polyps. These dyes can highlight different patterns on the surface of polyps called *pit patterns*. These patterns were described by Kudo and colleagues[15] using magnification endoscopy and have been shown to accurately differentiate hyperplastic and adenomatous polyps (**Fig. 1, Table 1**).[16]

Performance

A prospective study of 122 patients evaluated 206 polyps less than 10 mm using conventional colonoscopy, chromoendoscopy with indigo carmine, and chromoendoscopy with indigo carmine and magnification. The predicted histology was compared with the gold standard (ie, histopathologic diagnosis of endoscopically resected polyps). The overall sensitivity, specificity, and accuracy for distinguishing between neoplastic and nonneoplastic lesions using conventional colonoscopy were 88.8%, 67.4%, and 84.0%, respectively, although these were 93.1%, 76.1%, and 89.3%, respectively, for chromoendoscopy without magnification, and 96.3%, 93.5%, and 95.6%, respectively, for chromoendoscopy with magnification. Chromoendoscopy using indigo carmine with magnification was significantly superior in distinguishing neoplastic from nonneoplastic lesions, compared with conventional colonoscopy ($P<.0001$) and chromoendoscopy without magnification ($P = .0152$).[17] However, another study in 141 patients evaluating 175 polyps, of which 161 were less than 10 mm, showed somewhat lower accuracy in histologic characterization using chromoendoscopy with magnification. The overall sensitivity, specificity, and diagnostic accuracy for distinguishing between neoplastic and nonneoplastic lesions were 93.8%, 64.6%, and 80.1%, respectively.[18] Several other studies using chromoendoscopy with magnification have shown diagnostic accuracies between 80% and 96% for distinguishing neoplastic from nonneoplastic lesions.[19–21]

Feasibility

Chromoendoscopy has not been adopted widely in the western countries because it is perceived to be labor-intensive, cumbersome, and messy. It also increases the duration and cost of the procedure because of the use of dye and spray catheter. Magnification endoscopes were used to describe the pit patterns by Kudo and colleagues,[15] and these are not available in the United States. In addition, concerns exist regarding in vitro data showing that methylene blue can cause single-strand DNA breaks in epithelial cells.[22]

ELECTRONIC CHROMOENDOSCOPY

This technology provides a visual contrast akin to chromoendoscopy, without the need to spray dye. There are 3 different platforms: NBI (Olympus; Tokyo, Japan), Fujinon Intelligent Color Enhancement (FICE; Fujinon, Inc., Wayne, NJ, USA), and i-Scan (Pentax; Tokyo, Japan).

NARROW BAND IMAGING
Technology

NBI is by far the most extensively studied of the 3 electronic chromoendoscopy systems. In white light endoscopy, the entire spectrum of visible light (400–700 nm) is used, and therefore the mucosa is seen in its natural color. NBI uses optical filter in the endoscopy system to transmit an increased proportion of blue light (415 nm) and a decreased proportion of red light.[23,24] It narrows the white light spectrum into 2 different wavelengths: blue (390–445 nm) and green (530–550 nm) light.[25] These wavelengths correspond to the maximum or peak absorption spectrum of

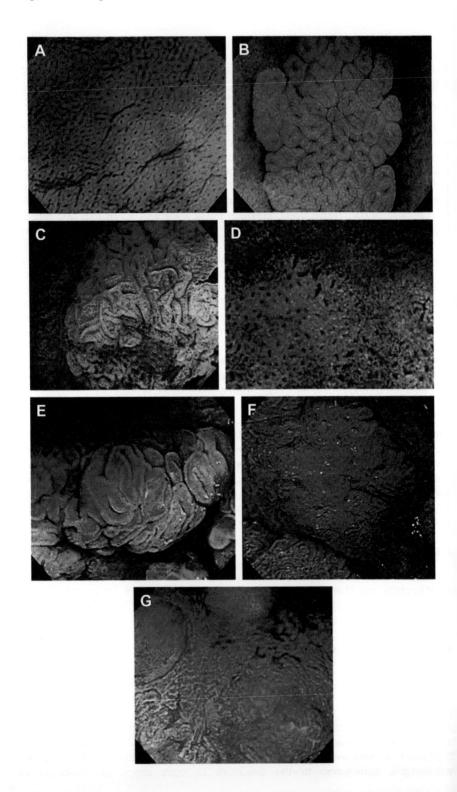

Table 1			
Kudo's classification of pit pattern for predicting histology using chromoendoscopy			
Type	Description	Most Likely Histology	Neoplastic/Nonneoplastic
I	Round crypts	Normal mucosa	Nonneoplastic
II	Regular wider or stellar crypts	Hyperplastic polyp	Nonneoplastic
III-L	Elongated or roundish crypts	Adenoma	Neoplastic
III-s	Tubular or roundish pits smaller than the normal crypts	Adenoma	Neoplastic
IV	Branch-like or gyrus-like crypts	Adenoma	Neoplastic
V-i	Irregular crypts	Superficial invasive/deep invasive cancer	Neoplastic
V-n	Non-structural crypts	Deep submucosal invasive cancer	Neoplastic

Adapted from Kudo S, Rubio CA, Teixeira CR, et al. Pit pattern in colorectal neoplasia: endoscopic magnifying view. Endoscopy 2001;33:371; with permission.

hemoglobin, which is the major tissue chromophore. Therefore, the vasculature appears dark. Also, blue light has a shorter wavelength and hence penetrates superficially compared with red light that has longer wavelength and penetrates deeper, which accentuates the mucosal architecture. These 2 principles combine to enhance superficial mucosal vasculature by optimizing absorbance and scattering of light. Because the vascular density and vascular patterns of adenomatous polyps are different from those of hyperplastic polyps, NBI can help distinguish them in real-time during colonoscopy.

Performance

Initial studies used the Kudo pit pattern to characterize polyp histology with NBI.[26,27] However, this extrapolation of the Kudo pit pattern to NBI was not believed to be reliable or accurate.[28] In one study, the agreement between the chromoendoscopic and NBI pit patterns was suboptimal, with a kappa of only 0.23.[28] Therefore, newer classifications have emerged, proposed by investigators from different parts of the world. East and colleagues[28] described the vascular pattern intensity classification with NBI. This system refers to the color intensity of the lines surrounding the mucosal pits on the surface of polyps on a 3-point scale. Strong vascular pattern intensity was suggestive of adenomas, and normal or weak pattern intensity was suggestive of hyperplastic polyps (**Fig. 2**, **Table 2**). Based on this classification, 116 polyps less than 10 mm in 62 patients were evaluated in a prospective study with NBI without magnification.[29] The

---

Fig. 1. Pit-pattern classification (A) The type I pit pattern of the normal mucosa consists of roundish pits, with a regular distribution. (B) The type II pit pattern consists of relatively large star-like or onion-like pits. (C) The type IIIL pit pattern is composed of tubular or roundish pits larger than normal ones. (D) The type III-s pit pattern is composed of tubular or roundish pits smaller than normal ones. (E) The type IV pit pattern is a branched or gyrus-like pattern. (F) The type V pit pattern is divided into VI and VN. The pit pattern VI ("I" for "irregular"), shown here, has pits, which are irregular in shape, size, and arrangement. (G) Type VN ("N" for "nonstructural") shows an absence of pit pattern. (*From* Kudo S, Rubio CA, Teixeira CR, et al. Pit pattern in colorectal neoplasia: endoscopic magnifying view. Endoscopy 2001;33:361; with permission.)

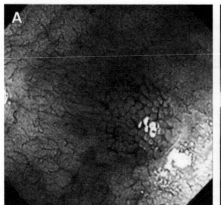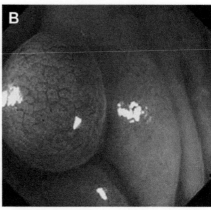

Fig. 2. (*A*) A 2-mm polyp with strong vascular pattern intensity. Histopathology showed it was an adenoma. (*B*) A 3-mm hyperplastic polyp showing weak pattern intensity. (*From* East JE, Suzuki N, Saunders BP. Comparison of magnified pit pattern interpretation with narrow band imaging vs chromoendoscopy for diminutive colonic polyps: a pilot study. Gastrointest Endosc 2007;66:311, 315; with permission.)

sensitivity, specificity, and accuracy were 94.0%, 89.0%, and 91.4%, respectively, in predicting histology. Similar results were seen for the subgroup analysis of diminutive (≤5 mm) polyps.[29] The authors' group described a simple classification system with NBI without magnification. Two patterns were described for hyperplastic polyps and 2 for adenomas (**Fig. 3, Table 3**).[30,31] These results showed a sensitivity, specificity, and accuracy of 96%, 89%, and 93%, respectively, for polyp histology prediction.[30] A similar classification was described by Rex[32] that showed an accuracy of 89% for characterizing adenomas. The meshed capillary pattern (CP) classification was proposed by investigators from Japan, using magnification NBI (**Fig. 4**).[33–35] CP I was suggestive of hyperplastic polyps, whereas CP II and CP III were diagnostic of adenomas. In a prospective study, the sensitivity, specificity, and accuracy for polyp histology prediction using this classification were 96.4%, 92.3%, and 95.3%, respectively. This Japanese classification was adapted for NBI without magnification in the United States, and showed a diagnostic accuracy of 91% with a sensitivity and negative predictive value of 93% and 91%, respectively. For lesions less than 5 mm, the sensitivity, negative predictive value, and accuracy were 87%, 91%, and 90%, respectively.[36] Another classification based on intensity and shape of small blood vessels on polyps was described from Europe.[37] A fine capillary pattern, with normal size and distribution of vessels, was characteristic of hyperplastic polyps, whereas adenomas showed an increased density, tortuous, corkscrew-type, and branching

Table 2
Classification based on microvascular density in predicting histology by narrow band imaging

	Nonneoplastic	Normal	Neoplastic
Vascular pattern	Weaker (paler) than the surrounding mucosa	The same as the surrounding mucosa	Stronger (darker) than the surrounding mucosa

Adapted from East JE, Suzuki N, Saunders BP. Comparison of magnified pit pattern interpretation with narrow band imaging versus chromoendoscopy for diminutive colonic polyps: a pilot study. Gastrointest Endosc 2007;66:312; with permission.

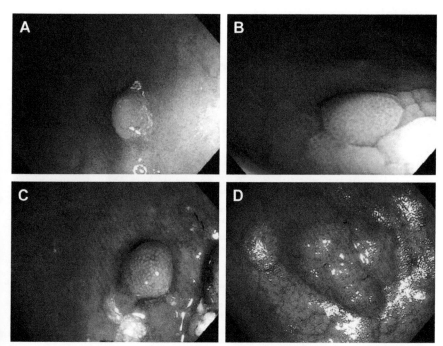

Fig. 3. (*A*) A 2-mm hyperplastic polyp showing fine capillary network but absent mucosal pattern (bland pattern). (*B*) A 4-mm hyperplastic polyp showing the circular pattern with dots. (*C*) A 4-mm adenoma showing the round or oval pattern. (*D*) A 6-mm adenoma showing the tubulogyrus pattern. (*From* Rastogi A. Optical diagnosis of small colorectal polyp histology with high-definition colonoscopy using narrow band imaging. Clin Endosc 2013;46(2):122; with permission.)

vascularization (**Fig. 5**). Using this classification on 200 polyps from 131 patients, NBI with and without magnification showed an accuracy of 91% and 89%, respectively, in differentiating neoplastic from nonneoplastic polyps.[37] Recently, a group of international experts unified various aspects of previously described NBI classifications and proposed and validated the NBI International Colorectal Endoscopic (NICE)

Table 3	
Surface mucosal and vascular pattern classification for predicting histology by narrow band imaging	
Histology	**Surface Mucosal and Vascular Pattern**
Hyperplastic	1. Circular pattern with dots: pattern with central dark dots surrounded by clear lighter area 2. Fine capillary network alone with absent mucosal pattern: bland appearance
Adenoma	1. Round/oval pattern: characterized by dark circular outline and a lighter central area 2. Tubulogyrus pattern: dark brown linear or convoluted tubular Structures

Adapted from Rastogi A, Bansal A, Wani S, et al. Narrow-band imaging colonoscopy: a pilot feasibility study for the detection of polyps and correlation of surface patterns with polyp histologic diagnosis. Gastrointest Endosc 2008;67:718; with permission.

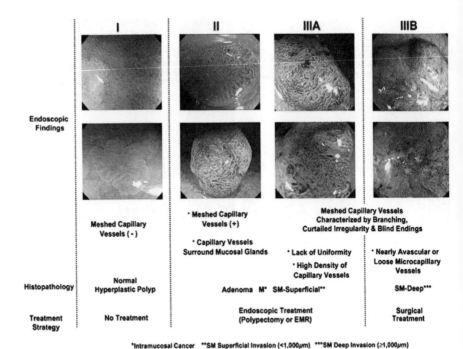

Fig. 4. Sano's capillary pattern classification (CP classification) of early colorectal lesions using NBI. EMR, endoscopic mucosal resection; M, mucosal; SM, submucosal. (*From* Uraoka T, Saito Y, Ikematsu H, et al. Sano's capillary pattern classification for narrow-band imaging of early colorectal lesions. Dig Endosc 2011;23(Suppl 1):113; with permission.)

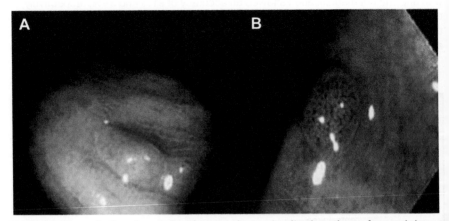

Fig. 5. (*A*) Hyperplastic polyp. Only a few vessels are visualized on the surface and do not show increased branching. (*B*) Polyp showing increased density of irregular, curved, and dilated blood vessels. Histologic examination showed adenoma. (*From* Tischendorf JJ, Schirin-Sokhan R, Streetz K, et al. Value of magnifying endoscopy in classifying colorectal polyps based on vascular pattern. Endoscopy 2010;42:24; with permission.)

classification to predict histology with NBI without magnification (**Fig. 6, Table 4**).[38] Using the NICE classification, 118 polyps less than 10 mm were evaluated. The sensitivity, negative predictive value, and accuracy for histology prediction were 98%, 95%, and 89%, respectively.[38]

A meta-analysis on real-time optical diagnosis of polyp histology by NBI included 35 studies and revealed encouraging results in distinguishing neoplastic and nonneoplastic polyps. The reported diagnostic performances were sensitivity, 91.5%; specificity, 85.2%; and negative predictive value, 82.5%. For the 5205 diminutive (<6 mm) polyps that were assessed, the sensitivity was 86.9% and specificity was 84.4%.[39] These results were similar to those of a previous meta-analysis of studies on NBI for differentiating neoplastic from nonneoplastic polyps in real-time that included 28 studies with 6280 polyps. The overall sensitivity was 91.0%, the specificity was 82.6%, and the negative predictive value exceeded 90%. When the diagnosis of diminutive polyps was made with high confidence, then the sensitivity was 93.4% and the specificity was 84.0%.[40]

Feasibility

NBI is a promising imaging technique for polyp histology prediction. It is hassle-free and easy to use, because it can be activated by the push of a button on the handle of the endoscope. Because it is incorporated in the newer and current generation of the Olympus endoscopy system, NBI will be associated with no added costs or extra capital investment once this system is acquired by an endoscopy unit.

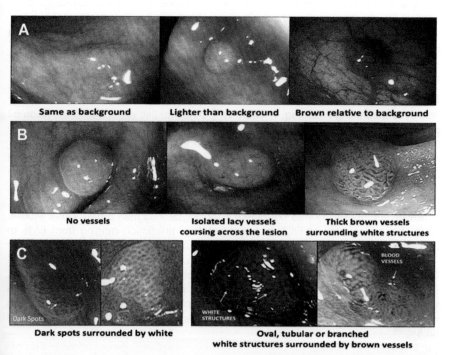

Fig. 6. Features of the Narrow-Band Imaging International Colorectal Endoscopic (NICE) criteria: (A) color, (B) vessels, and (C) surface pattern. (*From* Hewett DG, Kaltenbach T, Sano Y, et al. Validation of a simple classification system for endoscopic diagnosis of small colorectal polyps using narrow-band imaging. Gastroenterology 2012;143:607.e1; with permission.)

Table 4
Narrow band imaging classification of polyps based on international colorectal endoscopic classification

	Type 1	Type 2
Color	Same or lighter than background	Brown relative to background
Vessels	None or isolated lacy vessels	Brown vessels surrounding white structures
Surface pattern	Dark or white spots of uniform size or homogeneous absence of pattern	Oval, tubular, or branched white structures surrounded by brown vessels
Most likely histology	Hyperplastic polyp	Adenoma

From Hewett DG, Kaltenbach T, Sano Y, et al. Validation of a simple classification system for endoscopic diagnosis of small colorectal polyps using narrow-band imaging. Gastroenterology 2012;143:601; with permission.

Fujinon Intelligent Color Enhancement Technology

FICE uses a postprocessing technique in which the endoscopic image from the processor is altered by computerized spectral estimation technology. The reflected photons of the original image are arithmetically processed to reconstitute a virtual image. The system has 10 preprogrammed FICE settings using an optimal set of wavelengths that can be selected on the keyboard. Each one has a different setting for estimated red, green, and blue wavelength.[41] Image color varies as different wavelengths are applied (ie, shorter wavelengths for surface structures and longer for deeper vessels).[42,43] As a result, enhancement of the superficial mucosal vascular pattern on the polyp can be achieved, which can enable histology prediction.

Performance

An endoscopic capillary-vessel pattern classification for prediction of polyp histology was described using FICE (**Fig. 7**, **Table 5**).[43] Other studies extrapolated the Kudo pit pattern with chromoendoscopy to FICE, with types I and II suggestive of hyperplastic polyps and types III to V suggestive of adenomas.[44,45]

A randomized controlled study on 293 consecutive polyps[10] comparing FICE with standard colonoscopy reported better sensitivity (93% vs 83%; $P = .04$) but no difference in specificity (81% vs 82%; $P = .97$) or accuracy (89% vs 83%; $P = .13$) in distinguishing neoplastic and nonneoplastic polyps measuring less than 10 mm. However, the sensitivity was not different for polyps less than 5 mm. Other studies have shown accuracy of FICE in polyp histology prediction ranging from 85% to 98%.[44,46–48]

A recent meta-analysis included 14 studies with 4492 polyps that used FICE for distinguishing neoplastic from nonneoplastic polyps in real-time during colonoscopy. FICE showed a sensitivity of 92.5%, specificity of 85.1%, and negative predictive value of 83.7%. A subanalysis of the diagnostic performance of FICE from 4 studies with 937 diminutive polyps (<6 mm) showed a sensitivity of 83.6% and specificity of 86.5%.[39]

Feasibility

FICE is an easy-to-use technology that requires no extra cost or investment once the system has been acquired by an endoscopy unit.

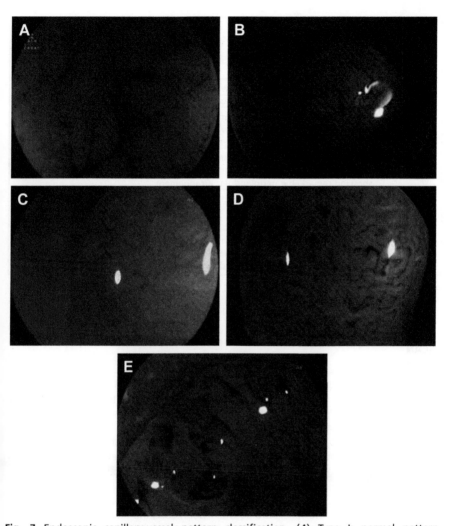

Fig. 7. Endoscopic capillary-vessel pattern classification. (*A*) Type I: normal pattern composed of thin subepithelial capillary vessels with a linear shape and regular arrangement surrounding the mucosal crypts. (*B*) Type II: this pattern exhibits hypovascularity or marginal capillaries of a thicker diameter, curved or straight but uniform, without dilatations, and the pericryptal arrangement is not remarkable. (*C*) Type III: numerous capillaries of thinner diameter, irregular and tortuous, with frequent point dilatations, and tapering like a spiral shape, showing remarkable periglandular arrangement. (*D*) Type IV: numerous long, spiral, or straight blood vessels with a thicker diameter, and sparse dilatations, running upright, surrounding the villous glands. (*E*) Type V: pleomorphism of capillaries and abnormal distribution and arrangement; numerous heterogeneous thick vessels with chaotic arrangement are the predominant feature. (*From* Teixeira CR, Torresini RS, Canali C, et al. Endoscopic classification of the capillary-vessel pattern of colorectal lesions by spectral estimation technology and magnifying zoom imaging. Gastrointest Endosc 2009;69:752; with permission.)

Table 5
Endoscopic capillary/vessel pattern classification for predicting histology using Fujinon Intelligent Color Enhancement

Types	Characteristics	Polyp
Type I	Thin subepithelial capillary vessels with a linear shape and regular arrangement surrounding the mucosal crypts	Hyperplastic
Type II	Hypovascularity or marginal capillaries of a thicker diameter, curved or straight but uniform, without dilatations, and the pericryptal arrangement is not remarkable	Hyperplastic
Type III	Numerous capillaries of thinner diameter, irregular and tortuous, with frequent point dilatations, and tapering like a spiral shape, showing remarkable periglandular arrangement	Adenoma
Type IV	Numerous long, spiral, or straight blood vessels with a thicker diameter, and sparse dilatations, running upright, surrounding the villous glands	Adenoma
Type V	Pleomorphism of capillaries and abnormal distribution and arrangement; numerous heterogeneous thick vessels with chaotic arrangement are the predominant feature	Neoplastic

Adapted from Teixeira CR, Torresini RS, Canali C, et al. Endoscopic classification of the capillary-vessel pattern of colorectal lesions by spectral estimation technology and magnifying zoom imaging. Gastrointest Endosc 2009;69:752; with permission.

i-SCAN
Technology

i-Scan is also a postprocessing technology that uses different software algorithms with real-time image mapping (RIM) to enhance different elements of the mucosa. This system has 3 adjustable modes of image enhancement: surface, contrast, and tone.[49] Surface enhancement highlights light to dark contrast, thereby enabling the edges of the lesion to be well demarcated, which can help identify subtle and flat lesions. Contrast enhancement highlights low-intensity areas, thereby helping to identify depressed lesions. Tone enhancement highlights vascular structures.[49]

Performance

As with NBI and FICE, the initial studies with i-Scan used the Kudo pit pattern.[50] More recently, however, different surface and vascular patterns have been described with i-Scan to predict polyp histology (**Fig. 8**, **Table 6**). Studies have shown accuracy with i-Scan ranging from 72% to 99%.[50–53] A meta-analysis of 9 studies using i-Scan for polyp histology prediction that included 984 polyps revealed a sensitivity of 89.5%, specificity of 89.3%, and negative predictive value of 86.5%.[39]

Feasibility

i-Scan is also an easy-to-use technology that incurs no extra investment once the endoscopy system is procured by an endoscopy unit.

AUTOFLUORESCENCE
Technology

Autofluorescence works on the principle that illumination of tissue by short-wavelength light stimulates endogenous fluorophores (eg, nicotinamide adenine dinucleotide [NAD], flavin, collagen). The electrons are excited to a higher energy level, and when they return to the ground state, fluorescence light of longer wavelength is

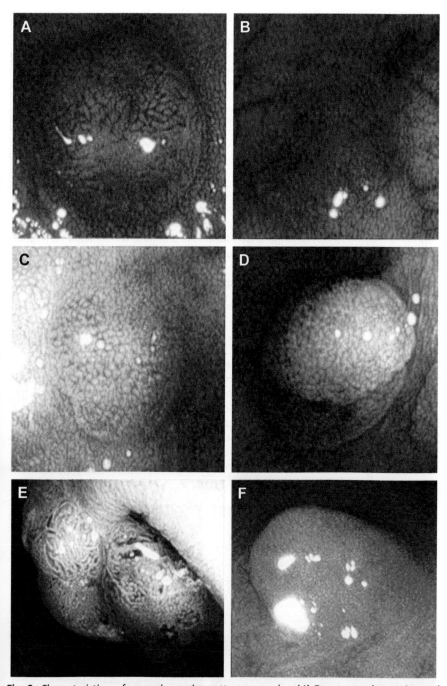

Fig. 8. Characteristic surface and vascular pattern examples. (*A*) Dense, regular, pericryptal vessels. (*B*) Several fine-thread vessels not following the edges of pits. (*C*) Small, compact, regular, round pits. (*D*) Large, noncompact pits. (*E*) Tubular and branched pits. (*F*) No visible surface patterns. (*From* Basford PJ, Longcroft-Wheaton G, Higgins B, et al. High-definition endoscopy with i-Scan for evaluation of small colon polyps: the HiSCOPE study. Gastrointest Endosc 2014;79:115; with permission.)

Table 6
Characteristic surface and vascular patterns in predicting histology by i-Scan

	Neoplastic	Nonneoplastic
Vascular pattern	Dense, regular, pericryptal vessels	No vessels or fine vessels not following edges of pits
Surface pattern	Small, compact, regular, round/ tubular/branched pits	No surface patterns or large noncompact pits

Adapted from Basford PJ, Longcroft-Wheaton G, Higgins B, et al. High-definition endoscopy with i-Scan for evaluation of small colon polyps: the HiSCOPE study. Gastrointest Endosc 2014;79:114; with permission.

emitted depending on the type of tissue and its fluorescent characteristics. This light is captured by sensitive cameras and displayed as a pseudo-color image of the tissue. Fluorophore composition among various tissues is different, which helps distinguish between neoplastic and nonneoplastic lesions. Neoplastic lesions are less autofluorescent because of a different distribution of collagen, increased mucosal thickness and glandular density.[41] Longer-wavelength light is emitted by adenomatous polyps and they appear purple (**Fig. 9**), whereas normal colonic mucosa and nonadenomatous polyps appear in green (**Fig. 10**).[54–57]

Performance

The diagnostic performance of autofluorescence for distinguishing neoplastic from nonneoplastic polyps, real-time, was summarized in a meta-analysis that included 9 studies with 1152 polyps. Summary estimates showed that the sensitivity was high at 88%, with a lower specificity and negative predictive value of 69.2% and 81.5%, respectively.[39] One study comparing NBI and autofluorescence in distinguishing neoplastic from nonneoplastic polyps showed similar sensitivity (90% vs 87%; $P = .79$) but lower specificity (37% vs 63%; $P<.001$) and accuracy (62% vs 75%; $P = .001$) for autofluorescence.[58] Another study revealed a fairly low diagnostic

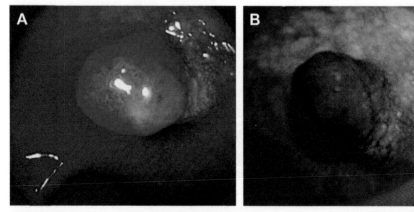

Fig. 9. Endoscopic images of colon adenoma. (*A*) High-resolution endoscopy. (*B*) Autofluorescence imaging. (*From* Sato R, Fujiya M, Watari J, et al. The diagnostic accuracy of high-resolution endoscopy, autofluorescence imaging and narrow-band imaging for differentially diagnosing colon adenoma. Endoscopy 2011;43:866; with permission.)

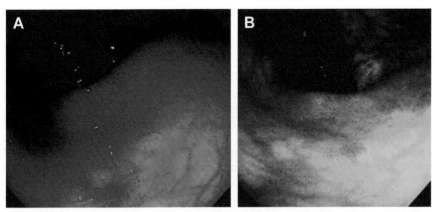

Fig. 10. Endoscopic images of a hyperplastic polyp. (*A*) High-resolution endoscopy. (*B*) Auto-fluorescence imaging. (*From* Sato R, Fujiya M, Watari J, et al. The diagnostic accuracy of high-resolution endoscopy, autofluorescence imaging and narrow-band imaging for differentially diagnosing colon adenoma. Endoscopy 2011;43:866; with permission.)

accuracy (55%) for autofluorescence in differentiating adenomas from hyperplastic polyps.[59]

Feasibility

Autofluorescence is a relatively easy-to-use technology, but is not yet commercially available in the United States.

CONFOCAL LASER ENDOMICROSCOPY
Technology

Confocal laser endomicroscopy (CLE) uses laser light and the application of a fluorescent agent (fluorescein sodium, acriflavine) to allow microscopic visualization of the tissue surface and structures below the surface. A magnification of up to 1000× allows visualization of subcellular details.[60,61] The confocal microscope consists of the light source, the sample plane, and the detector all in the same conjugate plane. A blue laser integrated with the light source is focused to a point on the colonic mucosa, which excites the mucosa at 488 nm, and the fluorescence emitted by the colonic mucosa is detected at 505 nm. This fluorescence is collected by an objective lens from that point and is forced through a pinhole to reach the detector. Light from out-of-focus planes in the colonic mucosa is blocked by the pinhole and does not reach the detector. This beam of light is scanned to build an image.[9,62] The principles of CLE are depicted in **Fig. 10**.

CLE is of 2 types: endoscopic-based confocal laser endomicroscopy (eCLE, Pentax), in which a miniaturized confocal scanner is integrated into the distal tip of a conventional endoscope, and a probe-based system (pCLE; Cellvizio, Mauna Kea Technologies, Paris, France), wherein a probe with a diameter of 2.5 mm and 30,000 optical fibers is passed through a working channel of the endoscope and attached to an external laser scanning unit. The 2 systems differ regarding the rate of image acquisition, field of view, resolution, and imaging depth. With eCLE, sections of 475 × 475 μm at variable imaging depths (range, 0–250 μm) are generated. The acquisition rate is 0.8 to 1.6 frames per second,[9] whereas the lateral and axial resolutions are 0.7 and 7.0 μm, respectively. With pCLE, the total field of view is 250 μm, with lateral and axial resolutions of 1.0 and 5.0 μm, respectively, and a image acquisition frame rate of 12 images per second.[9,63,64] Kiesslich and colleagues[65] described confocal criteria to characterize the histology of colon polyps (**Table 7**). The histology patterns are shown in **Figs. 11** and **12**.

Diagnostic Performance

A meta-analysis of 6 studies with 784 polyps revealed excellent performance characteristics of CLE in distinguishing neoplastic from nonneoplastic polyps. The sensitivity and specificity were 94.3% and 94.8%, respectively, with a negative predictive value of 94.8%.[39] The diagnostic performance was not significantly different between eCLE and pCLE (P = .53). In one study comparing the diagnostic ability of pCLE and FICE in distinguishing neoplastic and nonneoplastic polyps, pCLE had better sensitivity (91% vs 77%; P = .010) but similar specificity (76% vs 71%; P = .77). Accuracy was reported to be 86%.[66] However, not all studies have shown high accuracy rates in characterizing polyp histology using CLE. In the study by Kuiper and colleagues,[67] the accuracy for 2 endoscopists was 67% and 72% with pCLE, which were significantly lower than the accuracies with NBI (89%) and chromoendoscopy (89%).

Feasibility

Major disadvantages of CLE are that it is expensive and requires significant capital expenditure. It is also time-consuming, because extra time is required for image acquisition. Because of the very small field of view, stabilization of the endoscope or the probe over the polyp to acquire good-quality sequences and images can be challenging. Furthermore, for pCLE, intravenous administration of fluorescein sodium is required. The pCLE probe has a limited lifespan ($\approx$20 procedures), further increasing the cost burden. The best-quality images are obtained within 8 to 10 minutes of fluorescein dye injection, and therefore image quality can deteriorate in longer procedures, causing their interpretation to be challenging.[64,68] Lastly, contrast dye such as acriflavine is considered a carcinogen.[69,70]

Table 7
Confocal endomicroscopy criteria for prediction of histology

	Normal	Regenerative	Neoplastic
Vascular architecture	Hexagonal network delineating periluminal crypt stroma	Hexagonal network with no or mild increase in capillary density	Distorted/dilated vascular architecture with elevated leakage Irregular architecture with little/poor orientation to adjunct tissue
Crypt architecture	Regular luminal crypt openings/distribution Goblet cells visualized at normal density	Star-shaped luminal crypt openings ± focal aggregates of regular-shaped crypts ± goblet cell depletion	Ridge-lined irregular epithelial layer Crypt/goblet cell attenuation Irregular cell architecture with mucin depletion

Adapted from Kiesslich R, Burg J, Vieth M, et al. Confocal laser endoscopy for diagnosing intra-epithelial neoplasias and colorectal cancer in vivo. Gastroenterology 2004;127:708; with permission.

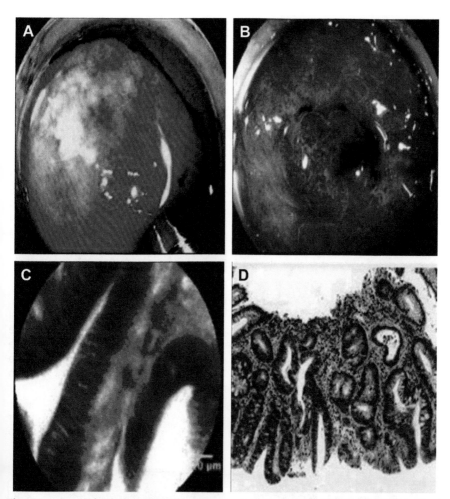

Fig. 11. Images of tubular adenoma. (*A*) Endoscopic image. (*B*) FICE image. (*C*) Confocal image. (*D*) Histopathology image (hamatoxylin-eosin [H&E]). (*From* Buchner AM, Shahid MW, Heckman MG, et al. Comparison of probe-based confocal laser endomicroscopy with virtual chromoendoscopy for classification of colon polyps. Gastroenterology 2010;138:836; with permission.)

ENDOCYTOSCOPY
Technology

Endocytoscopy provides ultra-high magnification images (up to 1400 times) after staining the mucosa with methylene blue (for nuclei) and crystal violet or toluidine blue (for cytoplasm). Endocytoscopy has 2 systems: an integrated system (iEC), which has a magnification lens integrated into the tip of the endoscope, and a probe-based system (pEC), wherein a probe with a magnification lens must be passed through a working channel of the endoscope. A mucolytic agent is first used to remove excess mucus from the colonic mucosa, after which the contrast agent is applied. Following this, the lens of either system is placed in contact with the mucosal surface to visualize cellular structures of the superficial epithelial layer of the colonic mucosa. Minute cellular details can be assessed, such as the size and shape of cells, nuclei, and the

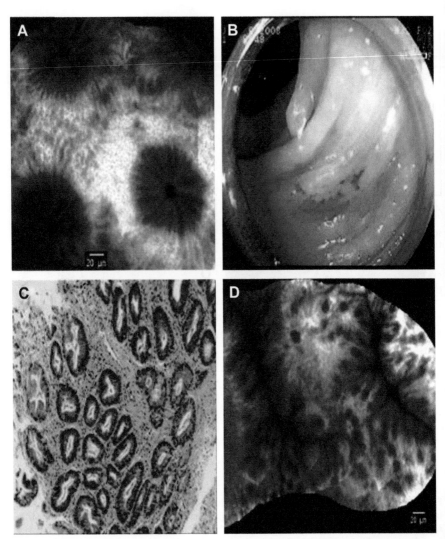

Fig. 12. Confocal images of colonic lesions. (*A*) Normal colon mucosa (pCLE view). (*B*) Hyperplastic lesion (endoscopic view). (*C*) Hyperplastic lesion (hematoxylin-eosin [H&E]). (*D*) Hyperplastic lesion (pCLE view, mosaic image). (*From* Buchner AM, Shahid MW, Heckman MG, et al. Comparison of probe-based confocal laser endomicroscopy with virtual chromoendoscopy for classification of colon polyps. Gastroenterology 2010;138:836; with permission.)

nucleus/cytoplasm ratio.[9,71,72] Based on the cellular details, Kudo and colleagues[73] and Sasajima and colleagues[74] proposed endocytoscopic criteria to predict the histology of colon polyps. Based on these 2 classification systems, newer revised Vienna classification categories have been proposed for predicting colon polyp histology (**Table 8**).[75,76] Various patterns observed with endocytoscopy are shown in **Fig. 13**.

Diagnostic Performance

A prospective study on 75 polyps revealed an accuracy of 93.3% by endocytoscopy in distinguishing neoplastic from nonneoplastic polyps.[74] Another study showed

Table 8 Revised Vienna classification categories for endocytoscopic prediction of polyp histology	
Normal (VCC 1 or 2)	Roundish lumens Fusiform nuclei
Hyperplastic polyp (VCC 1 or 2)	Narrow serrated lumens Small roundish granules
Low-grade adenoma (VCC 3)	Slit-like lumens Slightly swollen fusiform nuclei
High-grade adenoma (VCC 4 or 5)	Slit-like or irregular lumens Swollen roundish nuclei
Invasive cancer (VCC 4 or 5)	Unclear gland formation Agglomeration of distorted nuclei

Abbreviation: VCC, Vienna classification category.
Adapted from Mori Y, Kudo S, Ikehara N, et al. Comprehensive diagnostic ability of endocytoscopy compared with biopsy for colorectal neoplasms: a prospective randomized noninferiority trial. Endoscopy 2013;45:100; with permission.

endocytoscopy to have a better accuracy compared with conventional endoscopy in distinguishing neoplastic from nonneoplastic lesions (100% vs 97%, respectively; P<.01).[73] In a recent study, the diagnostic accuracy of endocytoscopy for the real-time discrimination of neoplastic lesions was 94%, which was noninferior to that of a pathologic evaluation of a standard biopsy specimen of the polyps.[75]

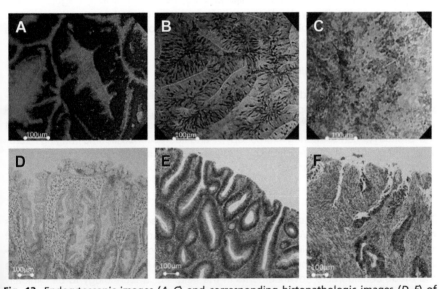

Fig. 13. Endocytoscopic images (*A–C*) and corresponding histopathologic images (*D–F*) of representative colorectal lesions. (*A, D*) Hyperplastic polyp: endocytoscopy shows narrow serrated lumens and small roundish granules (hamatoxylin-eosin [H&E]). (*B, E*) Low-grade dysplasia: endocytoscopy shows slit-like smooth lumens and uniform fusiform nuclei (hamatoxylin-eosin [H&E]). (*C, F*) Invasive submucosal cancer: endocytoscopy shows unclear gland formation and agglomeration of distorted nuclei (hamatoxylin-eosin [H&E]). (*From* Mori Y, Kudo S, Ikehara N, et al. Comprehensive diagnostic ability of endocytoscopy compared with biopsy for colorectal neoplasms: a prospective randomized noninferiority trial. Endoscopy 2013;45:99; with permission.)

Feasibility

Endocytoscopy is expensive and not available in United States. Because of the high magnification, even slight movements from breathing or contractions of the colon can impair the quality of the images, causing the use of this technology to be clinically challenging.[71]

SESSILE SERRATED ADENOMAS/POLYPS

Sessile serrated adenomas/polyps resemble hyperplastic polyps both morphologically and histologically.[77] They account for up to 20% of sporadic cancers because of a proposed alternative pathway of colorectal carcinogenesis: the serrated neoplasia pathway.[78,79] These lesions are easy to miss because of their subtle appearance. Therefore, it is important for endoscopists to familiarize themselves with the endoscopic appearance of these polyps. Tadepalli and colleagues[80] validated various endoscopic features of serrated polyps by reviewing previously recorded video clips. The most frequent sentinel signs that were suggestive of sessile serrated adenoma were the presence of a mucous cap, disruption of the contour of a fold by the polyp, the presence of a rim of debris or bubbles on the polyp, and the dome-shaped protrusion of the polyp above the mucosa. They concluded that NBI was superior in characterizing sessile serrated polyps compared with white light endoscopy. More recently, a group of international experts evaluated 150 images of polyps that were obtained from a retrospective database. They first identified and then validated specific endoscopic features of sessile serrated adenomas with NBI. These features included a cloud-like surface, indistinct borders, irregular shape, and dark spots inside crypts. The sensitivity, specificity, and accuracy of NBI for differentiating serrated polyps harboring either none or all 4 endoscopic features were 89%, 96%, and 93%, respectively.[81]

FUTURE ADVANCED IMAGING TECHNIQUES

Several other sophisticated imaging technologies are being evaluated for polyp histology prediction, including optical coherence tomography,[82,83] Raman endoscopy,[84–86] multiphoton microscopy,[87–90] second harmonic generation imaging,[91] coherent anti-Stokes Raman scattering microscopy,[92] and fluorescence lifetime imaging microscopy.[93] Limited data are available on these modalities, and hence their clinical application is yet to be determined.

SUMMARY

During the past several years, interest in the real-time prediction of polyp histology has increased tremendously. With the development of several imaging technologies that can assist with polyp histology characterization during colonoscopy have been developed, and investigators from different parts of the globe have tested these modalities and made considerable advancements in the field. For a technology to be clinically applicable and be embraced by the gastroenterology community, it should fulfill certain criteria. First and foremost it should be accurate in characterizing polyp histology. The technology should be easy to use, not too time-consuming, and the pattern recognition should be simple to learn. Furthermore, it should not require excessive capital expenditure; otherwise, the potential cost savings of real-time histology will be negated. Electronic chromoendoscopy fulfills these criteria. Of the 3 types of electronic chromoendoscopy, NBI has been the most extensively evaluated. Dye-based chromoendoscopy has not gained widespread use in Western countries.

Autofluorescence, albeit easy to use, has shown subpar performance characteristics and is not available in the United States. CLE and endocytoscopy have shown superior diagnostic performance but are expensive, challenging to use in clinical practice, and currently are mainly used as research tools for polyp histology prediction.

Real-time polyp histology prediction is here to stay. Additional work is needed to determine whether the performance of experts can be duplicated by nonexperts and community gastroenterologists. The technology that can show good performance when used by nonexperts and community gastroenterologists will ultimately win the race.

REFERENCES

1. Vogelstein B, Fearon ER, Hamilton SR, et al. Genetic alterations during colorectal-tumor development. N Engl J Med 1988;319:525–32.
2. Reya T, Clevers H. Wnt signalling in stem cells and cancer. Nature 2005;434: 843–50.
3. Butterly LF, Chase MP, Pohl H, et al. Prevalence of clinically important histology in small adenomas. Clin Gastroenterol Hepatol 2006;4:343–8.
4. Rex DK, Overhiser AJ, Chen SC, et al. Estimation of impact of American College of Radiology recommendations on CT colonography reporting for resection of high-risk adenoma findings. Am J Gastroenterol 2009;104:149–53.
5. Lieberman D, Moravec M, Holub J, et al. Polyp size and advanced histology in patients undergoing colonoscopy screening: implications for CT colonography. Gastroenterology 2008;135:1100–5.
6. Gupta N, Bansal A, Rao D, et al. Prevalence of advanced histological features in diminutive and small colon polyps. Gastrointest Endosc 2012;75:1022–30.
7. Hassan C, Pickhardt PJ, Rex DK. A resect and discard strategy would improve cost-effectiveness of colorectal cancer screening. Clin Gastroenterol Hepatol 2010;8:865–9, 869.e1–3.
8. Kessler WR, Imperiale TF, Klein RW, et al. A quantitative assessment of the risks and cost savings of forgoing histologic examination of diminutive polyps. Endoscopy 2011;43:683–91.
9. Coda S, Thillainayagam AV. State of the art in advanced endoscopic imaging for the detection and evaluation of dysplasia and early cancer of the gastrointestinal tract. Clin Exp Gastroenterol 2014;7:133–50.
10. Longcroft-Wheaton G, Brown J, Cowlishaw D, et al. High-definition vs standard-definition colonoscopy in the characterization of small colonic polyps: results from a randomized trial. Endoscopy 2012;44:905–10.
11. Rastogi A, Early DS, Gupta N, et al. Randomized, controlled trial of standard-definition white-light, high-definition white-light, and narrow-band imaging colonoscopy for the detection of colon polyps and prediction of polyp histology. Gastrointest Endosc 2011;74:593–602.
12. Rastogi A, Keighley J, Singh V, et al. High accuracy of narrow band imaging without magnification for the real-time characterization of polyp histology and its comparison with high-definition white light colonoscopy: a prospective study. Am J Gastroenterol 2009;104:2422–30.
13. Kato S, Fujii T, Koba I, et al. Assessment of colorectal lesions using magnifying colonoscopy and mucosal dye spraying: can significant lesions be distinguished? Endoscopy 2001;33:306–10.
14. Devuni D, Vaziri H, Anderson JC. Chromocolonoscopy. Gastroenterol Clin North Am 2013;42:521–45.

15. Kudo S, Tamura S, Nakajima T, et al. Diagnosis of colorectal tumorous lesions by magnifying endoscopy. Gastrointest Endosc 1996;44:8–14.

16. Kudo S, Rubio CA, Teixeira CR, et al. Pit pattern in colorectal neoplasia: endoscopic magnifying view. Endoscopy 2001;33:367–73.

17. Fu KI, Sano Y, Kato S, et al. Chromoendoscopy using indigo carmine dye spraying with magnifying observation is the most reliable method for differential diagnosis between non-neoplastic and neoplastic colorectal lesions: a prospective study. Endoscopy 2004;36:1089–93.

18. Tung SY, Wu CS, Su MY. Magnifying colonoscopy in differentiating neoplastic from nonneoplastic colorectal lesions. Am J Gastroenterol 2001;96:2628–32.

19. Konishi K, Kaneko K, Kurahashi T, et al. A comparison of magnifying and nonmagnifying colonoscopy for diagnosis of colorectal polyps: a prospective study. Gastrointest Endosc 2003;57:48–53.

20. Togashi K, Konishi F, Ishizuka T, et al. Efficacy of magnifying endoscopy in the differential diagnosis of neoplastic and non-neoplastic polyps of the large bowel. Dis Colon Rectum 1999;42:1602–8.

21. Hurlstone DP, Cross SS, Drew K, et al. An evaluation of colorectal endoscopic mucosal resection using high-magnification chromoscopic colonoscopy: a prospective study of 1000 colonoscopies. Endoscopy 2004;36:491–8.

22. Davies J, Burke D, Olliver JR, et al. Methylene blue but not indigo carmine causes DNA damage to colonocytes in vitro and in vivo at concentrations used in clinical chromoendoscopy. Gut 2007;56:155–6.

23. Gono K, Obi T, Yamaguchi M, et al. Appearance of enhanced tissue features in narrow-band endoscopic imaging. J Biomed Opt 2004;9:568–77.

24. Masaki T, Katada C, Nakayama M, et al. Narrow band imaging in the diagnosis of intra-epithelial and invasive laryngeal squamous cell carcinoma: a preliminary report of two cases. Auris Nasus Larynx 2009;36:712–6.

25. Zonios G, Perelman LT, Backman V, et al. Diffuse reflectance spectroscopy of human adenomatous colon polyps in vivo. Appl Opt 1999;38:6628–37.

26. Machida H, Sano Y, Hamamoto Y, et al. Narrow-band imaging in the diagnosis of colorectal mucosal lesions: a pilot study. Endoscopy 2004;36:1094–8.

27. Hirata M, Tanaka S, Oka S, et al. Magnifying endoscopy with narrow band imaging for diagnosis of colorectal tumors. Gastrointest Endosc 2007;65:988–95.

28. East JE, Suzuki N, Saunders BP. Comparison of magnified pit pattern interpretation with narrow band imaging versus chromoendoscopy for diminutive colonic polyps: a pilot study. Gastrointest Endosc 2007;66:310–6.

29. East JE, Suzuki N, Bassett P, et al. Narrow band imaging with magnification for the characterization of small and diminutive colonic polyps: pit pattern and vascular pattern intensity. Endoscopy 2008;40:811–7.

30. Rastogi A, Bansal A, Wani S, et al. Narrow-band imaging colonoscopy—a pilot feasibility study for the detection of polyps and correlation of surface patterns with polyp histologic diagnosis. Gastrointest Endosc 2008;67:280–6.

31. Rastogi A. Optical diagnosis of small colorectal polyp histology with high-definition colonoscopy using narrow band imaging. Clin Endosc 2013;46:120–9.

32. Rex DK. Narrow-band imaging without optical magnification for histologic analysis of colorectal polyps. Gastroenterology 2009;136:1174–81.

33. Sano Y, Ikematsu H, Fu KI, et al. Meshed capillary vessels by use of narrow-band imaging for differential diagnosis of small colorectal polyps. Gastrointest Endosc 2009;69:278–83.

34. Uraoka T, Saito Y, Ikematsu H, et al. Sano's capillary pattern classification for narrow-band imaging of early colorectal lesions. Dig Endosc 2011;23(Suppl 1):112–5.

35. Katagiri A, Fu KI, Sano Y, et al. Narrow band imaging with magnifying colonoscopy as diagnostic tool for predicting histology of early colorectal neoplasia. Aliment Pharmacol Ther 2008;27:1269–74.
36. Henry ZH, Yeaton P, Shami VM, et al. Meshed capillary vessels found on narrow-band imaging without optical magnification effectively identifies colorectal neoplasia: a North American validation of the Japanese experience. Gastrointest Endosc 2010;72:118–26.
37. Tischendorf JJ, Schirin-Sokhan R, Streetz K, et al. Value of magnifying endoscopy in classifying colorectal polyps based on vascular pattern. Endoscopy 2010;42:22–7.
38. Hewett DG, Kaltenbach T, Sano Y, et al. Validation of a simple classification system for endoscopic diagnosis of small colorectal polyps using narrow-band imaging. Gastroenterology 2012;143:599–607.e1.
39. Wanders LK, East JE, Uitentuis SE, et al. Diagnostic performance of narrowed spectrum endoscopy, autofluorescence imaging, and confocal laser endomicroscopy for optical diagnosis of colonic polyps: a meta-analysis. Lancet Oncol 2013;14:1337–47.
40. McGill SK, Evangelou E, Ioannidis JP, et al. Narrow band imaging to differentiate neoplastic and non-neoplastic colorectal polyps in real time: a meta-analysis of diagnostic operating characteristics. Gut 2013;62:1704–13.
41. Hussain ZH, Pohl H. Ancillary imaging techniques and adenoma detection. Gastroenterol Clin North Am 2013;42:547–65.
42. Longcroft-Wheaton GR, Higgins B, Bhandari P. Flexible spectral imaging color enhancement and indigo carmine in neoplasia diagnosis during colonoscopy: a large prospective UK series. Eur J Gastroenterol Hepatol 2011;23:903–11.
43. Teixeira CR, Torresini RS, Canali C, et al. Endoscopic classification of the capillary-vessel pattern of colorectal lesions by spectral estimation technology and magnifying zoom imaging. Gastrointest Endosc 2009;69:750–6.
44. Pohl J, Nguyen-Tat M, Pech O, et al. Computed virtual chromoendoscopy for classification of small colorectal lesions: a prospective comparative study. Am J Gastroenterol 2008;103:562–9.
45. Pohl J, Lotterer E, Balzer C, et al. Computed virtual chromoendoscopy versus standard colonoscopy with targeted indigocarmine chromoscopy: a randomised multicentre trial. Gut 2009;58:73–8.
46. Yoshida N, Naito Y, Inada Y, et al. The detection of surface patterns by flexible spectral imaging color enhancement without magnification for diagnosis of colorectal polyps. Int J Colorectal Dis 2012;27:605–11.
47. Santos CE, Pereira-Lima JC, Lopes CV, et al. Comparative study between MBI (FICE) and magnification chromoendoscopy with indigo carmine in the differential diagnosis of neoplastic and non-neoplastic lesions of the colorectum. Arq Gastroenterol 2009;46:111–5 [in Portuguese].
48. dos Santos CE, Lima JC, Lopes CV, et al. Computerized virtual chromoendoscopy versus indigo carmine chromoendoscopy combined with magnification for diagnosis of small colorectal lesions: a randomized and prospective study. Eur J Gastroenterol Hepatol 2010;22:1364–71.
49. Basford PJ, Longcroft-Wheaton G, Higgins B, et al. High-definition endoscopy with i-Scan for evaluation of small colon polyps: the HiSCOPE study. Gastrointest Endosc 2014;79:111–8.
50. Hoffman A, Sar F, Goetz M, et al. High definition colonoscopy combined with i-Scan is superior in the detection of colorectal neoplasias compared with

standard video colonoscopy: a prospective randomized controlled trial. Endoscopy 2010;42:827–33.

51. Lee CK, Lee SH, Hwangbo Y. Narrow-band imaging versus I-Scan for the real-time histological prediction of diminutive colonic polyps: a prospective comparative study by using the simple unified endoscopic classification. Gastrointest Endosc 2011;74:603–9.

52. Chan JL, Lin L, Feiler M, et al. Comparative effectiveness of i-SCAN and high-definition white light characterizing small colonic polyps. World J Gastroenterol 2012;18:5905–11.

53. Pigo F, Bertani H, Manno M, et al. i-Scan high-definition white light endoscopy and colorectal polyps: prediction of histology, interobserver and intraobserver agreement. Int J Colorectal Dis 2013;28:399–406.

54. van den Broek FJ, Fockens P, van Eeden S, et al. Endoscopic tri-modal imaging for surveillance in ulcerative colitis: randomised comparison of high-resolution endoscopy and autofluorescence imaging for neoplasia detection; and evaluation of narrow-band imaging for classification of lesions. Gut 2008; 57:1083–9.

55. Song LM, Banerjee S, Desilets D, et al. Autofluorescence imaging. Gastrointest Endosc 2011;73:647–50.

56. Falk GW. Autofluorescence endoscopy. Gastrointest Endosc Clin N Am 2009;19: 209–20.

57. Sato R, Fujiya M, Watari J, et al. The diagnostic accuracy of high-resolution endoscopy, autofluorescence imaging and narrow-band imaging for differentially diagnosing colon adenoma. Endoscopy 2011;43:862–8.

58. Kuiper T, van den Broek FJ, Naber AH, et al. Endoscopic trimodal imaging detects colonic neoplasia as well as standard video endoscopy. Gastroenterology 2011;140:1887–94.

59. Boparai KS, van den Broek FJ, van Eeden S, et al. Hyperplastic polyposis syndrome: a pilot study for the differentiation of polyps by using high-resolution endoscopy, autofluorescence imaging, and narrow-band imaging. Gastrointest Endosc 2009;70:947–55.

60. Goetz M. Endomicroscopy and targeted imaging of gastric neoplasia. Gastrointest Endosc Clin N Am 2013;23:597–606.

61. Goetz M, Malek NP, Kiesslich R. Microscopic imaging in endoscopy: endomicroscopy and endocytoscopy. Nat Rev Gastroenterol Hepatol 2014;11:11–8.

62. Goetz M, Kiesslich R. Advanced imaging of the gastrointestinal tract: research vs clinical tools? Curr Opin Gastroenterol 2009;25:412–21.

63. Humphris J, Swartz D, Egan BJ, et al. Status of confocal laser endomicroscopy in gastrointestinal disease. Trop Gastroenterol 2012;33:9–20.

64. Kantsevoy SV, Adler DG, Conway JD, et al. Confocal laser endomicroscopy. Gastrointest Endosc 2009;70:197–200.

65. Kiesslich R, Burg J, Vieth M, et al. Confocal laser endoscopy for diagnosing intra-epithelial neoplasias and colorectal cancer in vivo. Gastroenterology 2004;127: 706–13.

66. Buchner AM, Shahid MW, Heckman MG, et al. Comparison of probe-based confocal laser endomicroscopy with virtual chromoendoscopy for classification of colon polyps. Gastroenterology 2010;138:834–42.

67. Kuiper T, van den Broek FJ, van Eeden S, et al. Feasibility and accuracy of confocal endomicroscopy in comparison with narrow-band imaging and chromoendoscopy for the differentiation of colorectal lesions. Am J Gastroenterol 2012;107:543–50.

68. Becker V, von Delius S, Bajbouj M, et al. Intravenous application of fluorescein for confocal laser scanning microscopy: evaluation of contrast dynamics and image quality with increasing injection-to-imaging time. Gastrointest Endosc 2008;68: 319–23.
69. Polglase AL, McLaren WJ, Skinner SA, et al. A fluorescence confocal endomicroscope for in vivo microscopy of the upper- and the lower-GI tract. Gastrointest Endosc 2005;62:686–95.
70. Burleson GR, Caulfield MJ, Pollard M. Ozonation of mutagenic and carcinogenic polyaromatic amines and polyaromatic hydrocarbons in water. Cancer Res 1979; 39:2149–54.
71. ASGE Technology Committee, Kwon RS, Wong Kee Song LM, et al. Endocytoscopy. Gastrointest Endosc 2009;70:610–3.
72. Inoue H, Sasajima K, Kaga M, et al. Endoscopic in vivo evaluation of tissue atypia in the esophagus using a newly designed integrated endocytoscope: a pilot trial. Endoscopy 2006;38:891–5.
73. Kudo SE, Wakamura K, Ikehara N, et al. Diagnosis of colorectal lesions with a novel endocytoscopic classification—a pilot study. Endoscopy 2011;43:869–75.
74. Sasajima K, Kudo SE, Inoue H, et al. Real-time in vivo virtual histology of colorectal lesions when using the endocytoscopy system. Gastrointest Endosc 2006;63:1010–7.
75. Mori Y, Kudo S, Ikehara N, et al. Comprehensive diagnostic ability of endocytoscopy compared with biopsy for colorectal neoplasms: a prospective randomized noninferiority trial. Endoscopy 2013;45:98–105.
76. Dixon MF. Gastrointestinal epithelial neoplasia: Vienna revisited. Gut 2002;51: 130–1.
77. Torlakovic E, Skovlund E, Snover DC, et al. Morphologic reappraisal of serrated colorectal polyps. Am J Surg Pathol 2003;27:65–81.
78. Leggett B, Whitehall V. Role of the serrated pathway in colorectal cancer pathogenesis. Gastroenterology 2010;138:2088–100.
79. Snover DC. Update on the serrated pathway to colorectal carcinoma. Hum Pathol 2011;42:1–10.
80. Tadepalli US, Feihel D, Miller KM, et al. A morphologic analysis of sessile serrated polyps observed during routine colonoscopy (with video). Gastrointest Endosc 2011;74:1360–8.
81. Hazewinkel Y, Lopez-Ceron M, East JE, et al. Endoscopic features of sessile serrated adenomas: validation by international experts using high-resolution white-light endoscopy and narrow-band imaging. Gastrointest Endosc 2013;77: 916–24.
82. Tearney GJ, Brezinski ME, Bouma BE, et al. In vivo endoscopic optical biopsy with optical coherence tomography. Science 1997;276:2037–9.
83. Tearney GJ, Brezinski ME, Southern JF, et al. Optical biopsy in human gastrointestinal tissue using optical coherence tomography. Am J Gastroenterol 1997; 92:1800 4.
84. Bergholt MS, Zheng W, Lin K, et al. In vivo diagnosis of esophageal cancer using image-guided Raman endoscopy and biomolecular modeling. Technol Cancer Res Treat 2011;10:103–12.
85. Shao X, Zheng W, Huang Z. Near-infrared autofluorescence spectroscopy for in vivo identification of hyperplastic and adenomatous polyps in the colon. Biosens Bioelectron 2011;30:118–22.
86. Krafft C, Ramoji AA, Bielecki C, et al. A comparative Raman and CARS imaging study of colon tissue. J Biophotonics 2009;2:303–12.

87. Rivera DR, Brown CM, Ouzounov DG, et al. Compact and flexible raster scanning multiphoton endoscope capable of imaging unstained tissue. Proc Natl Acad Sci U S A 2011;108:17598–603.
88. Myaing MT, MacDonald DJ, Li X. Fiber-optic scanning two-photon fluorescence endoscope. Opt Lett 2006;31:1076–8.
89. Engelbrecht CJ, Johnston RS, Seibel EJ, et al. Ultra-compact fiber-optic two-photon microscope for functional fluorescence imaging in vivo. Opt Express 2008;16:5556–64.
90. Tang S, Jung W, McCormick D, et al. Design and implementation of fiber-based multiphoton endoscopy with microelectromechanical systems scanning. J Biomed Opt 2009;14:034005.
91. Campagnola P. Second harmonic generation imaging microscopy: applications to diseases diagnostics. Anal Chem 2011;83:3224–31.
92. Wang Z, Liu Y, Gao L, et al. Use of multimode optical fibers for fiber-based coherent anti-Stokes Raman scattering microendoscopy imaging. Opt Lett 2011;36:2967–9.
93. McGinty J, Galletly NP, Dunsby C, et al. Wide-field fluorescence lifetime imaging of cancer. Biomed Opt Express 2010;1:627–40.

New Paradigms in Polypectomy

Resect and Discard, Diagnose and Disregard

Ana Ignjatovic Wilson, MD, MRCP[a,b,*], Brian P. Saunders, MD, FRCP[a,b]

KEYWORDS

- Optical diagnosis • Colonic polyps • Colorectal cancer • Narrow band imaging

KEY POINTS

- There are major potential advantages for patients, clinicians, and health care providers if optical diagnosis rather than conventional histopathology is used to characterize small polyps at colonoscopy.
- Correct allocation of surveillance interval is the key outcome measure in assessing the accuracy and clinical acceptability of a Resect and Discard, Diagnose and Disregard strategy.
- Standards for achieving high-quality optical diagnosis have now been defined.
- High levels of accuracy in optical diagnosis of small polyps have been achieved at expert centers, but this has not been replicated in community practice.
- There is a need for improved training, assessment, and quality assurance of optical diagnosis for a resect-and-discard, diagnose-and-disregard strategy to become widely acceptable and a standard of care.

INTRODUCTION

Colorectal cancer (CRC) is one of the leading causes of morbidity and mortality in the Western world. In the United States alone, 135,260 people were diagnosed with and 51,783 died of CRC in 2011.[1] Most sporadic CRCs develop from adenomas in a well-described adenoma-carcinoma genetic sequence **Fig. 1**.[2] It involves a progression from normal epithelium to low-grade dysplastic adenoma to larger, protruding adenoma with high-risk features (high-grade dysplasia or villous component) and finally to invasive cancer as a result of mutations in several genes, including APC, KRAS, and p-53.[2] This pathway is thought to account for approximately two-thirds of all CRCs (see **Fig. 1**).

[a] Imperial College London, London SW7 2AZ, UK; [b] Wolfson Unit for Endoscopy, St. Mark's Hospital, Watford Road, Harrow, Middlesex HA1 3UJ, UK
* Corresponding author.
E-mail address: ana.wilson@nhs.net

Gastrointest Endoscopy Clin N Am 25 (2015) 287–302
http://dx.doi.org/10.1016/j.giec.2014.12.001
1052-5157/15/$ – see front matter © 2015 Elsevier Inc. All rights reserved.

giendo.theclinics.com

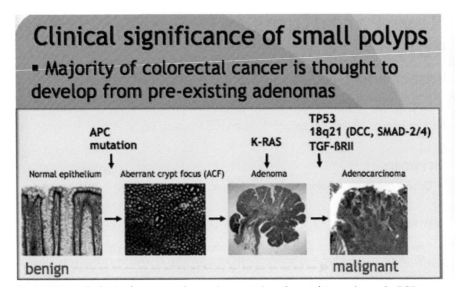

Fig. 1. Histopathologic changes and genetic events in colorectal tumorigenesis. TGF, transforming growth factor. (*Data from* Refs.[2,79–81])

Colonoscopy offers immediate therapeutic capability and resection of adenomas to halt the adenoma-carcinoma sequence, reducing the risk of CRC development. The evidence that colonoscopy prevents incident CRC and reduces mortality is indirect but substantial. Cohort studies of colonoscopy and polypectomy have suggested that, against Surveillance Epidemiology and End Results data, the rate of CRC detected was about 80% lower after polypectomy than expected for the population.[3,4] An Ontario population-based cohort study of 2,412,077 individuals 50 to 90 years of age followed over 14 years found that for every 1% increase in complete colonoscopy rate, the hazard of death from CRC decreased by 3%.[5] Additional evidence for a protective effect of colonoscopy with polypectomy can be extrapolated from flexible sigmoidoscopy trials, with the most recent randomized controlled trial[6] that enrolled 170,432 participants demonstrating that the incidence of CRC in people attending for screening was reduced by 33% (0.67; 95% confidence interval [CI] 0.60–0.76) and mortality by 43% (0.57; 95% CI 0.45–0.72). Therefore, population-based screening is widely recommended and implemented in Europe and the United States.[7,8] In the United States alone, more than 14 million screening colonoscopies are performed each year.[9]

Currently, most polyps seen at colonoscopy are removed by endoscopic resection and sent for histopathology. Bleeding and perforation are the most common complications of polypectomy, with risks of 0% to 4%[10,11] and 0% to 0.23%,[12,13] respectively, reported in the literature, although they are likely to be higher in routine and community clinical practice.

SIGNIFICANCE OF SMALL COLORECTAL POLYPS

Increased awareness of the importance of colonoscopic quality in addition to advanced technology available to operators has led to increased polyp detection rates, at least in the published literature. More than 90% of polyps detected at colonoscopy are small (6–9 mm) or diminutive (≤5 mm), with the latter making up the majority.[14–16] In a study of 13,992 asymptomatic patients who had a screening colonoscopy, 6360 (45%) patients had polyps and 83% of those had a largest polyp that was 9 mm or less in size.[14] Furthermore, only 2549 out of 4942 (52%) were neoplastic with the rest composed of hyperplastic and inflammatory polyps and lymphoid aggregates. Similar findings were reported in a retrospective study of 10,034 patients who underwent colonoscopy over a 5-year period.[16] Polyps that were 5 mm or less represented 81.6% of all polyps removed, and of those 47.9% were tubular adenomas. In a cumulative analysis[17] of 18,549 patients who had a screening colonoscopy, 51% of diminutive polyps were adenomas (range 49%–61%). However, this proportion might be even lower in the rectum and sigmoid colon where there is high prevalence of small hyperplastic polyps, reducing the reported prevalence of adenomas to less than 20%.[18]

Risk of cancer or advanced features (high-grade dysplasia or villous component >25%) in small and, particularly, in diminutive polyps is low (**Table 1**).

In a systematic review of 20,562 average-risk patients undergoing screening colonoscopy, advanced adenomas were detected in 1155 out 20,562 subjects (pooled prevalence of 5.6%, 95% CI 5.3–5.9). In addition, the study showed that 0.9% of patients with diminutive-only lesions had an advanced adenoma and 0.04% had cancer.[19] This finding led the investigators to conclude that, assuming a 5.6% prevalence of advanced adenomas and 3.3% per year progression of advanced adenoma to cancer,[20] the 5-year CRC risk associated with diminutive advanced adenomas would be 0.04% (compared with prescreening 5-year CRC risk of 0.92% for the general population). Recently there has been interest in serrated adenomas/polyps. These lesions are thought to be the precursors for the alternative serrated pathway to CRC development and are now considered premalignant similar to adenomas. Although surface appearances are often similar to simple hyperplastic polyps, the prevalence of serrated polyps/adenomas in diminutive polyps seems to be very low, 0.3% to 0.5%.[14,16,21]

As diminutive polyps are of such limited significance, some colonoscopic imaging tests, such as computed tomography colonography, do not report them.[16] Two prospective Scandinavian studies followed up 194 diminutive polyps after 2 and 3 years.[22,23] They showed that no diminutive polyp increased to a size of greater than 5 mm and no cases of high-grade dysplasia or cancer were detected.

As approximately 50% of small polyps are non-neoplastic,[16,24] many polypectomies are performed unnecessarily, increasing the risks of the procedure. Even small polyps, with little risk of harboring cancer, are currently resected and sent for histopathology as the number of adenomas is one of the best determinants of long-term risk of advanced neoplasia and allows an informed decision regarding future surveillance intervals.[25–27] Unlike the American and European guidelines on polyp surveillance, the British Society of Gastroenterology's guidelines use the size and number of adenomas as the main determinants of surveillance intervals and do not take into account the advanced histologic features (high-grade dysplasia or villous architecture), which have a low prevalence in diminutive polyps and have been questioned as predictors of subsequent advanced neoplasia.[28] Similarly, European guidelines for quality assurance in CRC screening and diagnosis recommend that local practice determines whether or not to use advanced features to determine surveillance intervals.[29]

An ability to correctly diagnose a diminutive polyp during colonoscopy (optical diagnosis) would allow for rectosigmoid hyperplastic polyps to be diagnosed and left in situ (diagnose and disregard) and for diminutive adenomas to be resected and discarded (resect and discard) without a need to retrieve the polyp for formal

Table 1
Proportion of small or diminutive adenomas with advanced histology

Study	Total Number of Diminutive Adenomas (Size Range)	Total Diminutive Advanced Histology (%)[a]	Total Number of Small Adenomas (Size Range)	Total Small Advanced Histology	Total Small Carcinoma
Shinya & Wolff,[82] 1979	—	—	1661 (5–9 mm)	249 (15.0%)[b]	8 (0.5%)
National Polyp Study,[83] 1990	1270 (<6 mm)	25 (2.0%)[b]	1230 (6–10 mm)	155 (12.6%)[b]	—
Gschwantler,[84] 2002	3016 (<5 mm)	104 (3.4%)[c] 561 (18.6%)[b]	2789 (5–10 mm)	350 (12.5%)[c] 1080 (38.7%)[b]	26 (0.9%)
Butterly et al,[24] 2006	1305 (<6 mm)	34 (2.6%)[b]	487 (6–9 mm) 921 (5–10 mm)	38 (7.8%)[b] 85 (9.2%)[b]	2 (0.4%) 8 (0.9%)
Sprung,[85] 2006 (abstract)	—	—	6694 (5–10 mm)	—	2 (0.03%)
Kim,[86] 2007	759 (≤5 mm)	3 (0.4%)	291 (6–9 mm)	11 (3.8%)[b]	0 (0%)
Lieberman et al,[14] 2008[d]	3744 (≤5 mm)	62 (1.7%)	1198 (6–9 mm)	79 (6.6%)	2 (0.2%)
Rex,[16] 2009	4211 (≤5 mm)	79 (0.87%)	689 (6–9 mm)	68 (5.3%)	4 (0.04%)
Bretagne,[87] 2010	520 (<5 mm)	2.8%			
Repici,[88] 2011	627 (<5 mm)	8.7%	388 (6–9 mm)	6.1%	—
Kolligs,[89] 2013	198,954 (<5 mm)	3.7%	106,270 (5–9 mm)	13.0%	—

[a] Butterly and colleagues[24] and Lieberman and colleagues[14] reported one invasive carcinoma at this size category; Gschwantler and colleagues reported zero.
[b] High-grade dysplasia, villous and tubulovillous morphology (>25% villous elements), not invasive carcinoma.
[c] High-grade dysplasia only.
[d] Screening population.

histopathology, especially as 7% to 19% of small polyps[30] may not be successfully retrieved or are unsuitable for histologic analysis because of diathermy artifact. In addition, small polyps may be misclassified at standard histopathology because of incorrect orientation and limited sectioning of the specimen (14% in a recent series[31]).

A frequently cited drawback of optical diagnosis is the lack of ability to distinguish between different grades of dysplasia (high vs low) and the presence of villous features. As mentioned earlier, both of these have been shown to be inconsistent in terms of ability to predict the risk of future neoplasia. Correlation between size and histology of adenomas mean that these two factors act as confounders.[14] Furthermore there is a wide interobserver variability between histopathologists when reporting on the degree of villous architecture.[32–34] A systematic review and meta-analysis on baseline risk factors for advanced adenomas found that there was no difference between villous versus tubular histology.[35] Although a few individual studies have suggested that high-grade dysplasia confers a higher risk of development of advanced adenomas,[27,36] this has not been confirmed by a large pooled study that used individual data from 6 other studies.[37] Therefore, optical diagnosis, which would be possible on all polyps seen, represents a paradigm change as it would enable surveillance intervals to be determined immediately after colonoscopy. This concept is attractive for physicians, patients, and health care providers as the management pathway is potentially streamlined and costs reduced.

Kessler and colleagues[38] performed modeling of real-time endoscopy histology followed by resection and discarding of less than 6 mm polyps versus resection and submission for histology on 4474 consecutive colonoscopies in which 10,400 polyps were removed, 9042 of them less than 6 mm (diminutive). They found that at $75 per specimen, at least $151,000 could be saved for each 1000 patients with at least one diminutive polyp and less than 1 in 1100 patients with diminutive polyps removed would have an undetected cancer in any removed polyp. If an assumption is made that 40% of 1.6 million annual colonoscopies performed in the United States detect at least one diminutive polyp, the potential savings from not sending these polyps for histopathologic assessment is greater than $95 million. Using a resect-and-discard policy for diminutive polyps would result in annual savings of $33 million when applied to colonoscopy screening of the US population (corresponding to overall savings of $330 million, assuming a cumulative period of 10 years to screen just less than a quarter of the US population).[39] Additional costs are incurred by bringing patients back for a follow-up appointment simply to determine the surveillance interval.

WHAT IS THE OPTIMAL MODALITY FOR OPTICAL DIAGNOSIS?

Table 2
Sensitivity, specificity, and accuracy for small polyp characterization using conventional white light colonoscopy

	No.	Mean Size (mm) (Range)	Sens (%)	Spec (%)	Acc (%)
Machida et al,[40] 2004	43	7.5 (2–25)	85.3	44.4	79.1
Apel et al,[41] 2006	273	2.95	93.0	60.0	81.0
De Palma et al,[43] 2006	240	3.0–4.0	91.4	68.3	76.3
Fu et al,[44] 2004	206	3.0–4.0	88.8	67.4	84.0
Su et al,[54] 2006	110	—	82.9	80.0	81.8
Tischendorf et al,[42] 2007	100	10.6 (2–50)	63.4	51.9	59.0
Chiu et al,[58] 2007	180	5.33 (2–20)	62.1–65.2	85.4–74.4	67.2–68.3
Ignjatovic et al,[90] 2011	80	4.5	69.0	60.0	64.0
Longcroft-Wheaton et al,[68] 2011	232	4.7 (2–9)	75.0	64.0	71.0

Abbreviations: Acc, accuracy; Sens, sensitivity; Spec, specificity.

White Light Colonoscopy

Conventional white light colonoscopy has been used to attempt to characterize colonic polyps, both in still images and in vivo. However, white light colonoscopy has a limited accuracy (59%–84%)[40–45] in differentiating neoplastic from non-neoplastic polyps (Table 2).

Chromoendoscopy

Chromoendoscopy has been in used in Japan to characterize small polyps during colonoscopy. By highlighting the shape of the colonic crypts, a pit pattern can be seen. Kudo pit-pattern is the most widely used classification system.[46] Kudo pit patterns I and II indicate non-neoplastic lesion, IIs, IIL and IV neoplastic lesion and V neoplastic lesion with submucosal invasion. This pattern is highly accurate with experts achieving accuracy of more than 90% for polyp characterization when using magnifying colonoscopes and chromoendoscopy. However, there is an appreciable learning curve of 200 to 300 histologically confirmed lesions to achieve that degree of accuracy.[47] The extra training, equipment, and time required for magnifying chromoendoscopy have not made it popular in the West, where it is rarely used outside academic centers (Table 3).

Table 3
Sensitivity, specificity, and accuracy for small polyp characterization using magnifying chromoendoscopy

	No. of Lesions	Mean Size (mm)	Sens (%)	Spec (%)	Acc (%)
Kato,[91] 2006	3438	>5	42.0	98.0	75.0
Togashi,[92] 2006	923	1–11	73.0	92.0	88.0
Konishi,[93] 2003	405	1–10	93.0	85.0	92.0
De Palma et al,[43] 2006	240	3–4	97.5	94.3	95.4
Tischendorf et al,[42] 2007	100	10.6 (2–50)	91.7	90.0	91.0
Chiu et al,[58] 2007	180	5.33 (2–20)	91.3–97.2	74.4–90.5	91.1–92.2

Abbreviations: Acc, accuracy; Sens, sensitivity; Spec, specificity.

Narrow Spectra Technologies

In recent years, several image-enhancing push-button technologies have been developed, such as Narrow Band Imaging (NBI, Olympus, Tokyo, Japan), i-SCAN (Pentax, Mississauga, ON), and Fujinon Intelligent Color Enhancement (FICE, Fujinon Inc, Wayne, NJ). These technologies have been integrated into the colonoscope and can achieve the benefits of chromoendoscopy in a quicker, cheaper, and more user-friendly way.

Most studies have assessed NBI, a blue light optical imaging modality that enhances mucosal detail and, in particular, vascular structures, allowing assessment of vascular pattern intensity[48] and the typical-appearing meshed brown capillary network of adenomas (Fig. 2).[49–51] As neoplastic tissue is characterized by increased angiogenesis, adenomas appear darker when viewed with NBI. Recently a consensus of experts developed and validated a classification system for the characterization of small colonic polyps: the NBI International Colorectal Endoscopic (NICE) classification.[52] This classification uses color, vessels, and surface pattern to differentiate between hyperplastic and adenomatous polyps and is applicable for nonmagnified NBI imaging (Table 4).

The use of microvascular assessment to differentiate between neoplastic and non-neoplastic lesions seems to have a short learning curve,[49,50,53] making it a potentially attractive, practical option for optical diagnosis. In previous academic studies, NBI (with and without magnification) has been shown to offer similar diagnostic accuracy to magnified chromoendoscopy in terms of sensitivity (92%–94%) and specificity (86%–88%) when performed by experienced endoscopists in academic centers.[40,53–58] Despite a recent large meta-analysis that showed an overall sensitivity of 91.0% and specificity of 82.6%,[59] the results from nonacademic centers have not replicated those values, with sensitivities ranging from 75% to 94% and specificities from 65% to 76%.[60–62]

However, beyond absolute sensitivity and specificity, the impact of these technologies on patient outcomes needs to be determined, before optical diagnosis becomes a routine clinical practice.

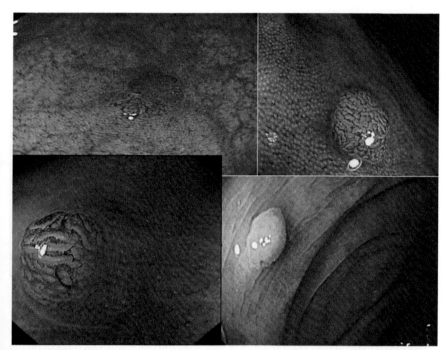

Fig. 2. NBI images of polyps - from top left clockwise - adenoma, adenoma, hyperplastic, adenoma.

IMPACT OF OPTICAL DIAGNOSIS FOR SMALL AND DIMINUTIVE COLORECTAL POLYPS

The first study to assess clinical implications of endoscopic diagnosis on surveillance intervals was performed by a single expert colonoscopist.[63] In this prospective study of 451 consecutively identified patients, high confidence predictions of adenoma were correct for 91% of diminutive polyps and only 1 out of 136 patients received different surveillance intervals when recommendations based on endoscopic and histopathologic diagnosis were compared.

Table 4
NICE classification

	Polyp Classification Using NBI	
Color	Same or lighter than background	Browner relative to background (verify color arises from vessels)
Vessels	None or isolated lacy vessels coursing across the lesion	Thick brown vessels surrounding white structures[a]
Surface pattern	Dark or white spots of uniform size or homogenous absence of pattern	Oval, tubular, or branched white structures[a] surrounded by brown vessels
Most likely pathology	Hyperplastic	Adenoma

[a] These structures may represent the pits and the epithelium of the crypt opening.
Adapted from Hewett DG, Kaltenbach T, Sano Y, et al. Validation of a simple classification system for endoscopic diagnosis of small colorectal polyps using narrow-band imaging. Gastroenterology 2012;143:599–607.e1; with permission.

A study from St Mark's assessed the accuracy of optical diagnosis and its impact on surveillance intervals in a prospective study that included 363 polyps from 130 patients.[64] The overall accuracy of NBI for small polyp characterization in this study, performed by 4 colonoscopists of varying degrees of experience, was 93% (with 6% of adenomas incorrectly diagnosed). In addition, optical diagnosis would have allowed 82 out of 130 (63%) patients to be given a follow-up colonoscopy date immediately after the procedure; only 2 patients would have had a different surveillance interval based on optical diagnosis compared with histopathology.

These initial studies suggested that optical diagnosis could be feasible and safe in routine clinical practice. However, before it could be translated into the community practice it was clear that certain parameters had to be set to serve as a benchmark of performance. Consequently American Society of Gastrointestinal Endoscopy (ASGE) developing a Preservation and Incorporation of Valuable Endoscopic Innovations (PIVI) statement for real-life endoscopic assessment of histology of diminutive polyps[65]:

1. In order for colorectal polyps 5 mm or less in size to be resected and discarded without pathologic assessment, endoscopic technology (when used with high confidence) used to determine histology of polyps 5 mm or less in size, when combined with the histopathologic assessment of polyps larger than 5 mm, should provide a greater than 90% agreement in assignment of postpolypectomy surveillance intervals when compared with decisions based on the pathology assessment of all identified polyps.
2. In order for a technology to be used to guide the decision to leave suspected rectosigmoid hyperplastic polyps 5 mm or less in size in place (without resection), the technology should provide at least 90% negative predictive value (NPV) (when used with high confidence) for adenomatous histology.

Although PIVI was developed to help direct the incorporation of endoscopic technologies into clinical practice rather than a legal standard of care, it has become a benchmark against which more recent resect-and-discard studies have been assessed. Again, the studies from academic centers performed well against this standard; Gupta and colleagues[66] analyzed the impact on surveillance intervals in a retrospective study of 410 patients with at least one polyp detected at colonoscopy. They could not determine the optical diagnosis in only 4 out of 1254 polyps (0.3%), and in vivo optical diagnosis for all polyps predicted the correct surveillance interval in 92.7% (95% CI 91.4%–96.2%) (based on the surveillance guidelines of 3 yearly colonoscopy for patients with 3 or more adenomas or with 1 or more advanced adenoma and 10 yearly for patients with 1 to 2 small adenomas or no adenomas). A total of 378 polyps were diagnosed as *not adenomas* by optical diagnosis, and of these 50 were found to be actually adenomas on histopathology resulting in NPV of 86.8% (95% CI 82.9%–90.0%). However, when optical diagnosis was limited to diminutive polyps in the rectosigmoid only, the NPV for diagnosing adenomas with NBI increased to 95.4% (95% CI 91.8%–97.7%) fulfilling both PIVI thresholds (albeit only when the surveillance interval for 1–2 adenomas is 10 years). This study, like the original DISCARD (Detect InSpect ChArcterise Resect and Discard) study, assessed both small and diminutive polyps and found no difference in accuracy between the two groups. Unsurprisingly when analyzing the cost reductions associated with a resect and discard policy, the greatest savings were possible if the strategy was used for all small and diminutive polyps, which in this study reduced the number of polyps sent to histopathology by 95% generating a potential total cost savings of $12,6681.95 or $309 per patient.

These results are similar to those reported by another academic unit using iSCAN instead of NBI to characterize small colonic polyps. Basford and colleagues[67] prospectively assessed 209 polyps in 84 patients and found it to have an accuracy of 94.7% and an NPV for diminutive adenomas in the rectosigmoid colon of 100%. In addition, iSCAN correctly predicted surveillance intervals in 97.2% of patients, comfortably fulfilling both PIVI performance thresholds. The same group[68] assessed the performance of FICE in the characterization of small polyps. They examined 232 polyps less than 10 mm in size and found that, although FICE correctly predicted surveillance intervals in 67 out of 69 patients, it had a lower NPV of 78%, less than the PIVI threshold of 90%.

As mentioned previously, the application of optical diagnosis to lesions 6 to 9 mm in size seems more controversial because advanced histologic features are more prevalent in this group. However, the much lower prevalence of 6 to 9 mm lesions compared with diminutive lesions in the general population would minimize their impact on the overall accuracy of optical diagnosis.[19]

The second clinical paradigm proposed by ASGE in PIVI involves leaving diminutive rectosigmoid hyperplastic polyps without resection (diagnose and disregard). This paradigm likely happens frequently in routine clinical practice with nonreporting of these lesions as hyperplastic polyps are thought to have no malignant potential. A recent survey of the American College of Gastroenterology confirmed wide variability in the management of diminutive polyps.[69] Although most responders (78.3%) reported that they never or rarely leave diminutive polyps in place in average-risk individuals, they were likely to leave them always or nearly always in certain scenarios, including patients with advanced age or comorbidities, those who are anticoagulated, in patients with history of nonadenomatous polyps in the same area, and when the appearances of polyp suggests nonadenomatous histology. Respondents with greater number of years in practice and those confident of being able to characterize polyps were more likely to leave polyps in place.

Hewett and colleagues[18] evaluated real-time histology of 235 rectosigmoid polyps using high-definition white light endoscopy and NBI. Most of the polyps (97.8%) were diminutive, and the accuracy of high-confidence predictions for those polyps was 99% (199 out of 201). The NPV for adenomatous histology was 75.6% (95% CI 60.5%–87.1%) overall for the diagnosis of all polyps. However, when only high-confidence predictions in diminutive polyps were analyzed, the NPV increased to 96.0% (95% CI 79.7%–99.9%) comfortably fulfilling the second PIVI threshold. This study confirmed that hyperplastic polyps are relatively easy to predict using NBI with a simple classification and that the diagnose-and-disregard paradigm may be easier to implement than resect and discard. The weakness of this study, however, is that it was performed by a single colonoscopist with great expertise and interest in optical diagnosis in an academic setting.

The fact that several studies based in community settings performed significantly less than the PIVI thresholds serves to illustrate that the resect-and-discard policy is not quite ready for general implementation. A prospective study from the United States involving community-based gastroenterologists[61] found that only 25% of gastroenterologists assessed polyps with 90% or greater accuracy using NBI. Although this study fulfilled the second PIVI threshold for diminutive rectosigmoid polyps, with NPV for adenomas of 91% (95% CI 86%–97%), it failed to satisfy the first threshold with the agreement of 80% (95% CI 77%–82%) for surveillance intervals based on optical diagnosis when compared with histopathology. Similarly, 2 other prospective studies from the Netherlands and Italy[60,62] showed the agreement between surveillance intervals of 81% and 83% respectively, well below the 90% PIVI threshold. Neither study analyzed the NPV for adenomas.

One of the postulates for this discrepancy may be insufficient training before studies in community settings.[70] Early studies of the impact of training suggested a short learning curve for using NBI for optical diagnosis. In a study by Raghavendra and colleagues,[71] 37 physicians (including medical residents, gastroenterology fellows, and faculty) participated in a 20-minute didactic teaching session on polyp characterization using still images of polyps seen with NBI without magnification. The participants completed a pretraining and post-training test; the accuracy of optical diagnosis had improved significantly, from 48% to 91% ($P = .001$). In addition, the interobserver agreement improved with training, from a pretest kappa coefficient of 0.05 to a post-test of 0.69 ($P<.001$).

As didactic teaching sessions are labor intensive and expensive, an alternative approach is to develop a computer-based teaching module for individual learning available on the Web or hospital intranet. Using such a module and with pretraining and post-training testing,[72] 21 participants of different levels of experience (novices, trainees, and experienced but not expert colonoscopists) evaluated NBI images of 30 small polyps. The accuracy of characterization improved significantly in the post-training test for all participants, with trainees achieving accuracy of 90%, comparable with experts. Similarly, there was an improvement in interobserver agreement following the training. However, the improvement in accuracy of optical diagnosis in both of these studies may have been driven largely by the artificial test setting in which the best polyp images were selected for inclusion in the test set, perhaps not representative of real-life performance.

When Rastogi and colleagues[73] developed a video-based teaching module, the accuracy of optical diagnosis achieved by nonexperts in both academic and community settings, although improved from pretraining testing, did not reach the level of accuracy of experts (81%). The fact that ex vivo training does not necessarily translate into clinical practice is further supported by the study by Ladabaum and colleagues[61] whereby 12 out of 13 community-based gastroenterologists identified adenomas with greater than 90% accuracy at the end of the training module and only 3 out of 12 did so at the end of in vivo study.

This finding suggests that a brief training module using still images and videos may not translate to high enough accuracy in routine clinical practice. It is likely that longer training will be required in vivo with feedback in order to achieve greater than 90% accuracy consistently.

The concept of degree of confidence of optical diagnosis may provide a solution for less experienced endoscopists. First introduced by Rex,[63] it essentially divides diagnoses into high and low confidence. It is accepted that polyps with any irregular features, such as central depression, irregular edges, or ulceration, would not be suitable for optical diagnosis and would be sent to histopathology as is the current practice. Polyps that do not have enough distinguishing features for an endoscopist to make the optical diagnosis with high confidence would also still be resected and sent for histopathology. In the study by Rex,[63] the accuracy of optical diagnosis was significantly higher when the diagnosis was made with high rather than low confidence. This finding was further supported by the findings of the study by Ladabaum and colleagues[61] whereby the adjusted odds ratio for high confidence as a predictor of accuracy was 1.8 (95% CI 1.3–2.5). It is anticipated that the percentage of high-confidence optical diagnoses would, therefore, increase with experience.

ARE WE READY TO IMPLEMENT A RESECT-AND-DISCARD, DIAGNOSE-AND-DISREGARD POLICY?

At present, it seems too early to suggest that this strategy is ready for routine clinical practice, especially in the community settings. Fundamental to the safe introduction of the strategy is the development of an enhanced and proven training program allied to a robust form of accreditation and then followed up by a process of audit and on-going quality assurance. A major obstacle to implementing optical diagnosis remains the fear of litigation as the responsibility for patient outcomes is no longer shared with histopathologists. Quality-assurance measures will need to be developed, including documentation of optical diagnosis. It is not yet clear whether high-definition still images or videos would be sufficient, but both present a storage problem for endoscopy units.

There is always resistance among medical professionals when dramatic changes to clinical practice are proposed.[74] The survey of the American College of Gastroenterology's members showed that around 50% of participants were not at all agreeable to a resect-and-discard approach, but less than 30% were not at all agreeable to leaving diminutive polyps in place if the guidelines endorsed this practice.

It does, however, seem as if the European guidelines are gently moving in support of this policy. The European Society of Gastrointestinal Endoscopy's guidelines[75] question the utility of surveillance for low-risk patients (1 or 2 adenomas). Several epidemiologic studies have assessed long-term CRC incidence/mortality in patients with 1 to 2 tubular adenomas with low-grade dysplasia and showed that these patients have a low long-term risk of developing CRC despite the lack of surveillance.[76,77] Accordingly, patients with 1 or 2 small polyps are advised to return to routine screening for both adenomas and hyperplastic lesions.

Furthermore, the recently published guidelines from the European Society of Gastrointestinal Endoscopy[78] on advanced imaging for the detection and differentiation of colorectal neoplasia suggest that virtual chromoendoscopy (NBI, iSCAN, and FICE) can be used under strictly controlled conditions for real-time optical diagnosis of diminutive colorectal polyps. The optical diagnosis has to be reported using validated scales, must be clearly photographically documented, and can be performed only by experienced endoscopists who are adequately trained and audited.

SUMMARY

Increased demand for colonoscopy combined with improved polyp detection rates has resulted in spiraling costs and increased needs for histopathology. An ability to correctly diagnose diminutive polyps optically at the time of colonoscopy would allow for small adenomas to be resected and discarded without the need for formal histopathology and for rectosigmoid hyperplastic polyps to be left in situ. This ability would allow surveillance intervals to be determined immediately after colonoscopy and, therefore, would potentially lead to significant time and cost savings with less patient risk from unnecessary polypectomies.

Routine implementation of a resect-and-discard policy based on optical diagnosis is still some way off in the future. A rigorous and efficacious training, accreditation, and quality-assurance program needs to be developed and validated. However, a carefully controlled resect-and-discard policy for diminutive polyps has now been endorsed in Europe, heralding the start of a fundamental and likely irresistible change in colonoscopic practice.

REFERENCES

1. U.S. Cancer Statistics Working Group. United States cancer statistics: 1999–2011 incidence and mortality web-based report. Atlanta (GA): Department of Health and Human Services, Centers for Disease Control and Prevention, and National Cancer Institute; 2014.

2. Vogelstein B, Fearon ER, Hamilton SR, et al. Genetic alterations during colorectal-tumor development. N Engl J Med 1988;319:525–32.

3. Citarda F, Tomaselli G, Capocaccia R, et al. Efficacy in standard clinical practice of colonoscopic polypectomy in reducing colorectal cancer incidence. Gut 2001; 48:812–5.

4. Winawer SJ, Zauber AG, Ho MN, et al. The National Polyp Study. Eur J Cancer Prev 1993;2(Suppl 2):83–7.

5. Rabeneck L, Paszat LF, Saskin R, et al. Association between colonoscopy rates and colorectal cancer mortality. Am J Gastroenterol 2010;105:1627–32.

6. Atkin WS, Edwards R, Kralj-Hans I, et al. Once-only flexible sigmoidoscopy screening in prevention of colorectal cancer: a multicentre randomised controlled trial. Lancet 2010;375:1624–33.

7. von Karsa L, Patnick J, Segnan N, et al. European guidelines for quality assurance in colorectal cancer screening and diagnosis: overview and introduction to the full supplement publication. Endoscopy 2013;45:51–9.

8. Levin B, Lieberman DA, McFarland B, et al. Screening and surveillance for the early detection of colorectal cancer and adenomatous polyps, 2008: a joint guideline from the American Cancer Society, the US Multi-Society Task Force on Colorectal Cancer, and the American College of Radiology. Gastroenterology 2008;134:1570–95.

9. Seeff LC, Richards TB, Shapiro JA, et al. How many endoscopies are performed for colorectal cancer screening? Results from CDC's survey of endoscopic capacity. Gastroenterology 2004;127:1670–7.

10. Wexner SD, Garbus JE, Singh JJ. A prospective analysis of 13,580 colonoscopies. Reevaluation of credentialing guidelines. Surg Endosc 2001;15:251–61.

11. Paspatis GA, Vardas E, Theodoropoulou A, et al. Complications of colonoscopy in a large public county hospital in Greece. A 10-year study. Dig Liver Dis 2008; 40:951–7.

12. Eckardt V, Kanzler G, Scmitt T, et al. Complications and adverse effects of colonoscopy with selective sedation. Gastrointest Endosc 1999;49:6.

13. Nelson D, McQuaid K, Bond J, et al. Procedural success and complications of large-scale screening colonoscopy. Gastrointest Endosc 2002;55:7.

14. Lieberman D, Moravec M, Holub J, et al. Polyp size and advanced histology in patients undergoing colonoscopy screening: implications for CT colonography. Gastroenterology 2008;135:1100–5.

15. Chen SC, Rex DK. Endoscopist can be more powerful than age and male gender in predicting adenoma detection at colonoscopy. Am J Gastroenterol 2007;102: 856–61.

16. Rex DK, Overhiser AJ, Chen SC, et al. Estimation of impact of American College of Radiology recommendations on CT colonography reporting for resection of high-risk adenoma findings. Am J Gastroenterol 2009;104:149–53.

17. Hassan C, Repici A, Zullo A, et al. Colonic polyps: are we ready to resect and discard? Gastrointest Endosc Clin N Am 2013;23:663–78.

18. Hewett DG, Huffman ME, Rex DK. Leaving distal colorectal hyperplastic polyps in place can be achieved with high accuracy by using narrow-band imaging: an observational study. Gastrointest Endosc 2012;76:374–80.

19. Hassan C, Pickhardt PJ, Kim DH, et al. Systematic review: distribution of advanced neoplasia according to polyp size at screening colonoscopy. Aliment Pharmacol Ther 2010;31:210–7.

20. Brenner H, Hoffmeister M, Stegmaier C, et al. Risk of progression of advanced adenomas to colorectal cancer by age and sex: estimates based on 840,149 screening colonoscopies. Gut 2007;56:1585–9.

21. Gupta N, Bansal A, Rao D, et al. Prevalence of advanced histological features in diminutive and small colon polyps. Gastrointest Endosc 2012;75:1022–30.
22. Hoff G, Foerster A, Vatn MH, et al. Epidemiology of polyps in the rectum and colon. Recovery and evaluation of unresected polyps 2 years after detection. Scand J Gastroenterol 1986;21:853–62.
23. Hofstad B, Vatn MH, Andersen SN, et al. Growth of colorectal polyps: redetection and evaluation of unresected polyps for a period of three years. Gut 1996;39:449–56.
24. Butterly LF, Chase MP, Pohl H, et al. Prevalence of clinically important histology in small adenomas. Clin Gastroenterol Hepatol 2006;4:343–8.
25. Levin B, Lieberman DA, McFarland B, et al. Screening and surveillance for the early detection of colorectal cancer and adenomatous polyps, 2008: a joint guideline from the American Cancer Society, the US Multi-Society Task Force on Colorectal Cancer, and the American College of Radiology. CA Cancer J Clin 2008;58:130–60.
26. Cairns SR, Scholefield JH, Steele RJ, et al. Guidelines for colorectal cancer screening and surveillance in moderate and high risk groups (update from 2002). Gut 2010;59:666–89.
27. Lieberman DA, Weiss DG, Harford WV, et al. Five-year colon surveillance after screening colonoscopy. Gastroenterology 2007;133:1077–85.
28. de Jonge V, Sint Nicolaas J, van Leerdam ME, et al. Systematic literature review and pooled analyses of risk factors for finding adenomas at surveillance colonoscopy. Endoscopy 2011;43:560–72.
29. Atkin WS, Valori R, Kuipers EJ, et al. European guidelines for quality assurance in colorectal cancer screening and diagnosis. First edition–colonoscopic surveillance following adenoma removal. Endoscopy 2012;44(Suppl 3):SE151–63.
30. Brooker J, Shah S, Saunders B. Current issues in the management of colonic polyps: a retrospective review of 2806 consecutive polypectomies [abstract]. Gut 2002;50(Suppl 2):1–125.
31. Yamada T, Tamura S, Onishi S, et al. A comparison of magnifying chromoendoscopy versus histopathology of forceps biopsy specimen in the diagnosis of minute flat adenoma of the colon. Dig Dis Sci 2009;54:2002–8.
32. Rex DK, Alikhan M, Cummings OW, et al. Accuracy of pathologic interpretation of colorectal polyps by general pathologists in community practice. Gastrointest Endosc 1999;50:468–74.
33. Turner JK, Williams GT, Morgan M, et al. Interobserver agreement in the reporting of colorectal polyp pathology among bowel cancer screening pathologists in Wales. Histopathology 2013;62:916–24.
34. Costantini M, Sciallero S, Giannini A, et al. Interobserver agreement in the histologic diagnosis of colorectal polyps. The experience of the multicenter adenoma colorectal study (SMAC). J Clin Epidemiol 2003;56:209–14.
35. Saini SD, Kim HM, Schoenfeld P. Incidence of advanced adenomas at surveillance colonoscopy in patients with a personal history of colon adenomas: a meta-analysis and systematic review. Gastrointest Endosc 2006;64:614–26.
36. Bonithon-Kopp C, Piard F, Fenger C, et al. Colorectal adenoma characteristics as predictors of recurrence. Dis Colon Rectum 2004;47:323–33.
37. Martinez ME, Baron JA, Lieberman DA, et al. A pooled analysis of advanced colorectal neoplasia diagnoses after colonoscopic polypectomy. Gastroenterology 2009;136:832–41.
38. Kessler WR, Imperiale TF, Klein RW, et al. A quantitative assessment of the risks and cost savings of forgoing histologic examination of diminutive polyps. Endoscopy 2011;43:683–91.

39. Hassan C, Pickhardt PJ, Rex DK. A resect and discard strategy would improve cost-effectiveness of colorectal cancer screening. Clin Gastroenterol Hepatol 2010;8:865–9, 869.e1–3.

40. Machida H, Sano Y, Hamamoto Y, et al. Narrow-band imaging in the diagnosis of colorectal mucosal lesions: a pilot study. Endoscopy 2004;36:1094–8.

41. Apel D, Jakobs R, Schilling D, et al. Accuracy of high resolution of chromoendoscopy in prediction of histologic findings in diminutive lesions of the rectosigmoid. Gastrointest Endosc 2006;63:824–8.

42. Tischendorf JJ, Wasmuth HE, Koch A, et al. Value of magnifying chromoendoscopy and narrow band imaging (NBI) in classifying colorectal polyps: a prospective controlled study. Endoscopy 2007;39:1092–6.

43. De Palma GD, Rega M, Masone S, et al. Conventional colonoscopy and magnified chromoendoscopy for the endoscopic histological prediction of diminutive colorectal polyps: a single operator study. World J Gastroenterol 2006;12:2402–5.

44. Fu KI, Sano Y, Kato S, et al. Chromoendoscopy using indigo carmine dye spraying with magnifying observation is the most reliable method for differential diagnosis between non-neoplastic and neoplastic colorectal lesions: a prospective study. Endoscopy 2004;36:1089–93.

45. Su MY, Ho YP, Chen PC, et al. Magnifying endoscopy with indigo carmine contrast for differential diagnosis of neoplastic and non-neoplastic colonic polyps. Dig Dis Sci 2004;49:1123–7.

46. Kudo S, Tamura S, Nakajima T, et al. Diagnosis of colorectal tumorous lesions by magnifying endoscopy. Gastrointest Endosc 1996;44:8–14.

47. Togashi K, Konishi F, Ishizuka T, et al. Efficacy of magnifying endoscopy in the differential diagnosis of neoplastic and non-neoplastic polyps of the large bowel. Dis Colon Rectum 1999;42:1602–8.

48. East JE, Suzuki N, Saunders BP. Comparison of magnified pit pattern interpretation with narrow band imaging versus chromoendoscopy for diminutive colonic polyps: a pilot study. Gastrointest Endosc 2007;66:310–6.

49. Konerding MA, Fait E, Gaumann A. 3D microvascular architecture of pre-cancerous lesions and invasive carcinomas of the colon. Br J Cancer 2001;84:1354–62.

50. Sano Y, Ikematsu H, Fu KI, et al. Meshed capillary vessels by use of narrow-band imaging for differential diagnosis of small colorectal polyps. Gastrointest Endosc 2009;69:278–83.

51. Hirata M, Tanaka S, Oka S, et al. Magnifying endoscopy with narrow band imaging for diagnosis of colorectal tumors. Gastrointest Endosc 2007;65:988–95.

52. Hewett DG, Kaltenbach T, Sano Y, et al. Validation of a simple classification system for endoscopic diagnosis of small colorectal polyps using narrow-band imaging. Gastroenterology 2012;143:599–607.e1.

53. Hirata M, Tanaka S, Oka S, et al. Evaluation of microvessels in colorectal tumors by narrow band imaging magnification. Gastrointest Endosc 2007;66:945–52.

54. Su MY, Hsu CM, Ho YP, et al. Comparative study of conventional colonoscopy, chromoendoscopy, and narrow-band imaging systems in differential diagnosis of neoplastic and nonneoplastic colonic polyps. Am J Gastroenterol 2006;101:2711–6.

55. Rogart JN, Jain D, Siddiqui UD, et al. Narrow-band imaging without high magnification to differentiate polyps during real-time colonoscopy: improvement with experience. Gastrointest Endosc 2008;68:1136–45.

56. Rastogi A, Pondugula K, Bansal A, et al. Recognition of surface mucosal and vascular patterns of colon polyps by using narrow-band imaging: interobserver and intraobserver agreement and prediction of polyp histology. Gastrointest Endosc 2009;69:716–22.

57. East JE, Suzuki N, Stavrinidis M, et al. Narrow band imaging for colonoscopic surveillance in hereditary non-polyposis colorectal cancer. Gut 2008;57:65–70.
58. Chiu HM, Chang CY, Chen CC, et al. A prospective comparative study of narrow-band imaging, chromoendoscopy, and conventional colonoscopy in the diagnosis of colorectal neoplasia. Gut 2007;56:373–9.
59. McGill SK, Evangelou E, Ioannidis JP, et al. Narrow band imaging to differentiate neoplastic and non-neoplastic colorectal polyps in real time: a meta-analysis of diagnostic operating characteristics. Gut 2013;62:1704–13.
60. Kuiper T, Marsman WA, Jansen JM, et al. Accuracy for optical diagnosis of small colorectal polyps in nonacademic settings. Clin Gastroenterol Hepatol 2012;10: 1016–20 [quiz: e79].
61. Ladabaum U, Fioritto A, Mitani A, et al. Real-time optical biopsy of colon polyps with narrow band imaging in community practice does not yet meet key thresholds for clinical decisions. Gastroenterology 2013;144:81–91.
62. Paggi S, Rondonotti E, Amato A, et al. Resect and discard strategy in clinical practice: a prospective cohort study. Endoscopy 2012;44:899–904.
63. Rex DK. Narrow-band imaging without optical magnification for histologic analysis of colorectal polyps. Gastroenterology 2009;136:1174–81.
64. Ignjatovic A, East JE, Suzuki N, et al. Optical diagnosis of small colorectal polyps at routine colonoscopy (Detect InSpect ChAracterise Resect and Discard; DISCARD trial): a prospective cohort study. Lancet Oncol 2009;10:1171–8.
65. Rex DK, Kahi C, O'Brien M, et al. The American Society for Gastrointestinal Endoscopy PIVI (Preservation and Incorporation of Valuable Endoscopic Innovations) on real-time endoscopic assessment of the histology of diminutive colorectal polyps. Gastrointest Endosc 2011;73:419–22.
66. Gupta N, Bansal A, Rao D, et al. Accuracy of in vivo optical diagnosis of colon polyp histology by narrow-band imaging in predicting colonoscopy surveillance intervals. Gastrointest Endosc 2012;75:494–502.
67. Basford PJ, Longcroft-Wheaton G, Higgins B, et al. High-definition endoscopy with i-Scan for evaluation of small colon polyps: the HiSCOPE study. Gastrointest Endosc 2014;79:111–8.
68. Longcroft-Wheaton GR, Higgins B, Bhandari P. Flexible spectral imaging color enhancement and indigo carmine in neoplasia diagnosis during colonoscopy: a large prospective UK series. Eur J Gastroenterol Hepatol 2011;23:903–11.
69. Gellad ZF, Voils CI, Lin L, et al. Clinical practice variation in the management of diminutive colorectal polyps: results of a national survey of gastroenterologists. Am J Gastroenterol 2013;108:873–8.
70. Rastogi A. Optical diagnosis of small colorectal polyp histology with high-definition colonoscopy using narrow band imaging. Clin Endosc 2013;46:120–9.
71. Raghavendra M, Hewett DG, Rex DK. Differentiating adenomas from hyperplastic colorectal polyps: narrow-band imaging can be learned in 20 minutes. Gastrointest Endosc 2010;72:572–6.
72. Ignjatovic A, Thomas-Gibson S, East JE, et al. Development and validation of a training module on the use of narrow-band imaging in differentiation of small adenomas from hyperplastic colorectal polyps. Gastrointest Endosc 2011;73:128–33.
73. Rastogi A, Rao DS, Gupta N, et al. Impact of a computer-based teaching module on characterization of diminutive colon polyps by using narrow-band imaging by non-experts in academic and community practice: a video-based study. Gastrointest Endosc 2014;79(3):390–8.
74. Hogan RB 3rd, Brill JV, Littenberg G, et al. Predict, resect, and discard... really? Gastrointest Endosc 2012;75:503–5.

75. Hassan C, Quintero E, Dumonceau JM, et al. Post-polypectomy colonoscopy surveillance: European Society of Gastrointestinal Endoscopy (ESGE) guideline. Endoscopy 2013;45:842–51.

76. Atkin WS, Morson BC, Cuzick J. Long-term risk of colorectal cancer after excision of rectosigmoid adenomas. N Engl J Med 1992;326:658–62.

77. Cottet V, Jooste V, Fournel I, et al. Long-term risk of colorectal cancer after adenoma removal: a population-based cohort study. Gut 2012;61:1180–6.

78. Kaminski MF, Hassan C, Bisschops R, et al. Advanced imaging for detection and differentiation of colorectal neoplasia: European Society of Gastrointestinal Endoscopy (ESGE) guideline. Endoscopy 2014;46:435–49.

79. Fearon ER, Vogelstein B. A genetic model for colorectal tumorigenesis. Cell 1990; 61(5):759–67.

80. Ignjatovic A. Recognition of colonic dysplasia at colonoscopy using advanced technology (MD res thesis). Imperial College London; 2011. p. 187.

81. Wilson JM. The role of macrophage migration inhibitory factor in intestinal tumorigenesis (PhD thesis). University of Leeds; 2005. p. 266.

82. Shinya H, Wolff WI. Morphology, anatomic distribution and cancer potential of colonic polyps. Ann Surg 1979;190:679–83.

83. O'Brien MJ, Winawer SJ, Zauber AG, et al, The National Polyp Study. Patient and polyp characteristics associated with high-grade dysplasia in colorectal adenomas. Gastroenterology 1990;98:371–9.

84. Gschwantler M, Kriwanek S, Langner E, et al. High-grade dysplasia and invasive carcinoma in colorectal adenomas: a multivariate analysis of the impact of adenoma and patient characteristics. Eur J Gastroenterol Hepatol 2002;14:183–8.

85. Sprung DJ. Prevalence of adenocarcinoma in small adenomas. American Journal of Gastroenterology 2006;S199.

86. Kim DH, Pickhardt PJ, Taylor AJ. Characteristics of advanced adenomas detected at CT colonographic screening: implications for appropriate polyp size thresholds for polypectomy versus surveillance. AJR Am J Roentgenol 2007; 188:940–4.

87. Bretagne JF, Manfredi S, Piette C, et al. Yield of high-grade dysplasia based on polyp size detected at colonoscopy: a series of 2295 examinations following a positive fecal occult blood test in a population-based study. Dis Colon Rectum 2010;53:339–45.

88. Repici A, Hassan C, Radaelli F, et al. Accuracy of narrow-band imaging in predicting colonoscopy surveillance intervals and histology of distal diminutive polyps: results from a multicenter, prospective trial. Gastrointest Endosc 2013; 78:106–14.

89. Kolligs FT, Crispin A, Graser A, et al. Risk factors for advanced neoplasia within subcentimetric polyps: implications for diagnostic imaging. Gut 2013;62:863–70.

90. Ignjatovic A, East JE, Guenther T, et al. What is the most reliable imaging modality for small colonic polyp characterization? Study of white-light, autofluorescence, and narrow-band imaging. Endoscopy 2011;43:94–9.

91. Kato S, Fu KI, Sano Y, et al. Magnifying colonoscopy as a non-biopsy technique for differential diagnosis of non-neoplastic and neoplastic lesions. World J Gastroenterol 2006;12:1416–20.

92. Togashi K, Konishi F. Magnification chromo-colonoscopy. ANZ J Surg 2006;76: 1101–5.

93. Konishi K, Kaneko K, Kurahashi T, et al. A comparison of magnifying and nonmagnifying colonoscopy for diagnosis of colorectal polyps: A prospective study. Gastrointest Endosc 2003;57:48–53.

Advanced Polypectomy and Resection Techniques

Amir Klein, BSc, MD[a], Michael J. Bourke, MBBS, FRACPS[b],*

KEYWORDS

- Polypectomy • Endoscopic mucosal resection (EMR)
- Endoscopic submucosal dissection (ESD) • Lateral spreading tumors (LSTs)
- Advanced mucosal neoplasia (AMN) • Submucosal invasion (SMI)

KEY POINTS

- Endoscopic mucosal resection (EMR) is a safe, cost-effective and curative intervention for most advanced mucosal neoplasms of the colon.
- Lesion morphology can be used to stratify for the risk of submucosal invasion (SMI).
- En bloc EMR is usually limited to lesions less than or equal to 20 mm. Larger lesions are best treated by piecemeal EMR or, if early invasive disease is suspected, endoscopic submucosal dissection (ESD).
- Real-time macroscopic assessment of lesion type and risk of SMI may be valuable in therapeutic strategy selection.
- Recurrence is seen in 10% to 20% of EMR at first surveillance after piecemeal resection but is effectively treated endoscopically with long-term remission.
- In the colon, ESD has little if any long-term advantage compared with EMR.
- ESD is associated with a longer procedure time, increased risk of perforation, mandatory multiday hospitalization, and increased costs compared with EMR.
- Bleeding and perforation can be adequately managed endoscopically. Careful assessment of the postresection mucosal defect is a vital component of the procedure.

INTRODUCTION

Most colorectal cancer (CRC) arises from adenomatous polyps through a process of accumulated molecular abnormalities, leading to increased cytologic dysplasia and eventually cancer.[1] The gradual nature of this process allows effective screening and intervention. Long-term follow-up clearly shows the effectiveness of colonoscopy and polypectomy in reducing the incidence and mortality of CRC.[2,3]

[a] Department of Gastroenterology and Hepatology, Westmead Hospital, Crn Hawkesbury & Darcy Rds, Sydney, Westmead New South Wales 2145, Australia; [b] Department of Gastroenterology and Hepatology, Westmead Hospital, University of Sydney, Crn Hawkesbury & Darcy Rds, Sydney, Westmead New South Wales 2145, Australia
* Corresponding author.
E-mail address: michael@citywestgastro.com.au

Gastrointest Endoscopy Clin N Am 25 (2015) 303–333
http://dx.doi.org/10.1016/j.giec.2014.11.005
1052-5157/15/$ – see front matter © 2015 Elsevier Inc. All rights reserved.

More than 80% to 90% of polyps encountered during routine colonoscopy are less than 10 mm in size, do not contain advanced disease, and can be readily treated with conventional snare polypectomy by an appropriately trained endoscopist.[4–6]

Approximately 5% of adenomatous polyps are flat and sessile lesions larger than 10 mm.[7] They may show extensive lateral growth along the bowel surface before developing an invasive component. The term advanced mucosal neoplasia (AMN) may be used to describe flat and sessile lesions larger than 20 mm.[6,8]

Treatment of colonic AMN may require the use of advanced polypectomy techniques such as endoscopic mucosal resection (EMR), endoscopic submucosal dissection (ESD), or hybrid techniques. Technique selection is influenced by lesion morphology, location, patient comorbidities, and local expertise. Prospective studies have shown that wide-field EMR is safe and effective.[9] Compared with surgery, it is substantially more cost-effective[10] and may confer a mortality benefit, particularly in elderly patients with comorbidities.[11]

Postprocedural complications are most common following complex endoscopic resection.[12,13] Bleeding (both immediate and delayed) and perforation are most commonly encountered. Also, incomplete resection leading to residual disease and luminal stenosis after circumferential resection may occur.

INDICATIONS/CONTRAINDICATIONS AND LIMITATIONS

Accepted indications and contraindications for advanced endoscopic resection in the colon are summarized in **Box 1**. In general, all patients found to have colonic AMN should be considered for endoscopic therapy with an experienced clinician. Modeling using the (CR) Physiologic and operative severity score for the enumeration of mortality and morbidity (POSSUM) and the Association of Coloproctology of Great Britain and Ireland score (ACPGBI) scores applied to a large prospective multicenter AMN cohort has shown this to be associated with less morbidity and mortality. In addition, markedly reduced costs with a predicted difference of approximately 6 days' hospital stay and approximately US$10,000 per patient savings were calculated compared with surgical resection.[10,11]

Box 1
Indications and contraindications for advanced endoscopic resection in the colon

Indications

Large sessile or laterally spreading adenomas or serrated lesions larger than 20 mm

Lesions in difficult locations: appendiceal orifice, ileocecal valve, lower rectum, behind folds

Polyps in difficult situations: following failed removal attempts, lesions over scars

Large thick-stalked pedunculated polyps

Large colonic lipomas

Lesions in chronic inflammatory bowel disease

Contraindications

Findings suggesting deep invasion (deep irregular depression, fold convergence, firm consistency, nonlifting, type Vn/Vi Kudo pit pattern, type IIIb Sano vascular pattern, type 3 Narrow-band Imaging International Colorectal Endoscopic [NICE] criteria)

Unavailability of supporting infrastructure (dedicated trained staff, tertiary level radiological and surgical support)

Inadequate experience and/or training

Endoscopic Versus Surgical Resection

Even extensive colonic lesions limited to the mucosa can be cured with endoscopic resection, because the unique absence of lymphatics in the colonic mucosa precludes lymph node metastasis (LNM).[14]

Submucosal invasion (SMI) is the hallmark of CRC, and is associated with LNM in 1% to 16% of endoscopically attempted resections.[14–18] The risk of LNM is related to the depth of invasion, the tumor grade, and the presence or absence of lymphovascular invasion (LVI). When invasion is limited to the submucosa (T1 lesions) further stratification into high-risk and low-risk groups can be performed.[14] Low-risk features include SMI depth less than 1 mm, well-differentiated tumor grade, and absence of LVI.[14,15,18] In such cases, endoscopic therapy may be considered adequate when resection is complete and the deep and lateral margins are negative.[14,18] High-risk features include tumor budding, LVI, poorly differentiated tumor grade, and SMI depth greater than 1 mm. If found in an EMR specimen or predicted by endoscopic assessment, surgical resection with lymph node dissection is appropriate.[14,18,19]

Real-time endoscopic prediction of SMI risk may be challenging. The hallmark of invasive disease is disorganization or loss of the pit pattern and/or microvascular pattern. Endoscopists may be alerted to this by a transition point in the surface structure of the lesion from the regular pits (type III or IV) to a disordered, less obvious pit structure (discussed later).

The decision to proceed with surgery or endoscopic therapy should also take into account factors such as patient comorbidities and lesion location. For example, surgery in the rectum compared with the right colon is more complicated and associated with higher morbidity, whereas EMR in the right colon is associated with an increased risk of delayed bleeding (Fig. 1).

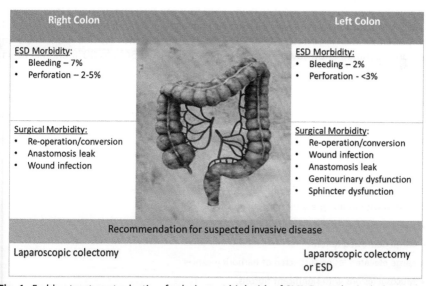

Fig. 1. En bloc treatment selection for lesions at high risk of SMI. Examples include nongranular lesions with depressed area (c component) or focal area of altered pit pattern (Vi [irregularly mixed pit types]). If careful lesion assessment predicts deep SMI, endoscopic treatment should not be considered.

Endoscopic Mucosal Resection Versus Endoscopic Submucosal Dissection

Performing ESD in the colon differs from gastric ESD. A narrow elongated lumen, a more difficult and less stable scope position, and a thinner wall all contribute to a more challenging procedure with a higher risk for perforation.[18,20] Consequently, colonic ESD requires careful consideration and should be reserved for specific indications. The Japan Colorectal ESD Standardization Implementation Working Group issued recommendations on the indications for colonic ESD. These recommendations are summarized in **Box 2**.[21–23] Most Western experts do not support the use of ESD for noninvasive disease.

The benefit of en bloc excision by ESD rather than piecemeal EMR is based on the potential for improved outcomes in 3 areas:

1. More accurate histologic assessment; this may be of benefit with subtle SMI that could be missed or misinterpreted by histopathologists when assessing multiple piecemeal specimens. In practice, this has not proved to be clinically relevant.
2. Reduced recurrence; however, recent long-term outcomes from large prospective EMR series show that recurrence is usually diminutive and easily treated in follow-up and does not affect the likelihood of long-term remission.[9,12,18,24,25]
3. The possibility of cure in low-risk SMI; based on large Japanese series to date, such cases are infrequent, comprising only approximately 10% of patients treated by ESD.[26]

Thus in most cases an initial ESD strategy to treat AMN offers little additional benefit to patients, but exposes them to increased procedural risks and the health service to increased costs, decreased colonoscopy capacity, and mandatory multiday hospital admission for these patients.[26]

Available data suggest that, compared with EMR, ESD has a higher rate of curative resection (91%–95% vs 79.6%).[9,12,18,25] In a systematic review of 22 studies with 2841 treated lesions[27] ESD en bloc resection rates of 96% with an R0 rate of 88% were observed. However, most of these studies were retrospective and thus subject to bias, because cases in which ESD was not possible or was technically unsuccessful are generally not reported. Moreover, recent prospective studies performed in Western countries show lower en bloc resection rates of 64% to 90% and R0 rates of 53% to 80%.[28–30]

Box 2
Indications for colonic ESD

- Large (>20 mm) lesion amenable to endoscopic treatment in which en bloc EMR resection is difficult
- Laterally spreading tumor-nongranular: particularly of the pseudodepressed type
- Lesions with Kudo type V pit pattern
- Carcinoma with known SMI
- Large depressed lesion
- Large elevated lesion suspected of harboring cancer
- Mucosal lesions with significant fibrosis
- Local residual early cancer after prior endoscopic resection
- Sporadic localized tumors in chronic inflammation, such as ulcerative colitis

ESD is also associated with a longer procedure time (75–121 minutes vs 25 minutes), increased risk of perforation (3%–7.4% vs 1%–2%), increased risk of hospitalization (100% vs 7.7%), and increased costs compared with EMR.[9,12,25,31]

Taken together, it seems that ESD confers little, if any, significant advantage compared with EMR in the colon and has not been proved thus far to be associated with better long-term outcome.[26]

Proficiency and Safety

Performing safe and effective endoscopic resection of AMN requires selective expertise and should preferably be performed in tertiary referral centers with a high volume of cases. Physician training in EMR and ESD requires dedicated training programs that incorporate clinical, interpretive, and technical skills. Equally important is the availability of highly trained nursing staff and surgical, radiological, and anesthetic support.

TECHNIQUE/PROCEDURE

Patient assessment and preparation
- Candidates for advanced endoscopic resection should fully consent to the procedure and its alternatives.
- A comprehensive medical history and medication list is essential. Newer generation anticoagulants and antiplatelets are increasingly used. These agents are highly potent, have a rapid onset of action, and physicians should be aware of the risks and recommendations regarding cessation and resumption of these medications in the extreme environment of advanced endoscopic resection (**Table 1**).[32–34]
- The patient's comorbidities need to be factored into the therapeutic process at all stages.
- Dedicated referral letters should include a description of the lesion location, size, Paris morphology, and color images.
- Biopsies are not mandatory because they rarely provide additional data relevant to treatment selection. Aggressive tunneling biopsies are best avoided because of their propensity to create submucosal fibrosis, which can require a more technically complicated procedure.
- Standard colonoscopic techniques and patient positioning are used to reach the lesion.
- The lesion should be positioned at 6 o'clock in the endoscopic field, preferably on the nondependent side. Ideally, the patient should also be positioned in a way that any fluid or resected specimens accumulate away from the lesion. Thus the working field is not obscured and, in the event of complications (bleeding or perforation), access is optimized and the risk of extraluminal contamination is minimized.
- Polyps in difficult positions (eg, around folds, ileocecal valve [ICV], flexures) may require multiple patient position and endoscope changes and ancillary devices such as a short distal cap attachment.

TECHNICAL PREPARATIONS
Submucosal Injectate

The submucosal injection solution is composed of 3 main elements: the colloid solution, diluted epinephrine, and an inert dye (indigo carmine or methylene blue).

- The colloid fluid creates a cushion between the mucosa and muscularis propria (MP), thus reducing the risk of deep tissue entrapment in the snare, transmural

Table 1
Recommendations on cessation and resumption of antiplatelets and anticoagulation medications in high-risk advanced endoscopic resection

	Mode of Action	Elimination/Metabolism Route	Cessation: Preprocedure		Resumption: Postprocedure	
			High-risk Thromboembolic Condition	Low-risk Thromboembolic Condition	High-risk Thromboembolic Condition	Low-risk Thromboembolic Condition
Aspirin	COX inactivation	—	No	7 d before	NA	POD 1
Clopidogrel	ADP receptor antagonist	Hepatic	7 d before[a]	7 d before	POD 1	POD 1
Prasugrel	ADP receptor antagonist	Hepatic	7 d before[a]	7 d before	POD 1	POD 1
Warfarin	Vitamin K antagonist	Hepatic	5 d before[b]	5 d before	POD 1[b]	POD 1
Dabigatran	Direct Thrombin inhibition	Renal	5 d before[c]	5 d before[c]	POD 2[d]	POD 7[d]
Rivaroxaban	Factor Xa inhibition	Renal	3 d before[c]	3 d before[c]	POD 2[d]	POD 7[d]
Apixaban	Factor Xa inhibition	Renal	3 d before[c]	3 d before[c]	POD 2[d]	POD 7[d]

Abbreviations: ADP, adenosine diphosphate; COX, cyclooxygenase; POD, postoperative day.

[a] High-risk conditions always warrant discussion with the patient's cardiologist (for clopidogrel, presence of coronary artery stents; for anticoagulants, prosthetic metal heart valve, atrial fibrillation plus mitral stenosis, <3 months following venous thromboembolism event, thrombophilia syndromes).

[b] For high-risk condition, start low-molecular-weight heparin (LMWH) 2 days after stopping warfarin; omit LMWH on day of procedure. On resumption of warfarin, continue LMWH until adequate International Normalized Ratio is reached.

[c] Recommendations are for patients with normal renal function. Impaired renal function warrants longer cessation of dabigatran and rivaroxaban.

[d] The ideal timing of resumption of newer anticoagulation agents following high-risk endoscopic procedures is not known. Expert opinions are presented here.

Data from Baron TH, Kamath PS, McBane RD. New anticoagulant and antiplatelet agents: a primer for the gastroenterologist. Clin Gastroenterol Hepatol 2014;12(2):187–95; and Veitch AM, Baglin TP, Gershlick AH, et al. Guidelines for the management of anticoagulant and antiplatelet therapy in patients undergoing endoscopic procedures. Gut 2008;57(9):1322–9.

thermal injury, and perforation. Normal saline (NS) is commonly used; however, in a randomized trial, the inexpensive colloid plasma volume expander succinylated gelatin (Gelofusine; Braun, Melsungen, Germany) was superior to NS, requiring significantly fewer injections, fewer resections, and an overall reduced EMR time.[35]

- Diluted epinephrine (adrenaline, 1:100,000) in the injectate may be used to reduce minute bleeding, keeping the EMR field dry and delaying the dispersion of the submucosal injectate. It does not seem to significantly alter clinically significant post-EMR bleeding (CSPEB).
- An inert dye (80 mg of indigo carmine or 20 mg of methylene blue in a 500-mL solution) avid for the connective tissue of the submucosa is also added to the solution. This dye facilitates better delineation of the lesion margins, especially in Paris 0-IIa/IIb, nongranular (NG), or serrated lesions. In addition, the extent of the submucosal cushion is defined and the correct plane of resection can be confirmed at all times.[6,8]

The Electrosurgical Unit Settings

Microprocessor-controlled electrosurgical generators delivering alternating cycles of high-frequency short-pulse cutting with more prolonged coagulation current are now most commonly used (VIO 300D; ERBE, Tübingen, Germany. ESG100; Olympus Medical, Tokyo, Japan). Tissue impedance is sensed via signals from the return electrode, adjusting power output in order to avoid deep tissue injury.

Carbon Dioxide Insufflation

The routine use of CO_2 for insufflation during endoscopic procedures has gained wide acceptance in recent years. Multiple studies comparing the use of CO_2 with air insufflation have consistently shown reduce postprocedural pain and bloating without any adverse effects.[36] The use of CO_2 insufflation during EMR of large colonic lesions has been shown to significantly reduce postprocedural admissions for pain,[37] which improves and clarifies postprocedural decision making, reducing unnecessary imaging and cross-team consultations.

Snares

A variety of snares are available for use in advanced colonic resection. The choice of a specific snare may be influenced by lesion size, morphology, and location; however, on many occasions it is a personal preference (**Fig. 2**). Stiff serrated (spiral) snares are preferred to increase tissue capture. The 20-mm spiral snare (wire diameter, 0.48 mm) is mainly used for large en bloc or wide-field piecemeal resections. The 15-mm braided snare is also commonly used for piecemeal EMR. Additional snares of various sizes (10–20 mm and occasionally larger) and shapes (oval, round, and hexagonal) are occasionally required. Small thin wire snares (wire diameter, 0.3 mm) are used to remove tissue in difficult locations and situations (periappendiceal, submucosal fibrosis) and small residual tissue within and at the margin of the defect.

APPROACH
Lesion Assessment

Endoscopic assessment before lesion resection is essential. This assessment entails an overview evaluation of lesion morphology, followed by targeted interrogation of any suspicious areas. A thorough assessment can identify lesions with significant scarring or inaccessibility and may also identify lesions with possible SMI, which may dictate a change in the endoscopic approach or referral for surgical treatment.

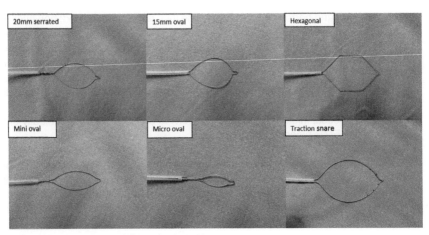

Fig. 2. Various snares used for colonic EMR.

Overview

The Paris classification of superficial neoplasia[38,39] should be used for morphologic classification (**Fig. 3**). Polypoid lesions are elevated more than 2.5 mm above the surrounding mucosa. They are divided into sessile (0-Is), pedunculated (0-Ip), or mixed (0-Isp) types. Nonpolypoid lesions may be slightly elevated (0-IIa), completely flat (0-IIb), or slightly depressed (0-IIc). Excavated lesions are labeled (0-III). Sessile lesions can be further categorized based on their surface topography into granular (G), nongranular (NG), or mixed morphologies (**Fig. 4**).

Paris classification and surface topography may be used to predict lesion histopathology and stratify the risk of SMI.[9,40–43] Low-risk lesions include homogeneous 0-IIa G types. The highest risk lesions are 0-IIa + c NG types. Intermediate risk lesions are

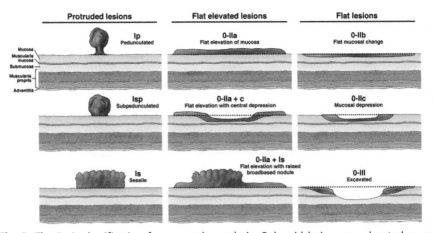

Fig. 3. The Paris classification for mucosal neoplasia. Polypoid lesions are elevated more than 2.5 mm above the surrounding mucosa. They are divided into sessile (0-Is), pedunculated (0-Ip) or mixed (0-Isp) types. Nonpolypoid lesions may be slightly elevated (0-IIa), completely flat (0-IIb), slightly depressed (0-IIc), or excavated (0-III). (*From* Holt BA, Bourke MJ. Wide field endoscopic resection for advanced colonic mucosal neoplasia: current status and future directions. Clin Gastroenterol Hepatol 2012;10(9):970; with permission.)

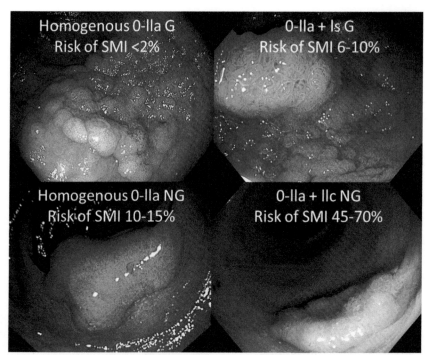

Fig. 4. Common morphologic types of AMN and their corresponding risk of SMI. (*Data from* Moss A, Bourke MJ, Williams SJ, et al. Endoscopic mucosal resection outcomes and prediction of submucosal cancer from advanced colonic mucosal neoplasia. Gastroenterology 2011;140(7):1909–18; and Wada Y, Kashida H, Kudo S, et al. Diagnostic accuracy of pit pattern and vascular pattern analyses in colorectal lesions. Dig Endosc 2010;22(3):192–9.)

heterogenous 0-IIa types with a depressed (IIc) or elevated (Is) component. Furthermore, the 0-Is nodule or 0-IIc depressed component in a flat lesion are the mostly likely sites to harbor SMI.[6,9] **Fig. 4** summarizes the relative risk of SMI in commonly encountered morphologic types. Recognition of these high-risk features should guide targeted surface assessment of the lesion and may ultimately dictate a change in the treatment strategy.

Focal interrogation
Focal interrogation is vital and involves assessing areas at risk of SMI, particularly nodules or depressed areas, evaluating the pit pattern and vascular patterns (VP). The mucosal pit pattern was initially described with the use of chromoendoscopy by Kudo and colleagues[40] 2 decades ago. The use of high-definition white-light endoscopy may now achieve sufficient accuracy in most situations.

AMN most commonly display pit pattern types III (large or elongated pits) or IV (branching gyruslike pits). Type III predicts tubular adenoma (TA) and type IV tubulovillous adenoma (TVA). Type V is associated with cancer. Vi (irregularly mixed pits) suggests at least intramucosal cancer (World Health Organization 2010 now terms this high-grade dysplasia) and Vn (nonstructural pit pattern) is predictive of submucosal invasive malignancy.[9,44]

Narrow-band imaging (NBI) and postprocessing imaging techniques, such as Fujinon intelligent chromoendoscopy and I-scan, highlight the mucosal VP. The modified Sano system classifies lesions by their mucosal microvasculature as seen with

NBI.[45] An organized brown capillary network surrounding the pits can be seen in tubular adenomas, whereas irregular complex branching capillaries or avascular areas suggest advanced histology and cancer.[45–48]

Pit pattern and VP have also been shown to accurately predict deep SMI (>1000 microm).[44,49,50] More recently, the Narrow-band Imaging International Colorectal Endoscopic (NICE) criteria, a composite score including lesion color, surface pattern, and capillary pattern, has been shown to accurately predict SMI in flat colonic lesions.[51] **Fig. 5** summarizes the various focal interrogation techniques.

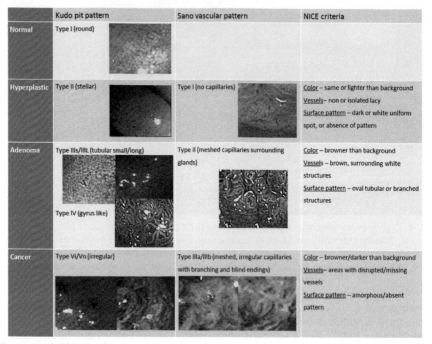

	Kudo pit pattern	Sano vascular pattern	NICE criteria
Normal	Type I (round)		
Hyperplastic	Type II (stellar)	Type I (no capillaries)	Color – same or lighter than background; Vessels – non or isolated lacy; Surface pattern – dark or white uniform spot, or absence of pattern
Adenoma	Type IIIs/IIIL (tubular small/long); Type IV (gyrus like)	Type II (meshed capillaries surrounding glands)	Color – browner than background; Vessels – brown, surrounding white structures; Surface pattern – oval tubular or branched structures
Cancer	Type Vi/Vn (irregular)	Type IIIa/IIIb (meshed, irregular capillaries with branching and blind endings)	Color – browner/darker than background; Vessels – areas with disrupted/missing vessels; Surface pattern – amorphous/absent pattern

Fig. 5. Available classification systems used for characterization and prediction of lesion histology and SMI in colonic AMN.

RESECTION TECHNIQUES
Endoscopic Mucosal Resection

Core injection principles

- An adequately performed injection is vital to successful resection. The injection should elevate the lesion into the lumen and toward the colonoscope, improving access.
- Excessive injection should be avoided because this may hinder adequate visualization and create excessive tension within the cushion, which makes snare capture of adequate tissue challenging. For large piecemeal EMR, we recommend an inject-and-resect technique with 1 to 3 resections per injection.
- Inadequate injection may be appreciated by (**Fig. 6**):
  - Ongoing injection without tissue elevation or intraluminal fluid escape; this indicates transmural placement of the needle tip with extramural injection. If excessive, this may cause postprocedural pain. Draw back gently to find the correct plane.

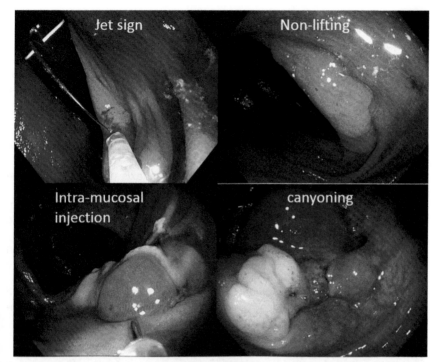

Fig. 6. Examples of inadequate submucosal injection.

- o Mucosal injection: the immediate appearance of a superficial blue bleb without lifting of the lesion.
- o Jet sign: when significant submucosal fibrosis is present, a jet of fluid exits the lesion at high pressure during injection.
- o A canyoning effect may occur as a result of central fibrosis. The lesion remains anchored in its original position, but the tissue of the perimeter elevates. This effect makes the lesion difficult to access, ensnare, and remove.
- Poor mucosal lifting usually indicates one of 2 things: invasive disease or submucosal fibrosis caused by previous aggressive biopsy or resection attempts. In some NG LSTs it may be caused by lesion biology. Sometimes at the flexures or in the rectosigmoid in lesions with a Is component it may be caused by repeated tumor prolapse.
- Position the needle tip tangentially to the mucosal surface and gently touch the surface. Ask an assistant to commence the injection while simultaneously stabbing the mucosa with the needle tip. The correct plane is confirmed by an immediate elevation of the mucosa.
- Use a dynamic injection technique: pull back slightly on the injection catheter or colonoscope and slowly deflect the tip of the colonoscope up while maintaining the position of the needle tip in the submucosal plane. The mucosa may even be gently rotated into the lumen by torquing the endoscope shaft.

Core snaring principles

- The lesion should be removed in as few pieces as safely possible. Provided safety is ensured, en bloc resection should be considered for lesions less than or equal to 20 mm, which may allow a more accurate histologic assessment and reduce the risk of recurrent/residual tissue compared with piecemeal resection.[6,8]

- Orient the lesion in the 5 to 6 o'clock position.
- Attempt to resect any large nodules (Is) first in 1 piece and submit them separately for pathologic analysis because these are most likely to harbor an invasive component (**Fig. 7**).[9]
- Include a 2-mm to 3-mm margin of normal mucosa.
- Use the edge of the defect as the base for the next snare placement, and align the snare along the defect margin to reduce the risk of adenoma islands (within the defect), which are subsequently difficult to remove.
- For large en bloc resections, align the longitudinal axis of the snare with the longest axis of the lesion to maximize tissue capture.
- Open the snare fully over the lesion, then angle down firmly with the up-down control onto the fluid cushion while aspirating air. This technique reduces colonic wall tension and maximizes tissue capture.
- Gradually close the snare while advancing the catheter or endoscope to maintain the snare base at the lesion edge. Monitor the lesion continuously, to ensure adequate trapping.
- Close the snare tightly to exclude muscularis propria from the captured tissue. If using a spiral (serrated) or any braided snare, it is not possible to transect ensnared tissue of more than 10-mm diameter without the use of diathermy.

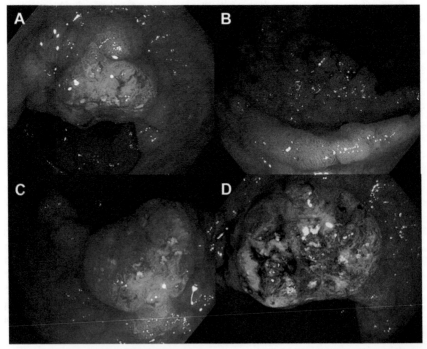

Fig. 7. Example of a Paris type 0-IIa + Is G LTS. (*A*, *B*) Overview of the lesion. (*C*, *D*) Focal interrogation with white light and NBI of the Is component raises concerns for an advanced disorder by the presence of a Kudo type Vi pit pattern and a Sano type IIIa vascular pattern. The final pathologic diagnosis showed poorly differentiated adenocarcinoma within TVA.

- We prefer to take the snare for the final transection phase. Sensory feedback is invaluable to inform the endoscopist on the safety and efficacy of the excision. Safe tissue capture is confirmed by 3 maneuvers:
  - Mobility: move the snare catheter quickly back and forth; it should move freely relative to the underlying colonic wall.
  - Degree of closure: the snare should close fully (a distance of no more than 1 cm between the thumb and the fingers). If the clinician is unsure, the snare is partially opened and tented into the lumen to release the deeper tissue before repeat closure.
  - Transection speed: transection should be fast. The snare is kept tightly closed while the foot pedal is depressed in short pulses. One to 3 pulses are usually sufficient to transect the tissue. A longer transection raises concerns of either MP entrapment or deeper neoplastic invasion.
- Fractionated current that alternates cutting and coagulating cycles is preferred (ENDO CUT mode Q, effect 3, cut duration 1, cut interval 6; ERBE, Tübingen, Germany). Low peak voltage coagulation (SOFT COAG effect 4, maximum 80 W, ERBE, Tübingen, Germany) may be used for vessel coagulation using the snare tip during EMR.[52]
- Adequate irrigation of the mucosal defect following each resection serves for assessment of residual adenomatous tissue within the mucosal defect, evidence of deep injury, and can assist in control of intraprocedural bleeding.

Fig. 8 shows sequential steps in EMR of a large colonic lesion.

ENDOSCOPIC SUBMUCOSAL DISSECTION

The ESD technique uses the principal of creating a submucosal cushion, using an injection catheter, in similar fashion to EMR, which is followed by controlled dissection within the submucosal plane beneath the lesion, permitting en bloc resection.[18,27,53]

A variety of endoscopic knives are available for ESD and the choice of a specific knife is usually a personal one. Few comparative studies are available, although certain knives may be advantageous in particular situations.[54,55] The procedure is performed by alternating between the knife and the injector. The hybrid knife has both injection and cutting capabilities, which greatly reduces the need for device exchange and substantially speeds up the procedure.[56]

- Colonic lesions are easily discerned endoscopically and, in contrast with gastric or esophageal ESD, preincision marking of the lesion is usually not necessary.
- Submucosal injection of fluid is performed using either an injection needle or a hybrid knife, and a circumferential mucosal incision is performed keeping a margin of 3 to 4 mm of normal mucosa around the lesion.
- Controlled submucosal dissection is then performed using additional submucosal injections as required as dissection progresses.
- A range of electrosurgical settings are used by different centers. The mucosal layer needs to be cut open, as opposed to the submucosal layer, which can be divided with more hemostatic current. For the mucosal incision, we use ENDO CUT Q (effect 3, cut duration 3, cut interval 3), whereas the submucosal dissection is performed with DRYCUT (effect 2, maximum 100 W, ERBE Tübingen, Germany). SOFT COAG (effect 4, maximum 80 W) may be used for vessel coagulation. Additional settings are available and there are no comparative data to suggest the optimal setting.

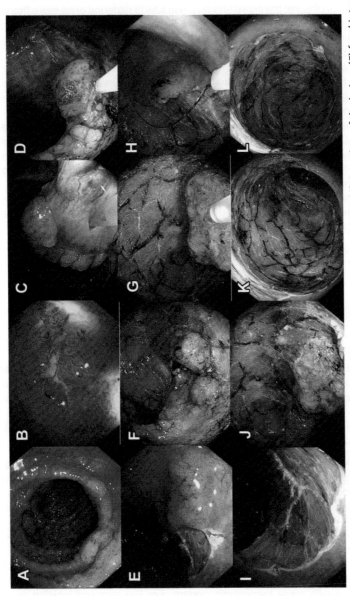

Fig. 8. Colonic piecemeal EMR of a large (80 mm) Paris 0-IIa mixed (G + NG) circumferential LST. (*A*) Overview of the lesion, (*B*) focal interrogation with NBI, (*C*) dynamic submucosal injection, (*D*) snaring of the specimen, (*E–J*) sequential resections using the inject-and-resect technique, (*K, L*) the final mucosal defect (no bleeding and no evidence of deep injury).

- A clear plastic cap on the tip of the endoscope is used to create traction on the lesion, which facilitates the submucosal dissection. It also allows stable knife position and better visibility.
- Correct patient positioning and the use of gravity to ensure lesion detachment away from the scope is useful.
- During resection, any bleeding vessels are coagulated before continuing resection.
- Prophylactic coagulation of large vessels in the final mucosal defect is commonly performed, although no evidence exists to support this practice in the colon.[18,53]
- Any possible perforations recognized during the procedure can be closed using endoclips.

Fig. 9 shows sequential steps in a rectal ESD.

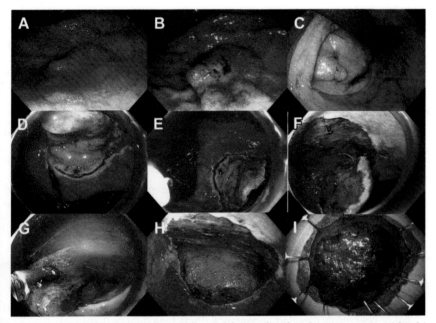

Fig. 9. Rectal ESD of a 20-mm Paris 0-IIa + c NG lesion. (*A, B*) Lesion assessment with white light and NBI, (*C*) initial submucosal injection, (*D, E*) circumferential submucosal incision; (*F*) controlled submucosal dissection, (*G*) prophylactic clipping of a large submucosal vessel, (*H*) the final mucosal defect, (*I*) the pinned en bloc specimen.

HYBRID TECHNIQUES

The hybrid ESD and EMR technique uses circumferential mucosal incision followed by en bloc snare resection of the lesion. This technique may lead to improved R0 resection rates for EMR with shorter procedure time than ESD.[57,58] Further study in the human colon is necessary to define its role. One limitation is the risk of MP entrapment with large lesions in the mobile intra-abdominal colon.

POLYPS IN UNIQUE AND DIFFICULT SITUATIONS
Anorectum

- The unique lymphovascular supply and innervation of the distal rectum and anus requires a modified approach.[6]

- Lymphovascular drainage from the distal rectum enters directly into the systemic circulation, bypassing the reticuloendothelial system operating with conventional portal drainage. Significant bacteremia is a risk with major resection. Prophylactic intravenous antibiotics for large or extensive (>30–40 mm) resections should be considered.[59]
- Sensory nerve supply distal to the dentate line is somatic, and a long-acting local anesthetic such as ropivacaine 0.5% to 0.75% added to the submucosal injectate is effective for postprocedural pain relief.[59] In this setting, continuous electrocardiographic monitoring is required.
- The hemorrhoidal vessels are thick walled and, when an adequate submucosal injection is made, they are resistant to snare entrapment and EMR can safely proceed over them.[59]

Periappendiceal Lesions

- Resection is challenging but can usually be achieved if circumferential involvement of the appendiceal orifice is less than 50% and the proximal margin within the appendix can be visualized and is accessible.
- The periappendiceal mucosa often elevates poorly and a small thin wire snare is preferred.[6]

Ileocecal Valve

- AMN involving the ICV have higher rates of recurrence after EMR (odds ratio [OR], 3.38).[9]
- Limited access and difficult scope position require both anterograde and retrograde approaches.
- Proximal extension into the terminal ileum presents difficulties in access and differentiation from the normal villiform ileal tissue, which may have a similar appearance.
- Extensive resections can be performed and ICV stenosis is uncommon.[6,60]

Sessile Serrated Polyps

- Sessile serrated polyps (SSPs) are premalignant lesions and represent approximately 10% of lesions greater than 20 mm referred for endoscopic resection.[9]
- Endoscopic detection and resection is difficult because of their bland and often flat or only mildly elevated appearance (Paris type 0-IIa or 0-IIb).
- The presence of adherent mucus or debris may alert endoscopists to their presence.
- The true margins can often only be correctly recognized after submucosal injection.
- Recognition of residual neoplastic tissue at the defect margin is often difficult and resection with a wide margin is recommended.
- SSPs may contain an area of dysplasia that can often be appreciated endoscopically. The presence of dysplasia represents a more advanced form of SSP with a higher risk for malignant transformation, so care should be taken to remove the entire lesion (**Fig. 10**).[61,62]

Previously Attempted Lesions

- Previous attempts at resection or aggressive biopsies can cause significant submucosal fibrosis.
- Submucosal fibrosis hinders effective and safe resection.
- To find the resection plane, submucosal injection should start away from the fibrotic area.
- Small, stiff, thin wire snares are preferred.

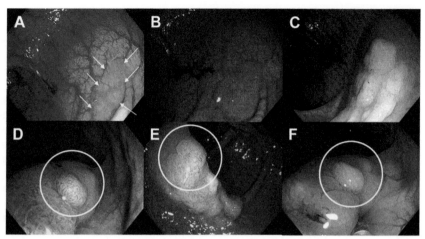

Fig. 10. Examples of SSPs. (*A*) Barely perceptible 0-IIb SSP in white light. The perimeter of the lesion (*Yellow arrow*). (*B, C*) The use of NBI or indigo carmine/methylene blue for the submucosal injection helps to discern the polyp's margins. (*D–F*) SSPs with a dysplastic nodule highlighted by NBI and the submucosal injectate.

Resection of Large, Thick-stalked Pedunculated Lesions

- Large pedunculated adenomas constitute most of these lesions in the colon. Submucosal lipomas account for a small percentage.
- Lesion size in relation to lumen diameter, and potential complications, such as bleeding and perforation, make resection challenging (**Fig. 11**).

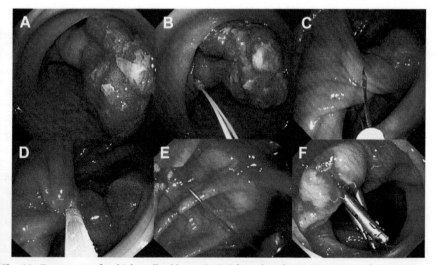

Fig. 11. Treatment of a thick-stalked large Paris 0-Ip polyp. (*A, B*) Placement of an Endoloop (this can be left with no further treatment to undergo slow transection in the case of a confirmed lipoma or resected with a snare above the Endoloop in case of an adenomatous polyp). (*C–F*) Snare resection of a large pedunculated polyp with no pretreatment of the stalk results in brisk arterial bleeding, which is successfully controlled with clips.

- Prophylactic measures to prevent postpolypectomy bleeding have been developed:
  - Endoloop placement has been shown to significantly reduce the risk of bleeding after polypectomy of large (≥2 cm) pedunculated polyps.[63,64] The Endoloop can be difficult to deploy and knowledge of its proper deployment is required by both endoscopists and their assistants.
  - Endoscopic clips have been used to ligate the stalk before resection with variable results. They are generally not large enough for very thick stalks (>10 mm). Multiple clips are required and postpolypectomy bleeding has been reported in up to 5.9% of cases.[65,66]
- Large colorectal lipomas are almost always benign. Resection of these lesions often requires large amounts of cautery because of the poor conduction of fatty tissue. This process may be associated with a significant risk of perforation. Prior ligation of the base affords some security against this. The ligate-and-let-go technique,[67] with placement of an Endoloop to cause slow tissue destruction by necrosis, avoids the potential risks of excision.

ENDOSCOPIC TATTOOING

Endoscopic tattooing in the colon serves 3 main purposes:

1. Tumor localization during laparoscopic surgery.
2. Localization of difficult-to-detect lesions (ie, medial wall ascending colon, transverse colon, lengthy left colon) referred for EMR.
3. Localization of the post-EMR scar for surveillance purposes.

The 2 most commonly used tattooing agents are Endomark (India ink; PMT/Permark Inc, Chanhassen, MN) and Spot (sterile carbon particle suspension; GI Supply Inc, Camp Hill, PA). Both are sterilized, ready-to-use products; however, currently only Spot is US Food and Drug Administration approved for tattooing.[68]

Injection of properly diluted and sterile agents is generally safe and complications are rare.[68,69] Localized peritonitis may result from inadvertent transmural injection. Injection in close proximity to the lesion may result in significant submucosal fibrosis, which makes the subsequent EMR more difficult and potentially prone to complications.[70] Steps to ensure adequate and safe injection include:

- Use of a double-injection technique.[70–72] First inject saline to confirm that the needle tip is in the submucosal space. Once the saline bleb appears, stop the injection, leaving the needle in the cushion, and change syringes. Inject the tattooing agent into the cushion. Additional saline is used to flush the remaining tattooing agent from the catheter.
- A total of 2 to 3 mL of tattooing agent per site should be used.
- A distance of approximately 3 cm between the tattoo and the lesion should be kept in order to avoid dispersion of the agent to the submucosal space under the lesion.
- A total of 2 to 3 sites are recommended to ensure adequate extraluminal visualization.

COMPLICATIONS AND THEIR MANAGEMENT

Advanced resection in the colon is associated with an increased risk of complications. These complications may include bleeding, nonspecific postprocedural pain, serositis, perforation, and recurrent/residual tissue. Careful evaluation of the mucosal defect, early recognition of the endoscopic and clinical signs, and prompt treatment are crucial for successful prevention and management.

Bleeding

Bleeding is the most common complication. Bleeding occurs in up to 7% and 9% of colonic EMR and ESD procedures, respectively,[12,31,73,74] and can be categorized as intraprocedural bleeding (IPB) or delayed bleeding. The term clinically significant post-endoscopic bleeding (CSPEB) has been used in an attempt to standardize the nomenclature. It is delayed bleeding occurring after the procedure and requiring presentation to an emergency department, hospitalization, or medical intervention.[73]

Intraprocedural bleeding

IPB is rarely serious. In a large prospective cohort of large (>20 mm) lesions managed by EMR,[73] IPB occurred at a rate of 11.3%. On multivariate analysis IPB was associated with larger lesion, Paris 0-IIa + Is morphology, villous or tubulovillous histology, and procedures performed at lower-volume centers. In this cohort, all cases were successfully controlled endoscopically.

Management of IPB can be achieved with hemostatic clips, coagulation forceps, and snare tip soft coagulation (STSC); however, there are no comparative data on efficacy and safety (**Fig. 12**). STSC has been shown to be a safe and effective technique for treatment of IPB.[52] The technique requires the use of a microprocessor-controlled generator capable of delivering fixed low-voltage output (<190 V) in a specific mode (SOFT COAG, 80 W, effect 4, ERBE VIO, Tübingen, Germany), which results in a dramatic reduction in current flow as resistance increases rapidly with desiccation of tissue during STSC application, theoretically limiting the potential for deep thermal injury. The thermal therapy is applied to active bleeding points using a light touch with 1 to 2 mm of exposed snare tip. Coagulating forceps are preferred for more severe bleeding or if STSC fails after 2 to 3 attempts. Clips tend to get in the way, may not adequately compress minor vessels, and are best avoided.

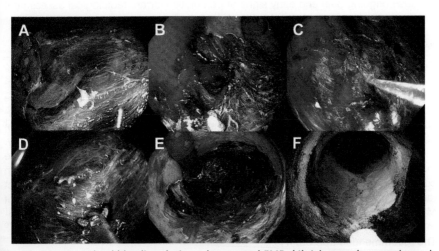

Fig. 12. Intraprocedural bleeding during a large rectal EMR. (*A*) A large submucosal vessel. (*B, C*) During active bleeding, vigorous irrigation assists in identifying the point of bleeding. (*D, E*) Coagulation forceps are used to control the bleeding. (*F*) A modified starch polymer (Endoclot; Vitramed Bioscience, Malaysia) is applied to the mucosal defect in an attempt to prevent delayed bleeding.

Clinically significant bleeding after endoscopic mucosal resection

Prospective data have shown that CSPEB occurs in 6.2% to 7% of patients undergoing EMR for large (>20 mm) lesions.[73,75] Risk factors associated with CSPEB on multivariate analysis include proximal colon location, age, aspirin use, IPB, and use of an electrosurgical current not controlled by a microprocessor. Most (68.5%) bleeding episodes occur within 48 hours and age is independently associated with bleeding after 48 hours.[73,75]

CSPEB is usually amenable to endoscopic therapy; however, occasionally angiography and surgery are needed. Endoscopic treatment may include adrenaline injection, use of coagulation forceps, hemostatic clips, or a combination of these methods. A recent retrospective case-control study of 524 lesion greater than 20 mm that underwent EMR[76] showed lower bleeding rates when partial or full clip closure of the resection defect was performed. In a large, multicenter, prospective cohort of lesions greater than 20 mm undergoing EMR (N = 1039; mean lesion size, 35.5 mm; 55% right colon),[77] 55% of the patients were able to avoid repeat colonoscopy because CSPEB settled spontaneously. When colonoscopy was performed, endoscopic therapy was only necessary in 21 of 27 (77%) cases. The need for endoscopic intervention for hemostasis was associated with frequent hematochezia, American Society of Anesthesiologists score greater than or equal to 2, and need for transfusion. Based on these data, the investigators suggested a risk-based algorithm for the management of CSPEB.

Further research into the role of clip closure and additional modalities, such as novel spray-on adherent pharmacologic agents or mechanical barriers, is required.

Postprocedural Pain

Nonspecific postprocedural pain is common following large, complex endoscopic resection. Excessive transmural injection, serositis, and gaseous distention are common causes that may be partially avoided by adequate injection techniques and the routine use of CO_2 for insufflation.[6,37] Ongoing clinical evaluation is mandatory because ongoing pain and early signs of peritonitis warrant radiological assessment with computed tomography and surgical consultation.

Perforation

Colonic perforation occurs in approximately 1% to 2% of EMR cases and in up to 5% to 10% of colonic ESD cases.[9,12,23,25] Immediate full-thickness perforation usually occurs following deep resection and is usually immediately appreciated and may be treated. Delayed perforation is most likely caused by coagulation necrosis or unrecognized partial MP injury.[6,20,74] These perforations may be more serious. Because of delayed presentation, peritonitis is often present and surgery is frequently necessary.

Real-time recognition of MP injury can be achieved by careful examination of the mucosal defect following each snare resection and at the end of the procedure. In colonic EMR, the recognition of the target sign on the resected specimen or the defect target sign within the mucosal defect[78] may assist physicians in early recognition of MP injury (**Fig. 13**). More recently, the novel approach of topical submucosal chromoendoscopy (TSC) was described and shown to improve detection of MP injury.[79] The recommended approach is:

- First look for areas of nonstaining. After EMR, the defect should have a homogeneous blue-mat appearance.
- A range of appearances, including visible uninjured MP, submucosal fibrosis, submucosal fat, and vessels that may be herniated, may be seen (**Fig. 14**).

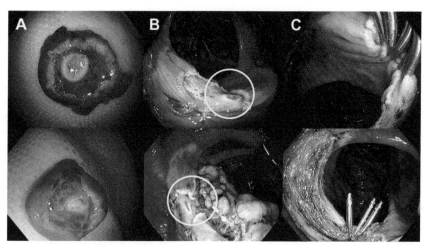

Fig. 13. Target sign (*A*)/mirror target sign (*B*), and successful clipping (*C*) of the muscularis propria injury.

- Nonstaining areas are further interrogated by TSC. The injection catheter is positioned gently against the mucosal defect with the needle withdrawn and dye is flushed. The dye is taken up by the connective tissue fibers of the submucosa.
- Any poorly staining areas suspicious for deep injury are recognized and treated by clip closure.

Recognition of deep or full-thickness perforation warrants immediate treatment, which can be achieved in most cases of EMR and ESD with clip closure.[78–80] Core principles include:

- Minimize luminal insufflation to reduce tension and prevent expansion of the defect.

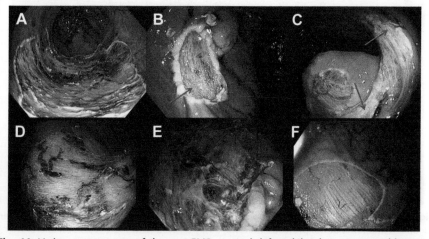

Fig. 14. Various appearances of the post-EMR mucosal defect. (*A*) A homogeneous blue-mat appearance, (*B*) presence of submucosal fat (*arrow*), (*C*) nonstaining submucosal fibrosis (*arrows*), (*D*) multiple large submucosal vessels, (*E*) a large herniating submucosal vessel, (*F*) visible noninjured MP fibers.

- Keep the defect clear of fluid; this can be achieved by changing the patient's position and administering antiperistaltic agents.
- If possible, remove any adenomatous tissue adjacent to the defect because it cannot be removed following application of the clips. Do not do this if there is an obvious hole; in those circumstances, prompt closure is crucial.
- Clip application should progress from one side of the defect to the other. Do not start in the middle. MP injuries or targets tend to be transversely oriented to the long axis of the colon. The edges of the defect are grasped with the clip arms; gentle suction is applied, the edges of the MP injury can be everted into the lumen by further suction, gentle pressure is applied, and then the assistant closes the clip. Adequate convergence of the defect edges is confirmed by gas insufflation if necessary and the clip is then deployed.

Recurrence

Recurrence following large EMR resection of AMN ranges from 10% to 30% and is usually small, unifocal, and easily treated at the first surveillance endoscopy **(Fig. 15)**.[9,18,24] Recurrence at first surveillance is likely to be residual disease from the index piecemeal EMR.[18] Long-term follow-up in the Australian colonic endoscopic resection (ACE) study has shown that following treatment, if necessary, of recurrence at first surveillance, subsequent recurrence is infrequent.[9,24] In this description of the

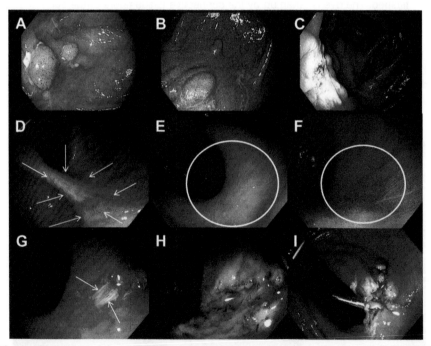

Fig. 15. Evaluation of the post-EMR scar and treatment of residual adenoma. (A–C) Residual/recurrent adenoma at the previous EMR site, easily treated with snare resection and/or thermal ablation to destroy possible microadenoma; (D) overview of a scar (arrows delineates scar margins); (E, F) no evidence of recurrence on white light, but NBI clearly shows residual adenomatous tissue in the center of the scar; (G, H) cold avulsion and STSC is performed with exposure of muscle fibers; (I) the defect is clipped.

first 1000 cases in this longitudinal cohort study, in which mean lesion size was 36.4 mm, if the initial EMR was successful, then 98% of patients were free of adenoma at 16-month follow-up. Main risk factors for recurrence were lesion size greater than 40 mm (OR, 8.2; $P<.001$) and use of argon plasma coagulation (OR, 2.4; $P<.001$).[24]

Treatment of residual tissue (not amenable to snare resection) at the index procedure or residual/recurrent tissue at surveillance colonoscopy can be achieved in most cases; however, the optimal technique has yet to be determined. Application of argon plasma coagulation to residual tissue at resection is suboptimal, with residual disease at surveillance evident in 14% to 50% of cases.[81,82] Additional techniques include cold avulsion with biopsy forceps and the use of soft coagulation with a snare tip to ablate remnant adenomatous tissue; however, these techniques are currently based on personal experience only and although investigation is ongoing, no prospective data are yet available (**Fig. 16**).

Table 2 summarizes the major complications of advanced endoscopic resection.

POSTOPERATIVE CARE

Patients undergoing advanced endoscopic resections require close monitoring following the procedure. Patient discomfort and developing clinical signs of complications should be recognized and treated early. We suggest a 2-stage evaluation scheme (**Fig. 17**).

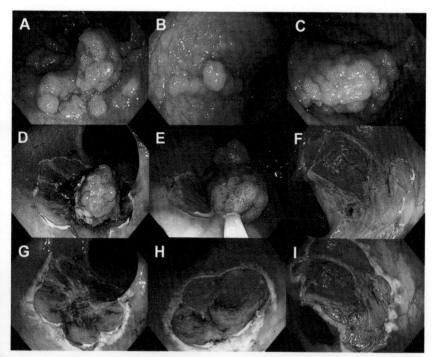

Fig. 16. (*A–C*) Three examples of large, laterally spreading polyps. (*D–F*) The lesions are resected by piecemeal EMR. (*G–I*) Once fully snare resected, ensuring no residual adenoma, the margins of the defects are treated by thermal ablation with STSC to ablate potential microadenoma.

Table 2
Major complications following advanced endoscopic resection in the colon

	EMR (%)	ESD (%)
Bleeding	0.4–7	0.5–9
Perforation	1–2	5–10
Recurrence	10–30	0–11

FOLLOW-UP

A repeat colonoscopy (surveillance colonoscopy 1 [SC1]) is recommended at 4 to 6 months after the index procedure to assess the scar area for any residual/recurrent tissue. The optimal timing of this procedure is not precisely known and it may be possible for those with only low-grade dysplasia to have SC1 at 12 months. The scar is carefully interrogated using both high-definition white light and NBI. Residual/recurrent tissue is treated with hot snare resection or cold avulsion followed by thermal ablation. Second surveillance colonoscopy is performed after an additional 12 months and then the patient can be followed according to the current postpolypectomy recommendations for CRC screening and prevention.[83]

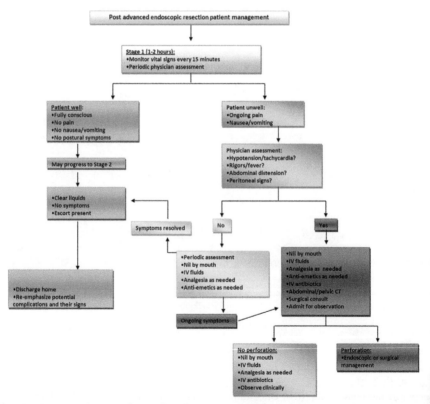

Fig. 17. Suggested post–advanced endoscopic resection management scheme. CT, computed tomography; IV, intravenous.

CURRENT CONTROVERSIES/FUTURE CONSIDERATIONS
Treatment of T1 Cancers

Optimal treatment of early (T1) CRC remains an active area of debate and research. Low-risk T1 cancers (SMI <1 mm, no LVI, well-differentiated tumor) may be suitable for endoscopic therapy alone. En bloc resection is a prerequisite and, if that is the case, then the risk of recurrence and lymph node metastasis is low.[19] High-risk T1 lesions (SMI >1 mm, LVI, or poor tumor differentiation) traditionally require surgery because the risk of LNM in those that can be endoscopically resected may reach 16%.[14,15] However, multiple factors, including patient personal preference, comorbidities, surgical risk profile, location of the lesion, and potential adverse outcomes of surgery, may make endoscopic treatment a viable option in selected cases. Endoscopically removed high-risk lesions carry a significant risk of local and regional recurrence and this treatment cannot be considered adequate in surgically fit patients.[84,85] Additional comparative prospective data are needed to better define selection criteria for endoscopic versus surgical treatment.

Individualized Treatment

Personalized medicine is gaining acceptance in various medical fields. Specific genetic abnormalities associated with the adenoma-to-carcinoma pathway have been correlated with lesion location and morphology.[86,87] Further research into the genetic subtypes of AMN may allow risk stratification, treatment selection, and surveillance recommendations.

Prediction of Histology and Complications

Accurate real-time endoscopic prediction of lesion histology and depth of invasion is currently limited to selected experts in the field. Results are difficult to duplicate. Further improvements in endoscopic imaging accompanied by dedicated training programs may allow improved sensitivity and specificity among colonoscopists. Recent studies in large prospective cohorts have highlighted risk factors for complications, such as bleeding perforation and recurrence.[9,73,78] Qualitative or quantitative analysis of the mucosal defect following endoscopic resection may provide additional insights regarding the risk of delayed complications.

SUMMARY

- EMR is safe and effective for noninvasive AMN because no risk of LNM exists.
- AMN with SMI is associated with a risk of LNM that may be stratified into high and low risk. Low-risk lesions may be managed endoscopically, whereas high-risk lesions mandate consideration of surgery.
- En bloc EMR is usually limited to lesions less than or equal to 20 mm. Larger lesions that are deemed to be endoscopically manageable are best treated by piecemeal EMR.
- Colonic ESD seems to confer little if any long-term advantage compared with EMR. ESD is also associated with a longer procedure time, increased risk of perforation, multiday hospitalization, and increased costs compared with EMR.
- Real-time macroscopic assessment of lesion type and risk of SMI may be valuable in therapeutic strategy selection; however, further validation in nontertiary practice is required.
- Recurrence is seen in 10% to 30% of EMR at first surveillance after piecemeal resection, but is effectively treated endoscopically with long-term remission. The first surveillance colonoscopy may be considered part of the primary

EMR treatment protocol, with complete eradication assessed at second surveillance.

- EMR and ESD share common complications. Bleeding and perforation can be adequately managed endoscopically. Careful assessment of the postresection mucosal defect may allow for early recognition and treatment of deep mural injury.
- The further development and promulgation of lesion-specific management guidelines for colonic AMN are likely to further improve outcomes and reduce costs.

REFERENCES

1. Levin B, Lieberman DA, McFarland B, et al. Screening and surveillance for the early detection of colorectal cancer and adenomatous polyps, 2008: a joint guideline from the American Cancer Society, the US Multi-Society Task Force on Colorectal Cancer, and the American College of Radiology. Gastroenterology 2008;134(5):1570–95.
2. Winawer SJ, Zauber AG, Ho MN, et al. Prevention of colorectal cancer by colonoscopic polypectomy. The National Polyp Study Workgroup. N Engl J Med 1993; 329:1977–81.
3. Kahi CJ, Imperiale TF, Juliar BE, et al. Effect of screening colonoscopy on colorectal cancer incidence and mortality. Clin Gastroenterol Hepatol 2009;7(7): 770–5 [quiz: 711].
4. Gupta N, Bansal A, Rao D, et al. Prevalence of advanced histological features in diminutive and small colon polyps. Gastrointest Endosc 2012;75(5):1022–30.
5. Repici A, Hassan C, Vitetta E, et al. Safety of cold polypectomy for <10mm polyps at colonoscopy: a prospective multicenter study. Endoscopy 2012;44:27–31.
6. Holt BA, Bourke MJ. Wide field endoscopic resection for advanced colonic mucosal neoplasia: current status and future directions. Clin Gastroenterol Hepatol 2012;10(9):969–79.
7. Rotondano G, Bianco MA, Buffoli F, et al. The Cooperative Italian FLIN Study Group: prevalence and clinico-pathological features of colorectal laterally spreading tumors. Endoscopy 2011;43:856–61.
8. Bourke M. Endoscopic mucosal resection in the colon: a practical guide. Tech Gastrointest Endosc 2011;13:35–49.
9. Moss A, Bourke MJ, Williams SJ, et al. Endoscopic mucosal resection outcomes and prediction of submucosal cancer from advanced colonic mucosal neoplasia. Gastroenterology 2011;140(7):1909–18.
10. Swan MP, Bourke MJ, Alexander S, et al. Large refractory colonic polyps: is it time to change our practice? A prospective study of the clinical and economic impact of a tertiary referral colonic mucosal resection and polypectomy service (with videos). Gastrointest Endosc 2009;70(6):1128–36.
11. Ahlenstiel G, Hourigan LF, Brown G, et al. Actual endoscopic versus predicted surgical mortality for treatment of advanced mucosal neoplasia of the colon. Gastrointest Endosc 2014;1:1–9.
12. Saito Y, Uraoka T, Yamaguchi Y, et al. A prospective, multicenter study of 1111 colorectal endoscopic submucosal dissections (with video). Gastrointest Endosc 2010;72(6):1217–25.
13. Ahmad NA, Kochman M, Long WB, et al. Efficacy, safety, and clinical outcomes of endoscopic mucosal resection: a study of 101 cases. Gastrointest Endosc 2002; 55:390–6.

14. Watanabe T, Itabashi M, Shimada Y, et al. Japanese Society for Cancer of the Colon and Rectum (JSCCR) guidelines 2010 for the treatment of colorectal cancer. Int J Clin Oncol 2012;17(1):1–29.
15. Bosch S, Teerenstra S, De Wilt JW, et al. Predicting lymph node metastasis in pT1 colorectal cancer: a systematic review of risk factors providing rationale for therapy decisions. Endoscopy 2013;45:827–34.
16. Kitajima K, Fujimori T, Fujii S, et al. Correlations between lymph node metastasis and depth of submucosal invasion in submucosal invasive colorectal carcinoma: a Japanese collaborative study. J Gastroenterol 2004;39(6):534–43.
17. Ikematsu H, Matsuda T, Emura F, et al. Efficacy of capillary pattern type IIIA/IIIB by magnifying narrow band imaging for estimating depth of invasion of early colorectal neoplasms. BMC Gastroenterol 2010;10:33.
18. Tutticci N, Bourke MJ. Advanced endoscopic resection in the colon: recent innovations, current limitations and future directions. Expert Rev Gastroenterol Hepatol 2014;8(2):161–77.
19. Ikematsu H, Yoda Y, Matsuda T, et al. Long-term outcomes after resection for submucosal invasive colorectal cancers. Gastroenterology 2013;144(3):551–9 [quiz: e14].
20. Sanchez-Yague A, Kaltenbach T, Raju G, et al. Advanced endoscopic resection of colorectal lesions. Gastroenterol Clin North Am 2013;42(3):459–77.
21. Tanaka S, Terasaki M, Hayashi N, et al. Warning for unprincipled colorectal endoscopic submucosal dissection: accurate diagnosis and reasonable treatment strategy. Dig Endosc 2013;25(2):107–16.
22. Takeuchi Y, Ohta T, Matsui F, et al. Indication, strategy and outcomes of endoscopic submucosal dissection for colorectal neoplasm. Dig Endosc 2012; 24(Suppl 1):100–4.
23. Nakajima T, Saito Y, Tanaka S, et al. Current status of endoscopic resection strategy for large, early colorectal neoplasia in Japan. Surg Endosc 2013;27(9):3262 70.
24. Moss A, Williams SJ, Hourigan LF, et al. Long-term adenoma recurrence following wide-field endoscopic mucosal resection (WF-EMR) for advanced colonic mucosal neoplasia is infrequent: results and risk factors in 1000 cases from the Australian Colonic EMR (ACE) study. Gut 2015;64(1):57–65.
25. Tanaka S, Oka S, Chayama K. Colorectal endoscopic submucosal dissection: present status and future perspective, including its differentiation from endoscopic mucosal resection. J Gastroenterol 2008;43(9):641–51.
26. Bourke MJ, Neuhaus H. Colorectal endoscopic submucosal dissection: when and by whom? Endoscopy 2014;46(8):677–9.
27. Repici A, Hassan C, De Paula Pessoa D, et al. Efficacy and safety of endoscopic submucosal dissection for colorectal neoplasia: a systematic review. Endoscopy 2012;44:137–50.
28. Probst A, Golger D, Anthuber M, et al. Endoscopic submucosal dissection in large sessile lesions of the rectosigmoid: learning curve in a European center. Endoscopy 2012;44:660–7.
29. Repici A, Hassan C, Pagano N, et al. High efficacy of endoscopic submucosal dissection for rectal laterally spreading tumors larger than 3 cm. Gastrointest Endosc 2013;77:96–101.
30. Rahmi G, Hotayt B, Chaussade S, et al. Endoscopic submucosal dissection for superficial rectal tumors: prospective evaluation in France. Endoscopy 2014; 46:670–6.
31. Saito Y, Uraoka T, Matsuda T, et al. Endoscopic treatment of large superficial colorectal tumors: a case series of 200 endoscopic submucosal dissections (with video). Gastrointest Endosc 2007;66:966–73.

32. Baron TH, Kamath PS, McBane RD. New anticoagulant and antiplatelet agents: a primer for the gastroenterologist. Clin Gastroenterol Hepatol 2014;12(2):187–95.

33. Veitch AM, Baglin TP, Gershlick AH, et al. Guidelines for the management of anti-coagulant and antiplatelet therapy in patients undergoing endoscopic proce-dures. Gut 2008;57(9):1322–9.

34. Feagins LA, Iqbal R, Harford WV, et al. Low rate of postpolypectomy bleeding among patients who continue thienopyridine therapy during colonoscopy. Clin Gastroenterol Hepatol 2013;11:1325–32.

35. Moss A, Bourke MJ, Metz AJ. A randomized, double-blind trial of succinylated gelatin submucosal injection for endoscopic resection of large sessile polyps of the colon. Am J Gastroenterol 2010;105:2375–82.

36. Dellon ES, Hawk JS, Grimm IS, et al. The use of carbon dioxide for insufflation during GI endoscopy: a systematic review. Gastrointest Endosc 2009;69:843–9.

37. Bassan MS, Holt B, Moss A, et al. Carbon dioxide insufflation reduces number of postprocedure admissions after endoscopic resection of large colonic lesions: a prospective cohort study. Gastrointest Endosc 2013;77(1):90–5.

38. Lambert R, Lightdale CJ. The Paris endoscopic classification of superficial neoplastic lesions: esophagus, stomach, and colon - Paris, France November 30 to December 1, 2002: foreword. Gastrointest Endosc 2003;58(6 Suppl):S3–43.

39. Axon A, Diebold MD, Fujino M, et al. Update on the Paris classification of super-ficial neoplastic lesions in the digestive tract. Endoscopy 2005;37:570–8.

40. Kudo S, Hirota S, Nakajima T, et al. Colorectal tumours and pit pattern. J Clin Pathol 1994;47:880–5.

41. Hurlstone DP, Sanders DS, Cross SS, et al. Colonoscopic resection of lateral spreading tumours: a prospective analysis of endoscopic mucosal resection. Gut 2004;53(9):1334–9.

42. Uraoka T, Saito Y, Matsuda T, et al. Endoscopic indications for endoscopic mucosal resection of laterally spreading tumours in the colorectum. Gut 2006; 55:1592–7.

43. Burgess NG, Hourigan LF, Zanati SA, et al. Gross morphology and lesion location stratify the risk of invasive disease in advanced mucosal neoplasia of the colon: results from a large multicenter cohort. Gastrointest Endosc 2014;79(5):AB556.

44. Wada Y, Kashida H, Kudo S, et al. Diagnostic accuracy of pit pattern and vascular pattern analyses in colorectal lesions. Dig Endosc 2010;22(3):192–9.

45. Katagiri A, Fu KI, Sano Y, et al. Narrow band imaging with magnifying colonos-copy as diagnostic tool for predicting histology of early colorectal neoplasia. Aliment Pharmacol Ther 2008;27:1269–74.

46. Rastogi A, Keighley J, Singh V, et al. High accuracy of narrow band imaging without magnification for the real-time characterization of polyp histology and its comparison with high-definition white light colonoscopy: a prospective study. Am J Gastroenterol 2009;104:2422–30.

47. Singh R, Nordeen N, Mei SL, et al. West meets East: preliminary results of narrow band imaging with optical magnification in the diagnosis of colorectal lesions: a multicenter Australian study using the modified Sano's classification. Dig Endosc 2011;23(Suppl 1):126–30.

48. Henry ZH, Yeaton P, Shami VM, et al. Meshed capillary vessels found on narrow-band imaging without optical magnification effectively identifies colorectal neoplasia: a North American validation of the Japanese experience. Gastrointest Endosc 2010;72(1):118–26.

49. Matsuda T, Saito Y, Nakajima T, et al. Macroscopic estimation of submucosal in-vasion in the colon. Tech Gastrointest Endosc 2011;13(1):24–32.

50. Matsuda T, Fujii T, Saito Y, et al. Efficacy of the invasive/non-invasive pattern by magnifying chromoendoscopy to estimate the depth of invasion of early colorectal neoplasms. Am J Gastroenterol 2008;103:2700–6.
51. Hayashi N, Tanaka S, Hewett DG, et al. Endoscopic prediction of deep submucosal invasive carcinoma: validation of the Narrow-band Imaging International Colorectal Endoscopic (NICE) classification. Gastrointest Endosc 2013; 78(4):625–32.
52. Fahrtash-Bahin F, Holt BA, Jayasekeran V, et al. Snare tip soft coagulation achieves effective and safe endoscopic hemostasis during wide-field endoscopic resection of large colonic lesions (with videos). Gastrointest Endosc 2013;78(1):158–63.e1.
53. Saito Y, Matsuda T, Fujii T. Endoscopic submucosal dissection of non-polypoid colorectal neoplasms. Gastrointest Endosc Clin N Am 2010;20(3):515–24.
54. Takeuchi Y, Uedo N, Ishihara R, et al. Efficacy of an endo-knife with a water-jet function (Flushknife) for endoscopic submucosal dissection of superficial colorectal neoplasms. Am J Gastroenterol 2010;105:314–22.
55. Lingenfelder T, Fischer K, Sold MG, et al. Combination of water-jet dissection and needle-knife as a hybrid knife simplifies endoscopic submucosal dissection. Surg Endosc 2009;23(7):1531–5.
56. Zhou PH, Schumacher B, Yao LQ, et al. Conventional vs waterjet-assisted endoscopic submucosal dissection in early gastric cancer: a randomized controlled trial. Endoscopy 2014;46(10):836–43.
57. Moss A, Bourke MJ, Tran K, et al. Lesion isolation by circumferential submucosal incision prior to endoscopic mucosal resection (CSI-EMR) substantially improves en bloc resection rates for 40-mm colonic lesions. Endoscopy 2010;42:400–4.
58. Terasaki M, Tanaka S, Oka S, et al. Clinical outcomes of endoscopic submucosal dissection and endoscopic mucosal resection for laterally spreading tumors larger than 20 mm. J Gastroenterol Hepatol 2012;27:734–40.
59. Holt BA, Bassan MS, Sexton A, et al. Advanced mucosal neoplasia of the anorectal junction: endoscopic resection technique and outcomes (with videos). Gastrointest Endosc 2014;79(1):119–26.
60. Nanda KS, Tutticci NJ, Burgess NG, et al. Endoscopic mucosal resection of advanced mucosal neoplasia involving the ileocecal valve with ileal infiltration: endoscopic features and outcome. Gastrointest Endosc 2014;79(5s):AB547.
61. Nanda KS, Tutticci N, Burgess N, et al. Caught in the act: endoscopic characterization of sessile serrated adenomas with dysplasia. Gastrointest Endosc 2014; 79(5):864–70.
62. Burgess NG, Tutticci NJ, Pellise M, et al. Sessile serrated adenomas/polyps with cytologic dysplasia: a triple threat for interval cancer. Gastrointest Endosc 2014; 80(2):307–10.
63. Di Giorgio P, De Luca L, Calcagno G, et al. Detachable snare versus epinephrine injection in the prevention of postpolypectomy bleeding: a randomized and controlled study. Endoscopy 2004;36:860–3.
64. Iishi H, Tatsuta M, Narahara H, et al. Endoscopic resection of large pedunculated colorectal polyps using a detachable snare. Gastrointest Endosc 1996;44:594–7.
65. Boo SJ, Byeon JS, Park SY, et al. Clipping for the prevention of immediate bleeding after polypectomy of pedunculated polyps: a pilot study. Clin Endosc 2012;45(1):84–8.
66. Luigiano C, Ferrara F, Ghersi S, et al. Endoclip-assisted resection of large pedunculated colorectal polyps: technical aspects and outcome. Dig Dis Sci 2010;55: 1726–31.

67. Kaltenbach T, Milkes D, Friedland S, et al. Safe endoscopic treatment of large colonic lipomas using endoscopic looping technique. Dig Liver Dis 2008;40: 958–61.
68. Kethu SR, Banerjee S, Desilets D, et al. Endoscopic tattooing. Gastrointest Endosc 2010;72(4):681–5.
69. Nizam R, Siddiqi N, Landas SK, et al. Colonic tattooing with India ink: benefits, risks, and alternatives. Am J Gastroenterol 1996;91:1804–8.
70. Moss A, Bourke MJ, Pathmanathan N. Safety of colonic tattoo with sterile carbon particle suspension: a proposed guideline with illustrative cases. Gastrointest Endosc 2011;74(1):214–8.
71. Fu KI, Fujii T, Kato S, et al. A new endoscopic tattooing technique for identifying the location of colonic lesions during laparoscopic surgery: a comparison with the conventional technique. Endoscopy 2001;33:687–91.
72. Sawaki A, Nakamura T, Suzuki T, et al. A two-step method for marking polypectomy sites in the colon and rectum. Gastrointest Endosc 2003;57:735–7.
73. Burgess NG, Metz AJ, Williams SJ, et al. Risk factors for intraprocedural and clinically significant delayed bleeding after wide-field endoscopic mucosal resection of large colonic lesions. Clin Gastroenterol Hepatol 2014;12(4):651–61.e1-3.
74. Kaltenbach T, Soetikno R. Endoscopic resection of large colon polyps. Gastrointest Endosc Clin N Am 2013;23(1):137–52.
75. Metz AJ, Bourke MJ, Moss A, et al. Factors that predict bleeding following endoscopic mucosal resection of large colonic lesions. Endoscopy 2011;43:506–11.
76. Liaquat H, Rohn E, Rex DK. Prophylactic clip closure reduced the risk of delayed postpolypectomy hemorrhage: experience in 277 clipped large sessile or flat colorectal lesions and 247 control lesions. Gastrointest Endosc 2013;77(3):401–7.
77. Burgess NG, Williams SJ, Hourigan LF, et al. A management algorithm based on delayed bleeding after wide-field endoscopic mucosal resection of large colonic lesions. Clin Gastroenterol Hepatol 2014;12(9):1525–33.
78. Swan MP, Bourke MJ, Moss A, et al. The target sign: an endoscopic marker for the resection of the muscularis propria and potential perforation during colonic endoscopic mucosal resection. Gastrointest Endosc 2011;73(1):79–85.
79. Holt BA, Jayasekeran V, Sonson R, et al. Topical submucosal chromoendoscopy defines the level of resection in colonic EMR and may improve procedural safety (with video). Gastrointest Endosc 2013;77(6):949–53.
80. Raju GS, Saito Y, Matsuda T, et al. Endoscopic management of colonoscopic perforations (with videos). Gastrointest Endosc 2011;74(6):1380–8.
81. Zlatanic J, Waye JD, Kim PS, et al. Large sessile colonic adenomas: use of argon plasma coagulator to supplement piecemeal snare polypectomy. Gastrointest Endosc 1999;49:731–5.
82. Regula J, Wronska E, Polkowski M, et al. Argon plasma coagulation after piecemeal polypectomy of sessile colorectal adenomas: long-term follow-up study. Endoscopy 2003;35:212–8.
83. Hassan C, Quintero E, Dumonceau JM, et al. Post-polypectomy colonoscopy surveillance: European Society of Gastrointestinal Endoscopy (ESGE) guideline. Endoscopy 2013;45(10):842–51.
84. Meining A, von Delius S, Eames TM, et al. Risk factors for unfavorable outcomes after endoscopic removal of submucosal invasive colorectal tumors. Clin Gastroenterol Hepatol 2011;9:590–4.
85. Kim MN, Kang JM, Yang JI, et al. Clinical features and prognosis of early colorectal cancer treated by endoscopic mucosal resection. J Gastroenterol Hepatol 2011;26:1619–25.

86. Metz AJ, Bourke MJ, Moss A, et al. A correlation of the endoscopic characteristics of colonic laterally spreading tumours with genetic alterations. Eur J Gastroenterol Hepatol 2013;25(3):319–26.
87. Kaji E, Kato J, Suzuki H, et al. Analysis of K-ras, BRAF, and PIK3CA mutations in laterally-spreading tumors of the colorectum. J Gastroenterol Hepatol 2011;26: 599–607.

Management of Polypectomy Complications

Selvi Thirumurthi, MD, MS, Gottumukkala S. Raju, MD*

KEYWORDS

- Colonoscopy • Polypectomy • Complications • Postpolypectomy bleeding
- Perforation • Prevention • Management

KEY POINTS

- The major complications of colonoscopy with polypectomy are postpolypectomy bleeding and colon perforation.
- Risk factors for postpolypectomy bleeding can be categorized as polyp-related, patient-related, and technique/device-related factors.
- Postpolypectomy bleeding can be controlled with injectable solutions and thermal and mechanical hemostatic devices.
- Risk factors for colon perforation can be polyp-related or technique/device-related.
- Methods of closure of colon perforation include endoclip placement, suturing, and others; appropriate management of patients with perforation is essential.

INTRODUCTION

Approximately 1.27 million colonoscopies are performed annually for colorectal cancer sreening. The risk of complications increases in patients who undergo colonoscopy with polypectomy (**Figs. 1** and **2**). The rate of serious complications (ie, requiring hospitalization within 30 days of colonoscopy) is 10-fold higher (7.0 per 1000 examinations) if biopsy or polypectomy is performed compared with colonoscopy without these interventions.[1] The 2 most significant complications include postpolypectomy bleeding (PPB) and colon perforation. The goal of this article is to review these complications in detail, assess risk factors for bleeding and perforation, and make recommendations regarding prevention and management.

No financial disclosures.
Department of Gastroenterology, Hepatology and Nutrition, University of Texas MD Anderson Cancer Center, 1515 Holcombe Boulevard, Unit 1466, Houston, TX 77030, USA
* Corresponding author.
E-mail address: gsraju@mdanderson.org

Gastrointest Endoscopy Clin N Am 25 (2015) 335–357
http://dx.doi.org/10.1016/j.giec.2014.11.006
1052-5157/15/$ – see front matter © 2015 Elsevier Inc. All rights reserved.
giendo.theclinics.com

POSTPOLYPECTOMY BLEEDING

The expected incidence of PPB ranges from 0.1% to 0.6%.[2] A rate greater than 1% in a practice should prompt a review of endoscopist technique.[3] PPB can be classified as immediate (intraprocedural or within 24 hours of the examination) or delayed (between 1 day to 14 days after the examination) and the severity of bleeding can be graded as follows: grade 1 (spontaneous hemostasis within 1 minute); grade 2 (continuous oozing but decreases over 1 minute); grade 3 (continuous oozing over 1 minute that requires endoscopic treatment); or grade 4 (active spurting) (**Box 1**).[4]

Most bleeding episodes are clinically trivial, whereas those episodes that require hospitalization, blood transfusion, repeat endoscopic intervention, or surgery are considered true complications.

Risk Factors for Postpolypectomy Bleeding

Polyp-related factors

Risk factors include polyp size, location, and morphology. Polyp size is the main factor and is consistently linked to higher bleeding rates. Polyps that are 1 cm or larger in size have a 2.0-fold to 4.5-fold increased risk of PPB[5,6]; this risk grows by 9% to 13% per millimeter increase in polyp size greater than 1 cm.[7,8] Polyps located in the right hemicolon are associated with a 2.6-fold to 4.6-fold increased risk of PPB.[5,7,9,10] Polyp morphology (pedunculated with a thick stalk or laterally spreading lesions) and histology (adenoma, villous features, and presence of adenocarcinoma) are associated with an increase in PPB.[4,5,11–13] In a prospective Australian Colonic Endoscopic Resection Study of patients undergoing wide field endoscopic mucosal resection (EMR) of large sessile colonic polyps, intraprocedural bleeding was associated with larger lesions, lesion histology, and Paris endoscopic classification of type 0–IIa + Is.[14]

Patient-related factors

Patient-related factors, such as age greater than 65, hypertension, cardiac disease, and renal disease, have been associated with a higher risk for PPB.[4,6,11] Older patients and those with cardiovascular disease are often on antithrombotic therapy when they present for colonoscopy. The use of anticoagulants before polypectomy and resumption of therapy afterward have been associated with a 3.7-fold and 5.2-fold increased risk for PPB, respectively.[4,8] Risks for PPB vary based on the type of antithrombotic agent, whether an anti-platelet agent (aspirin, nonsteroidal anti-inflammatory drugs [NSAIDs], clopidogrel, ticlopidine) or an anticoagulant (warfarin, heparin), and these are reviewed later in this article (**Table 1**).

Box 1
Grading scale of immediate postpolypectomy bleeding

Grade 1: Spontaneous hemostasis within 1 minute of observation

Grade 2: Continuous oozing but decreases over 1 minute of observation

Grade 3: Continuous oozing over 1 minute of observation and requires endoscopic therapy

Grade 4: Active spurting, requires endoscopic therapy, possible hospital admission, and transfusion

Adapted from Kim HS, Kim TI, Kim WH, et al. Risk factors for immediate postpolypectomy bleeding of the colon: a multicenter study. Am J Gastroenterol 2006;101:1333–41; with permission.

Table 1
Management of antithrombotic agents and risk of postpolypectomy bleeding

Antithrombotic Agent	Effect on Postpolypectomy Bleeding	Current Guidelines for Periprocedural Management[a]	Suggested Endoscopic Intervention
Aspirin/NSAIDs (antiplatelet)	No compelling data	Continue	Consider holding if large EMR planned
Clopidogrel (antiplatelet)	Mixed data: suggestion of increased delayed PPB. Increases risk of PPB in combination with aspirin	Hold for 7–10 d preprocedure and restart the next day postprocedure (depending on intervention performed)	Consider prophylactic clip placement over polypectomy site(s)
Warfarin (anticoagulation)	Increases risk of PPB	Hold for 3–5 d preprocedure and 1 d postprocedure	
Heparin (anticoagulation)	Increases risk of PPB	Hold for 4–6 h (unfractionated heparin) 12–24 h (low molecular weight heparin)	
SSRIs (antiplatelet)	Increased risk of *upper* GI bleeding; no studies with colonoscopy or polypectomy. Risk is further increased with simultaneous aspirin and NSAID use	N/A	Consider holding aspirin ± NSAIDs
Novel oral anticoagulants	Likely increased risk although no data available	No data available	Discontinue agents based on half-life and with input from cardiologist

[a] ASGE guidelines: Management of antithrombotic agents for endoscopic procedures. NB: The decision to discontinue antithrombotic therapy for endoscopy should be individualized to balance the risk of the planned endoscopic intervention and with the risk of the underlying condition for which the patient is on therapy.[20]

Aspirin and nonsteroidal anti-inflammatory drugs Although aspirin exposure results in a prolonged bleeding time of normal colonic mucosa, studies evaluating the impact of aspirin use on PPB reveal mixed results.[15] An increased risk for PPB with aspirin use before colonoscopy has been described in one small study (odds ratio [OR] 6.7). Another group reported increased risk of bleeding after EMR of lesions 2 cm or larger in patients with aspirin use within 7 days of the procedure (OR 6.3).[10,16] However, most data show that aspirin use, alone or in combination with other NSAIDs, does not increase the risk of PPB.[17–19] Variation in the aspirin dosage (81 mg vs 325 mg) may be a confounding factor.

Clopidogrel Current guidelines recommend holding thienopyridines (clopidogrel and ticlopidine) for at least 7 days before polypectomy based on the indication for antithrombotic therapy and the risk to the patient.[20] In a recent meta-analysis of PPB in patients on continued clopidogrel therapy, the overall pooled relative risk (RR) for PPB was 2.5 ($P<.05$).[21] The RR for delayed bleeding was 4.6 ($P<.05$) with the RR for immediate PPB 1.76 (however, $P>.05$).[21] Other studies have also reported higher rates of delayed PPB with uninterrupted clopidogrel therapy compared with controls, but the rates of PPB were low (less than 1%) and applied mainly to large polyps (greater than 1 cm in size).[22–24] Interestingly, clopidogrel monotherapy was not identified as an independent risk factor for PPB, but only increased the risk of PPB when used in combination with aspirin.[24] The risk of delayed PPB can be mitigated during colonoscopy by the application of through-the-scope clips (TTSC; endoclips) to the polypectomy site in patients who are on clopidogrel therapy during colonoscopy or are expected to resume it after the procedure.

Warfarin It is recommended that patients anticoagulated with warfarin should hold therapy for 3 to 5 days before colonoscopy.[20] Although there is no clearly established target international normalized ratio (INR) that is safe for polypectomy, an INR of 1.6 or less is generally considered acceptable. However, preprocedure INR is not routinely obtained in clinical practice. Some studies showed that patients on warfarin therapy had a higher risk of PPB (OR 11.6–13.3), whereas those on aspirin, NSAIDs, thienopyridines, and low-molecular-weight heparin did not.[25,26] Other predictors of PPB were the number of polyps removed (OR 1.2) and male gender (OR 9.2).[26]

Bridging therapy with heparin When evaluating the risk of warfarin therapy on PPB, it is important to consider the risk of thromboembolic events after temporary discontinuation of the drug. Patients at high risk for thromboembolic events are bridged with heparin while anticoagulation is suspended. In a CORI database study, the use of periprocedural heparin was not a risk factor for PPB.[27] In another study, patients on warfarin or antiplatelet agents were either bridged with heparin or simply discontinued antithrombotic therapy.[28] In patients on heparin bridge therapy, the risk of PPB was not only higher but also delayed in onset and recurrent, resulting in prolonged hospitalization. Warfarin use, bridging with heparin, and pedunculated polyps were independent predictors of PPB.[28] Endoscopists should consider empiric placement of endoclips at polypectomy sites in patients on warfarin therapy. Patients with an average INR of 2.3 and polyps ranging from 3 mm to 10 mm in size were successfully clipped and experienced no PPB when warfarin was held for only 36 hours preprocedure.[29]

Thrombocytopenia and selective serotonin reuptake inhibitors Endoscopists often hesitate to perform polypectomy on patients with cancer with thrombocytopenia or cirrhosis of the liver because of a perceived increased risk of PPB. In a study of patients with cancer with platelet counts of 75×10^3 or less, the risk of bleeding was 1.5% after biopsy and 4% after polypectomy for lesions 1 cm in size or smaller.[30] In addition, hemostasis was successfully achieved in 95% of actively bleeding patients, resulting in a decreased need for transfusion of blood products.[30]

Patients with early-stage liver cirrhosis (Child-Pugh score A or B) with an INR of 1.5 or less and platelet counts ranging between 30×10^3 and 242×10^3 had immediate PPB in 3% of patients; immediate hemostasis was achieved with clips, and there was no delayed bleeding.[31] Biopsy and polypectomy may be safe in patients with thrombocytopenia or early-stage cirrhosis with appropriate precautions. Patients with more advanced cirrhosis (Child-Pugh score B or C) were at increased risk for PPB (hazard ratio [HR] 3.5) along with polyp size (HR 3.6) and pedunculated type polyps (HR 2.4).[32]

The use of selective serotonin reuptake inhibitors (SSRIs) has been associated with an increased risk of both organ hemorrhage and adverse outcomes of surgery. SSRIs are thought to inhibit platelet adhesion by up to 50%, an effect that varies by agent and dosage.[33] Multiple studies have demonstrated an increased risk of *upper* gastrointestinal (GI) bleeding in patients using SSRIs (OR 1.6).[34–36] This effect is compounded by the concomitant use of NSAIDs (OR 4.2–8.0) and even more so when aspirin is added to the mix (OR 28.0).[34,35] There are little data evaluating the effect of SSRIs on lower GI bleeding to make recommendations at this time.

Technique/Device-Related Factors

There is wide variation in endoscopic resection techniques among gastroenterologists, specifically with the type of cut (cold vs hot snare resection) and type of current (pure cut vs pure coagulation vs blended current).

Polyps less than 1 cm in size are often removed with a biopsy forceps or a cold snare. Although "cold" snare resection of polyps increases risk of intraprocedural bleeding, it is easily controlled; it is not associated with delayed PPB as observed in a prospective multicenter trial of more than 1000 polypectomies.[37] There is no difference in PPB between cold-snare and hot-snare resection of polyps less than 1 cm.[38,39] However, rates of PPB were higher in hot-snare polypectomy in patients on warfarin.[40]

Cautery is generally used to resect polyps greater than 1 cm in size. There is variability among gastroenterologists in the electrosurgical settings used for snare resection in the United States: 46% use pure coagulation, 46% use blended current, and 3% use pure cut for polypectomy.[41] Pure cutting current increases the risk of bleeding, while pure coagulation current increases the risk of perforation. Hence, a blended cutting and coagulation current is used to minimize both of these complications.[2] Although there was no difference in the rate of PPB, immediate bleeding was more common after blended current use, whereas delayed bleeding was frequent in anticoagulated patients.[42] This area needs further investigation to help standardize endoscopic practice.

Prevention of Postpolypectomy Bleeding

Several studies report outcomes of the different techniques available to prevent PPB. These techniques include injectable solutions, placement of endoclips, deployment of a detachable loop, and application of thermal energy (with coagulation forceps or argon plasma coagulation) as well as a combination of these techniques (**Box 2**).

Solutions—epinephrine injection

Submucosal injection of fluid underneath a polyp elevates the lesion, separates it from the deeper layers, prevents transmural thermal injury, and thus improves the safety of

> **Box 2**
> **Evidence for prophylaxis of postpolypectomy bleeding**
>
> Early bleeding
>
>   Epinephrine injection superior to control (OR 0.37)
>
>   Combination therapy superior to monotherapy (OR 0.12)
>
>   Detachable loop superior to epinephrine or control (OR 0.25)
>
> Delayed bleeding
>
>   Epinephrine versus control: no difference in bleeding rates
>
>   Combination therapy versus monotherapy: no difference in bleeding rates
>
>   Neither detachable loops nor endoclips versus other techniques: no difference in bleeding rates

polypectomy. Dilute epinephrine offers the additional advantage of shrinking polyp size and reducing the risk of bleeding. This principle has been used to remove large pedunculated polyps with the injection of dilute epinephrine into the head and into the stalk of the polyp for volume reduction (epinephrine volume reduction).[43] Compared with saline injection or no preinjection, epinephrine injection results in lower PPB.[44,45] Saline tends to dissipate quickly from the submucosal cushion in highly vascularized areas like the rectum. Although this could be minimized by hypertonic saline (3.0%–4.7%) in combination with epinephrine or 50% dextrose, these solutions can result in local inflammation and delayed tissue damage. A 0.5% hyaluronic acid solution provides the most durable cushion but is also associated with an inflammatory reaction. A combination of saline and methylene blue or indigo carmine dye stains the submucosal space and provides visual confirmation of the depth of resection. Use of other solutions have been reported (fibrinogen, albumin, glycerol), but these are expensive and there are little data to support their use.[41]

Endoclips
Endoclips are frequently used to prevent PPB. Although clips have not been shown to be useful in the prevention of PPB after resection of smaller lesions, a recent study demonstrated that clips prevent delayed bleeding after EMR of lesions greater than 2 cm.[46,47] When endoclips were placed before polypectomy in patients on uninterrupted antithrombotic therapy, there was no PPB in either the endoclip or the control groups.[48] It is cost-effective in patients planning to resume antithrombotic therapy after the procedure, as shown in a decision analysis.[49] Clip application may be ineffective if the clip is unable to span across a thick stalk and occlude all the feeding blood vessels and may cause counterburn during snare resection if applied to a short stalk.[50]

Detachable loops
Detachable loops applied to the stalk of a pedunculated polyp result in vasoconstriction of feeding blood vessels and reduce the risk of PPB. The efficacy of endoloops in the prevention of PPB is similar to other mechanical hemostatic devices such as clips.[51] Endoloop ligation is particularly useful in the prevention of PPB from large polyps (>2 cm).[52]

Cautery
Cautery can be applied to treat and prevent PPB. However, neither argon plasma coagulation nor coagulation forceps treatment of nonbleeding vessels has been effective in the prevention of PPB.[53,54]

Combination therapy

Combination hemostatic therapy with epinephrine injection and application of mechanical devices (detachable loop or endoclip or both) reduces rates of PPB as well as severity of PPB in large polyps (>2 cm) compared with epinephrine injection alone.[55,56]

A meta-analysis and systematic review summarizes the data from available quality studies.[57] Both monotherapy (epinephrine injection or mechanical hemostasis) and a combination of epinephrine injection and mechanical hemostasis reduce early PPB; combination therapy is superior to monotherapy in the prevention of early PPB. Epinephrine injection alone is ineffective in the prevention of delayed PPB, whereas monotherapy with mechanical devices and a combination of epinephrine and mechanical devices are effective in the prevention of delayed PPB.[57]

Management of Postpolypectomy Bleeding

Three options are currently available to manage PPB depending on the timing and severity of bleeding: injectable solutions, thermal devices, and mechanical devices. A decision of whether to treat bleeding during or immediately after resection can be made and implemented promptly (**Box 3**).

Intraprocedural bleeding is associated with clinically significant delayed PPB after wide field EMR, and it should be treated aggressively and immediately.[58] One could consider injection of epinephrine or application of clips, loops, or cautery to control bleeding immediately depending on the source of bleeding.

Delayed PPB requires careful assessment of the patient and the severity of bleeding. The best course of action should be determined based on clinical features, such as hemodynamic instability, frequency of bloody bowel movements, comorbid conditions, patient age, resumption of antithrombotic agents, and so on. If resuscitation measures fail, patients should undergo urgent intervention: colonoscopy with hemostasis, angioembolization, or surgery. If resuscitation measures are successful, patients should be admitted to hospital for observation and monitoring of hemoglobin, platelets,

---

Box 3
Hemostatic devices

Thermal (contact)

- Heater probe

- Gold probe

- Snare tip cautery

- Hemostatic forceps

Thermal (noncontact)

- Argon plasma coagulation

Mechanical

- TTSC or endoclips

- Detachable loop

- OTSC

- Grasp bleeding stalk with snare device and constrict

- Band ligation

- Endoscopic suturing device

and coagulation profile. More than half of all bleeding subsides spontaneously and does not need any further intervention. Risk factors for ongoing bleeding or recurrence of bleeding that requires intervention include hematochezia hourly or every few minutes, hemodynamic instability, low hemoglobin on admission (<12 g/dL), transfusion requirement, and American Society of Anesthesiologists class of II or higher. If bleeding resolves spontaneously, the patients should be observed for 24 hours before discharge. If it continues or recurs, urgent intervention with colonoscopy is required.[14]

Injectable solutions for hemostasis
In the setting of active bleeding, injection of a 1:10,000 epinephrine-saline solution into the site will help achieve temporary hemostasis by a tamponade effect as well as vasoconstriction of the bleeding vessel.

Thermal hemostatic devices
Thermal devices generate heat and cause edema, coagulation, and vessel constriction through direct contact with the tissue (heater probe, gold probe, snare tip, hemostatic forceps) or indirectly (argon plasma coagulation). Bipolar devices, such as the heater probe and gold probe, complete the circuit within the device and no grounding pad is needed. Although tissue contact is necessary, pressure should not be applied in the colon, unlike when these devices are used in the stomach, because the colon wall is thinner and the settings should also be reduced accordingly (15 J heater probe, 10–15 W gold probe).[59]

When bleeding occurs after polypectomy, the snare is often readily available and the tip of snare can be applied to the bleeding site and soft coagulation applied. The snare is extended out of the sheath by 1 to 2 mm and the wire tip is applied to the bleeding point. Soft coagulation is applied until hemostasis occurs. The coagulation setting allows for desiccation of the tissue, which creates resistance to further current flow, thus limiting injury. This method alone (80 W, effect 4) was successful in 91% of cases when immediate PPB was seen.[60] Studies have also demonstrated the use of hemostatic forceps or graspers in pinching and retracting bleeding points to stop postpolypectomy and diverticular bleeding.[61]

Noncontact thermal energy can be applied with argon plasma coagulation where electron flow through ionized argon gas results in tissue desiccation. Again, desiccated tissue limits further energy flow, and the argon stream will shift to adjacent conductive tissue, allowing for hemostasis of the bleeding vessel.[62]

Mechanical hemostatic devices
The most popular method for endoscopic hemostasis is the application of endoclips or TTSC. In a survey of United States Department of Veteran Affairs gastroenterologists, placement of an endoclip was the preferred method to achieve hemostasis in cases of PPB in 76% of respondents (as well as for bleeding prophylaxis in patients on anticoagulation). For persistent bleeding after cold forceps biopsy, 55% of gastroenterologists would not apply any therapy.[63] Multiple studies have demonstrated that application of TTSC to the bleeding vessel achieves successful hemostasis. A novel technique of endoscopic clip tamponade has been described for bleeding in the midst of an EMR. The endoclip is closed over the lesion for 3 minutes to control bleeding; then the clip is opened so that resection may continue.[64] TTSC placement has also been used in combination with a detachable loop, which is placed to lasso the deployed endoclips together and provide an additional level of mechanical force.[65]

Other devices for mechanical hemostasis include the detachable loop, which is placed more easily over protuberant lesions like a bleeding polypectomy stalk. Endoscopic band ligation can be used in these situations.[66] Although over-the-scope clips

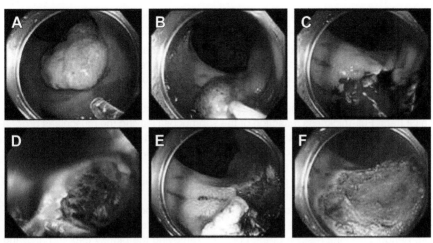

Fig. 1. Endoscopic hemostasis. (*A*) A large sessile polyp in the rectum. (*B*) Endoscopic mucosal resection. (*C*) Brisk arterial bleeding. (*D, E*) Hemostasis achieved with coagulation grasping forceps. (*F*) Clean resection base after APC with complete hemostasis. APC, argon plasma coagulation.

(OTSC) play a greater role in closing perforations, they been effective in PPB in small studies.[67,68] The precise placement of an OTSC may be challenging in the face of an active arterial bleed and would also require the scope to be withdrawn from the patient after localizing the site to retrofit the clip on to the scope. There have been no comparative studies of TTSC with OTSC for hemostasis in humans. The endoscopist should use the device that they are most familiar with and that is readily available in the setting of an acute arterial PPB.

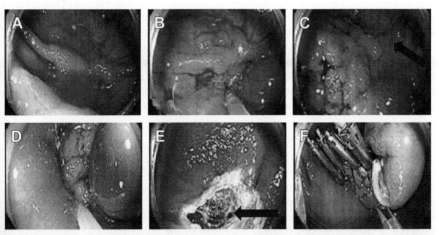

Fig. 2. Endoscopic clip closure of perforation and red flags suggestive of impending perforation. (*A*) Large flat lesion in the cecum with converging folds and central depression suggests submucosal fibrosis. (*B*) Mucosal bleb after injection of dilute indigo carmine solution without a submucosal lift indicates submucosal fibrosis. (*C*) A separate injection lifts the lesion, but the converging fold in the right upper corner (*arrow*) suggests submucosal fibrosis. (*D*) Inability to lift the lesion entrapped by snare is another sign of submucosal fibrosis ("sunken snare sign"). (*E*) Perforation in the middle of submucosal fibrosis (*arrow*). (*F*) Clip closure successful.

COLON PERFORATION

Colon perforation, a dreaded complication of polypectomy, is rare with routine polyp removal. The incidence of colonoscopic perforation varies from 0.7% to 0.9%.[1,69,70] However, the incidence of perforation has certainly increased with the introduction of endoscopic submucosal dissection (ESD) in the colon. The rates of perforation with ESD are 4% to 10%.[71]

The colon wall is approximately 3 mm thick. The submucosa is the strongest layer in the GI tract. Full-thickness resection of the submucosa leaving the muscularis propria intact results in postpolypectomy syndrome and delayed perforation[72]; this could be avoided by prophylactic clip closure of deep resections where the muscularis propria is exposed.

Once a perforation occurs, air escapes into the peritoneum. A massive air leak could result in tension pneumoperitoneum and cardiovascular arrest[73]; this could be prevented by the routine use of carbon dioxide instead of room air for colon insufflation, because carbon dioxide gets reabsorbed into the body faster than room air. In addition, periodic decompression of the colon by removing the biopsy cap and allowing the gas in the colon to vent out reduces this risk. Tension pneumoperitoneum presents with pulseless electrical activity. Once recognized, this requires immediate treatment. It involves insertion of a wide-bore needle or angiocath into the peritoneal cavity after confirming the presence of pneumoperitoneum by insertion of a smaller-gauge needle attached to a syringe filled with saline and observing air bubbles come up the syringe.[74] One could leave the endoscope in the colon as abdominal decompression is performed, so that the perforation could be closed once the patient is stabilized.

Within minutes of perforation, fluid leaks out of the colon and peritonitis sets in. If stool escapes, fecal peritonitis sets in. Hence, it is important to have a clean colon and aim for an excellent colon preparation.[75] In addition, making an effort to suction and dry up the colon segment where a resection is performed as well segments proximal and distal to the site of resection avoids the risk of flooding the site of resection if colon perforation were to occur. Placing the lesion in a nondependent position minimizes the risk of flooding of fluid and avoids fluid escape in case of perforation.

Once a perforation occurs, one should be ready to close it immediately if needed. Small perforations without peritoneal leakage of gas or fluid can be closed after extending and completing the resection; hurried closure and entrapment of polyp in the clip closed defect may result in a refractory recurrence that may be difficult to eradicate. Closure can be undertaken with TTSC or OTSC.

Microperforation and Macroperforation

Colonic perforations can be categorized based on the size of perforation and the timing of detection. Microperforations occur because of colonic wall thinning after the application of cautery and dissection of the submucosal layer that is not detected during endoscopy. These microperforations are detected when free air is seen on imaging studies done routinely after ESD in some centers.[76] Macroperforations occur because of deep and full-thickness resection of the colon wall and are obvious to the endoscopist in real time. These macroperforations result from inadequate injection of submucosal solution that fails to lift the lesion adequately, resection of the lesion into deep submucosa, or submucosal fibrosis from prior manipulation of the lesion (ie, attempted polypectomy).

Although immediate perforation detected during colonoscopy may be addressed endoscopically, delayed perforation often requires surgery. Patients presenting within 24 hours after the procedure are likely to have minimal peritoneal contamination and can successfully undergo surgical repair compared to patients with delayed presentation where fecal peritonitis has occurred and require a diversion procedure.[75,77] Risk factors for postoperative morbidity include blunt injury, poor bowel preparation, corticosteroid use, and age less than 67.[75,77]

Risk Factors for Perforation

Polyp-related factors
Polyp-related risk factors include location, size, and morphology of the lesion. Cecal location is an important risk factor for perforation. A nonpedunculated polyp in the cecum is associated with a 12-fold increased risk of perforation over a similar sized polyp in the distal colon.[78] Nonpolypoid or laterally spreading lesions are at risk for perforation (OR 4.1).[79] Lesions that may involve deeper tissue layers (Vienna classification 4: noninvasive high-grade dysplasia and Vienna classification 5: invasive neoplasia) were an independent risk factor for perforation.[70] Submucosal fibrosis from prior polypectomy attempts will impair successful lifting of the lesion with submucosal injection and increase the risk of perforation (OR 4.5).[80] Submucosal injection of hyaluronic acid solution is protective against perforation because of its ability to prolong the submucosal cushion effect for several minutes (OR 0.3).[79] It is critical to evaluate the morphology of the lesion in terms of their risk for perforation when contemplating resection so that adequate precautions can be taken (**Box 4**).

Technique/device-related factors
Colon perforation can result from mechanical injury (blunt force or torque-related) (55%), polypectomy (27%), or thermal injury (18%).[75,77]

Mechanical injury may occur while negotiating the colonoscope through a sigmoid colon that may be fixed by adhesions or extremely redundant.[77] It can also occur with retroflexion of the colonoscope in a small rectum, which is frequently observed in patients with severe proctitis or after pelvic radiation therapy. Blunt trauma results in large perforations (mean size 2 cm) of the rectosigmoid colon and may not be amenable to endoscopic closure.[81]

Box 4
Risk factors for colonic perforation

Polyp-related

- Morphology (laterally spreading, nonpedunculated)

- Location (cecum)

- Nonlifting with submucosal fluid injection (deeper layer involvement, prior attempted polypectomy)

Technique-related

- Mechanical injury (retroflexion in a small rectum, redundant sigmoid, or fixed angulation)

- Polypectomy injury

  o Resection of polyps greater than 1 cm in the right colon

  o Resection of polyps greater than 2 cm in the left colon

  o Multiple polyps

  o Thermal injury (argon plasma coagulation, electrocautery)

- Barotrauma (routinely decompress the colon, use carbon dioxide for insufflation)

Perforation related to polypectomy is due to unintentional deep thermal injury, full-thickness resection of the submucosa, or dissection through the muscularis propria. The incidence of perforation varies with type of resection: 0.01% with hot biopsy, 0.17% with polypectomy, 0.91% with EMR, and 3.3% with ESD.[69] Right hemicolon polyps larger than 1 cm, left hemicolon polyps larger than 2 cm, and multiple polyps all increase the risk for perforation.[9] Polypectomy perforations, EMR perforations, and ESD perforations tend to be smaller than those from blunt injury and are usually amenable to endoscopic closure.

Thermal injury from electrocautery or argon plasma coagulation used to ablate tissue or control bleeding may cause perforation. Unlike the perforations resulting from mechanical injury and polypectomy, perforations from thermal injuries tend to be small (1 cm) and are often located in the cecum.[81]

Skilled gastroenterologists with high procedural volume have a lower rate of perforation compared with non-GI endoscopists (surgeons, family physicians, and others). Additional risk factors include procedures performed at ambulatory surgery centers, older patients, female patients, and those with multiple comorbidities. Use of propofol for sedation does not increase the risk of perforation (see **Box 4**).[81–85]

Prevention of Colon Perforation

Several precautions can be taken by an endoscopist to minimize the risk of perforation and its consequences during polypectomy (**Box 5**).

Preprocedure counseling

Patients should be adequately counseled about the risks of EMR, especially if a large or complicated polypectomy is planned. Although this can be accomplished in patients referred for EMR by a preprocedure clinic visit, this may not be possible when one incidentally encounters a large flat lesion during a screening colonoscopy. This lesion could be managed by opting for one of these 3 approaches: (1) reschedule the patient on a separate day, which gives an opportunity to counsel the patient about the risks and benefits of EMR; (2) refer the patient to an EMR expert, who will counsel the patient and perform the procedure; or (3) resect during the same session. Take the opportunity to counsel the patient during the informed consent process that you may be removing a large polyp if encountered during a screening examination to avoid the need for a second procedure. As long as the patient understands the differences in risks between screening colonoscopy and colonoscopy with EMR, it is appropriate to proceed. This approach may avoid sampling the lesion, which increases the risk of turning the lesion into a defiant polyp, and make resection safer.[86]

Box 5
Prevention of colonic perforation

- Polyp is accessible and scope position can be maintained
- Lesion is positioned in a nondependent location
- Bowel preparation is excellent; residual feces and liquid are removed from the entire colon
- Appropriate volume of solution is injected into the submucosal space
- Adequate submucosal lift is achieved (especially if polypectomy has previously been attempted)
- Carbon dioxide used for insufflation

Bowel preparation

Colonoscopy should be deferred in patients with a poor bowel preparation because escape of feces and luminal contents into the peritoneal cavity results in fecal peritonitis. In those cases, colostomy with fecal diversion will be required and simple closure may not suffice.[75] Colon explosion can occur in patients undergoing polypectomy in the presence of poor colon preparation and accumulation of methane gas when combined with cautery.

Excellent bowel preparation reduces the risk of serious complications if a perforation were to occur. A split dose preparation with 2 L of PEG (polyethylene glycol) solution consumed over a period of 2 hours both the day before the procedure and the morning of the procedure, with the preparation completed 4 hours before procedure start time to ensure excellent colon preparation, is critical. One should aim for a Boston Bowel Preparation Scale score of 7 or greater.[87] The bowel preparation should be individualized based on the patient's need to travel to the facility, comorbid conditions (ie, diabetes, renal insufficiency), quality of previous bowel preparations, and tolerance of preparation solution.

Management of antithrombotic agents

The American Society of Gastrointestinal Endoscopy guidelines offer recommendations for the appropriate interval for discontinuing these agents and resuming them postprocedure. The decision to modify antithrombotic therapy should be individualized and optimally made in conjunction with the patient's primary care physician or cardiologist (see **Table 1**).[20]

Room setup and checklist

The endoscopy room should be set up to ensure patient safety and procedural efficiency and to minimize injury to the gastroenterologist. This setting is especially important when performing prolonged or complicated polypectomy or EMR.[88] Procedural efficiency lessens the strain on the endoscopist and can be critical in rescuing therapeutic misadventures when they occur. Therefore, all necessary equipment, supplies, and personnel should be readily available in the endoscopy room to minimize and manage complications of polypectomy. It is important to review the case with the team and ensure all equipment, including the ones required for rescue from complications, is available in the room. Recommendations to optimize the ergonomics of endoscopy are outlined in **Box 6**.

Patient positioning

It is important to position the patient such that it allows the lesion to be kept in a nondependent position. This position avoids escape of fluid into the peritoneum if a perforation were to occur. All residual fluid in the upstream and downstream segments of the colon should be suctioned before polypectomy to minimize the risk of peritoneal soiling.[81]

Endoscope setup—distal cap attachment, carbon dioxide

Although studies have not demonstrated the benefit of a cap-fitted colonoscope, the authors use it routinely for all polyp resections. The cap helps in accessing the lesion hidden under folds. In addition, the cap could be used to achieve tamponade if bleeding were to occur and helps to optimize endoclip placement. Carbon dioxide insufflation is preferable to room air especially with prolonged and high-risk procedures. It gets reabsorbed into the body faster than air if it escapes through a perforation and minimizes the risk of tension pneumoperitoneum that may otherwise require needle puncture of the abdomen and decompression. In addition, it reduces

---

Box 6
Room setup for colonoscopy with polypectomy

- Monitor positioned directly in front of endoscopist and just below eye level
- Monitors must be adjustable to accommodate endoscopists of varying heights (optimal viewing angle of 15°–25° below the horizon, viewing distance 52–182 cm)
- Examination table at or 0–10 cm below elbow level of endoscopist
- Adequate recovery time between procedures to rest endoscopist muscle groups
- Availability of both pediatric and adult colonoscopes and distal cap attachment
- Polypectomy devices (different shapes and sizes of snares, cold snares, injection needles, polyp retrieval nets)
- Agents to mix solutions for safe polypectomy (saline, indigo carmine, epinephrine)
- Hemostatic and closure devices (clips, hemostatic forceps, argon plasma coagulation (APC) machine, endoloop, and so on)
- Functioning argon plasma coagulation machine, probes, and grounding pads
- Capability to use carbon dioxide insufflation
- Technician/assistant with competency in using all necessary devices

Adapted from Shergill AK, McQuaid KR, Rempel D. Ergonomics and GI endoscopy. Gastrointest Endosc 2009;70:145–53; with permission.

---

postprocedure abdominal pain and hospitalizations.[89] The authors decompress the colon by removing the biopsy valve to allow passive venting of the colon, which may reduce the risk of a massive gas leak out of an otherwise distended colon through a perforation if it were to occur.

Management of Colon Perforations

During the last couple of decades, knowledge in assessing the depth of resection and identification of perforation during endoscopy has allowed management of these complications with prompt endoscopic closure, thus avoiding the need for surgery (**Box 7**).

Assessing the depth of resection

It is important to assess the depth of resection right after the cut is made. If a dye solution (like methylene blue or indigo carmine) is used to form a cushion underneath the polyp before resection, the submucosal space is tinted blue and confirms an appropriate depth. What if there are areas that are unstained in the polypectomy defect site? The technique of topical submucosal chromoendoscopy will help in these situations.[90] The injection catheter is positioned over the unstained area and irrigated with dye solution with the needle withdrawn. If this area absorbs the stain, submucosal

---

Box 7
Assessing depth of resection and defect closure devices

- Topical submucosal chromoendoscopy, target sign, stain resistance
- TTSC or endoclips
- OTSC
- Endoscopic suturing device, T-tags

depth is confirmed. Persistent nonstaining represents deep injury (white cautery ring indicating disruption of the muscularis propria layer), exposed muscle (uninterrupted concentric muscular rings), or submucosal fibrosis (dense white to yellow tissue).[90] The white cautery ring indicating disruption of the muscularis layer resembles a target sign surrounded by blue-stained submucosa. A corresponding target sign will also be present on the underside of the resected specimen.[72] These advances allow early detection of perforation during the procedure and well before the patient develops clinical signs of perforation or free air is seen on radiographic imaging and stresses the importance of methodically examining the polypectomy defect. Full-thickness resections and deep resection with exposure of the muscle should be closed with clips.

Through-the-scope clips

Binmoeller and colleagues[91] reported successful closure of a gastric perforation with endoscopic clips in the 1990s. Compared with the original clip, current versions allow one to rotate the clip to a desired angle for accurate placement and reopen the clip if the application is not satisfactory.[92] These clips are widely used for endoscopic closure of perforations and large defects.[46,93] Although TTSC are an effective method in closing polypectomy defects, they are limited by a smaller wingspan and lower closure force that can compromise tissue apposition and often necessitate the placement of multiple clips that adds to procedural cost and time.[94]

Over-the-scope clips

OTSC (Ovesco Endoscopy AG, Tubingen Germany) were first introduced in 2007. These clips are made of nitinol (nickel titanium alloy) and are housed on a metal applicator cap that fits over the distal tip of the endoscope, much like a band ligator. OTSC with rounded teeth are used for hemostasis, while those with pointed teeth are useful in closure of perforations. Compared with TTSC, OTSC grasp more tissue and offer a durable closure because of its higher grip force. The main disadvantage of OTSC is that they need to be loaded on to the scope before it can be deployed.[95–97]

Endoscopic suturing

Several endoscopic plicating devices have been introduced but are only used in a few specialized centers. Examples include the Eagle Claw VIII (Olympus Corporation, Tokyo, Japan), purse-string suturing device (LSI Solutions, Victor NY, USA), Flexible Endostitch (Covidien, North Haven, CT, USA), and Plicator (NDO Surgical Inc, Mansfield, MA, USA). Much of the experience with suturing devices comes from experimental models with only a few in vivo studies.[98] Other suture closure devices include T-tags, where a needle loaded with a metal T-tag and thread is inserted into the endoscope channel. Tissue is punctured, and the T-tag is ejected. This process is repeated on the opposite side of the defect, and the threads are cinched together.[99] More clinical work needs to be done using these devices, but they may offer a role in endoscopic closure of perforations in the future.

Endoscopic clip closure techniques

TTSC is the most popular device and can be used to safely close defects smaller than 2 cm in diameter by most endoscopists. These endoclips can successfully approximate the mucosal and submucosal layers in a partial thickness closure.[100] Endoscopists and their technicians should be familiar with the operation of the endoclips available in their endoscopy suite. When applying TTSC to a perforation site, it is important to keep the endoclip close to the tip of the scope for maximal control. The open wings of the endoclips should be positioned perpendicular to the defect and the lower edge of a transverse perforation captured with the lower wing. Gentle suction is applied to collapse the lumen to the endoclip to engage the opposite edge of the defect and capture maximal tissue. Once the endoclip is closed, optimal placement must be confirmed before deployment. An improperly positioned endoclip will hinder further endoclip placement. This process should begin at one end of the defect and be repeated until complete closure has been achieved.[81]

Proficiency with endoclip placement can be achieved with real-time experience in clinical practice. There are also hands-on courses held by major gastroenterology organizations worldwide where the technique can be perfected. In addition, DVDs are available from gastroenterology societies wherein this technique and others can be observed as performed by experts in the field.

OTSC is helpful in larger defects and in full-thickness resection of the colon but requires removal of the colonoscope to retrofit the device. In these circumstances, the patient should be positioned so the defect is in a nondependent location and the colon is fully decompressed before scope withdrawal to attach the OTSC. Over-the-scope suturing devices have been successful in the closure of 8 colonic perforations after ESD (Apollo Endosurgery, Austin, TX, USA) without any adverse events.[101]

Patient management after perforation

Patients should be admitted with strict nothing per mouth and given broad spectrum intravenous antibiotics and fluids. Blood counts should be monitored every 6 to 8 hours. Baseline imaging can be helpful in patients that deteriorate clinically. The surgical service should be involved at the outset in cases even when endoscopic closure has been achieved. Tension pneumoperitoneum should be decompressed with an 18-gauge or 20-gauge needle to prevent cardiopulmonary compromise.[74] Patients should be closely monitored and oral intake can be resumed once pain and fever subside, appetite and bowel function return, and leukocytosis has resolved.

Surgery is indicated for large perforations, for generalized peritonitis or ongoing sepsis, and in those who clinically deteriorate after apparently successful endoscopic clip closure of the defect. In one series, the technical success rate of TTSC closure was 91% (29/32) with 7 patients requiring surgery. TTSC was clinically unsuccessful in 5 patients who went on to require surgical intervention. Risk factors associated with the need for early surgical treatment (within 24 hours of endoscopic closure) were perforations greater than 1 cm, persistent leukocytosis, fever, severe abdominal pain, and a large amount of free intraperitoneal air (extending more than 3 cm below the diaphragm).[102] Laparoscopic approach may be possible based on local expertise and for patients that present early in their clinical course.[100] Greater delay to time of surgery resulted in an open surgical approach and need for diversion colostomy,[102] stressing the need for close clinical observation in the postendoscopic closure period.

How do outcomes for endoscopic clipping compare to surgical outcomes? One study compared the outcomes of patients with endoscopic closure for perforation versus surgery for those presenting with delayed perforation. Patients with failed clipping (either technical failure or clinical failure) that went on to surgery were excluded from analysis. Although the defects were significantly smaller in the clipping group, patient outcomes in terms of duration of fasting, treatment with antibiotics, and length of hospital stay were comparable to the surgical group.[103]

Postpolypectomy Syndrome

Postpolypectomy syndrome is due to transmural thermal injury resulting in localized peritonitis without perforation.[104,105] The incidence varies from 1.0 in 1000 to 3.0 per 100,000 examinations.[105] Risk factors for postpolypectomy syndrome include lesions larger than 1 cm (OR 2.8), nonpolypoid morphology (OR 3.3), and hypertension

(OR 3.0).[106] Large flat lesions require higher prolonged thermal energy, which increases the risk of transmural injury. Patients present with fever, localized abdominal pain and tenderness, and leukocytosis 1 to 5 days after polypectomy.[105] Management includes hospitalization, close monitoring, nothing by mouth, intravenous fluids, and antibiotics until clinical recovery is achieved. Typically, patients require fasting for 3 days, hospitalization for 5 days, and antibiotics for 7 days.[106] Postpolypectomy syndrome can be prevented by careful selection of appropriate endoscopic technique.

SUMMARY

Advances in the understanding of the risk factors for bleeding and perforation after endoscopic resection of polyps as well as the technology and techniques to prevent and manage these complications help shift the pendulum away from the need for surgical repair and toward endoscopic solutions.

REFERENCES

1. Levin TR, Zhao W, Conell C, et al. Complications of colonoscopy in an integrated health care delivery system. Ann Intern Med 2006;145:880–6.
2. Ko CW, Dominitz JA. Complications of colonoscopy: magnitude and management. Gastrointest Endosc Clin N Am 2010;20:659–71.
3. Rex DK, Petrini JL, Baron TH, et al. Quality indicators for colonoscopy. Gastrointest Endosc 2006;63:S16–28.
4. Kim HS, Kim TI, Kim WH, et al. Risk factors for immediate postpolypectomy bleeding of the colon: a multicenter study. Am J Gastroenterol 2006;101:1333–41.
5. Kim JH, Lee HJ, Ahn JW, et al. Risk factors for delayed post-polypectomy hemorrhage: a case-control study. J Gastroenterol Hepatol 2013;28:645–9.
6. Watabe H, Yamaji Y, Okamoto M, et al. Risk assessment for delayed hemorrhagic complication of colonic polypectomy: polyp-related factors and patient-related factors. Gastrointest Endosc 2006;64:73–8.
7. Buddingh KT, Herngreen T, Haringsma J, et al. Location in the right hemi-colon is an independent risk factor for delayed post-polypectomy hemorrhage: a multi-center case-control study. Am J Gastroenterol 2011;106:1119–24.
8. Sawhney MS, Salfiti N, Nelson DB, et al. Risk factors for severe delayed postpolypectomy bleeding. Endoscopy 2008;40:115–9.
9. Heldwein W, Dollhopf M, Rosch T, et al. The Munich Polypectomy Study (MUPS): prospective analysis of complications and risk factors in 4000 colonic snare polypectomies. Endoscopy 2005;37:1116–22.
10. Metz AJ, Bourke MJ, Moss A, et al. Factors that predict bleeding following endoscopic mucosal resection of large colonic lesions. Endoscopy 2011;43:506–11.
11. Consolo P, Luigiano C, Strangio G, et al. Efficacy, risk factors and complications of endoscopic polypectomy: ten year experience at a single center. World J Gastroenterol 2008;14:2364–9.
12. Dobrowolski S, Dobosz M, Babicki A, et al. Blood supply of colorectal polyps correlates with risk of bleeding after colonoscopic polypectomy. Gastrointest Endosc 2006;63:1004–9.
13. Gimeno-Garcia AZ, de Ganzo ZA, Sosa AJ, et al. Incidence and predictors of postpolypectomy bleeding in colorectal polyps larger than 10 mm. Eur J Gastroenterol Hepatol 2012;24:520–6.

14. Burgess NG, Williams SJ, Hourigan LF, et al. A management algorithm based on delayed bleeding after wide-field endoscopic mucosal resection of large colonic lesions. Clin Gastroenterol Hepatol 2014;12(9):1525–33.
15. Nakajima H, Takami H, Yamagata K, et al. Aspirin effects on colonic mucosal bleeding: implications for colonic biopsy and polypectomy. Dis Colon Rectum 1997;40:1484–8.
16. Pan A, Schlup M, Lubcke R, et al. The role of aspirin in post-polypectomy bleeding–a retrospective survey. BMC Gastroenterol 2012;12:138.
17. Manocha D, Singh M, Mehta N, et al. Bleeding risk after invasive procedures in aspirin/NSAID users: polypectomy study in veterans. Am J Med 2012;125: 1222–7.
18. Shiffman ML, Farrel MT, Yee YS. Risk of bleeding after endoscopic biopsy or polypectomy in patients taking aspirin or other NSAIDS. Gastrointest Endosc 1994; 40:458–62.
19. Yousfi M, Gostout CJ, Baron TH, et al. Postpolypectomy lower gastrointestinal bleeding: potential role of aspirin. Am J Gastroenterol 2004;99:1785–9.
20. ASGE Standards of Practice Committee, Anderson MA, Ben-Menachem T, et al. Management of antithrombotic agents for endoscopic procedures. Gastrointest Endosc 2009;70:1060–70.
21. Gandhi S, Narula N, Mosleh W, et al. Meta-analysis: colonoscopic post-polypectomy bleeding in patients on continued clopidogrel therapy. Aliment Pharmacol Ther 2013;37:947–52.
22. Feagins LA, Iqbal R, Harford WV, et al. Low rate of postpolypectomy bleeding among patients who continue thienopyridine therapy during colonoscopy. Clin Gastroenterol Hepatol 2013;11:1325–32.
23. Feagins LA, Uddin FS, Davila RE, et al. The rate of post-polypectomy bleeding for patients on uninterrupted clopidogrel therapy during elective colonoscopy is acceptably low. Dig Dis Sci 2011;56:2631–8.
24. Singh M, Mehta N, Murthy UK, et al. Postpolypectomy bleeding in patients undergoing colonoscopy on uninterrupted clopidogrel therapy. Gastrointest Endosc 2010;71:998–1005.
25. Hui AJ, Wong RM, Ching JY, et al. Risk of colonoscopic polypectomy bleeding with anticoagulants and antiplatelet agents: analysis of 1657 cases. Gastrointest Endosc 2004;59:44–8.
26. Witt DM, Delate T, McCool KH, et al. Incidence and predictors of bleeding or thrombosis after polypectomy in patients receiving and not receiving anticoagulation therapy. J Thromb Haemost 2009;7:1982–9.
27. Gerson LB, Michaels L, Ullah N, et al. Adverse events associated with anticoagulation therapy in the periendoscopic period. Gastrointest Endosc 2010;71: 1211–7.e2.
28. Inoue T, Nishida T, Maekawa A, et al. Clinical features of post-polypectomy bleeding associated with heparin bridge therapy. Dig Endosc 2014;26:243–9.
29. Friedland S, Soetikno R. Colonoscopy with polypectomy in anticoagulated patients. Gastrointest Endosc 2006;64:98–100.
30. Krishna SG, Rao BB, Thirumurthi S, et al. Safety of endoscopic interventions in patients with thrombocytopenia. Gastrointest Endosc 2014;80:425–34.
31. Jeon JW, Shin HP, Lee JI, et al. The risk of postpolypectomy bleeding during colonoscopy in patients with early liver cirrhosis. Surg Endosc 2012;26:3258–63.
32. Lee S, Park SJ, Cheon JH, et al. Child-Pugh score is an independent risk factor for immediate bleeding after colonoscopic polypectomy in liver cirrhosis. Yonsei Med J 2014;55:1281–8.

33. Hallback I, Hagg S, Eriksson AC, et al. In vitro effects of serotonin and noradrenaline reuptake inhibitors on human platelet adhesion and coagulation. Pharmacol Rep 2012;64:979–83.

34. Anglin R, Yuan Y, Moayyedi P, et al. Risk of upper gastrointestinal bleeding with selective serotonin reuptake inhibitors with or without concurrent nonsteroidal anti-inflammatory use: a systematic review and meta-analysis. Am J Gastroenterol 2014;109:811–9.

35. Dall M, Schaffalitzky de Muckadell OB, Lassen AT, et al. An association between selective serotonin reuptake inhibitor use and serious upper gastrointestinal bleeding. Clin Gastroenterol Hepatol 2009;7:1314–21.

36. Jiang HY, Chen HZ, Hu XJ, et al. Use of selective serotonin reuptake inhibitors and risk of upper gastrointestinal bleeding: a systematic review and meta-analysis. Clin Gastroenterol Hepatol 2015;13(1):42–50.e3.

37. Repici A, Hassan C, Vitetta E, et al. Safety of cold polypectomy for <10mm polyps at colonoscopy: a prospective multicenter study. Endoscopy 2012;44: 27–31.

38. Aslan F, Camci M, Alper E, et al. Cold snare polypectomy versus hot snare polypectomy in endoscopic treatment of small polyps. Turk J Gastroenterol 2014;25: 279–83.

39. Paspatis GA, Tribonias G, Konstantinidis K, et al. A prospective randomized comparison of cold vs hot snare polypectomy in the occurrence of postpolypectomy bleeding in small colonic polyps. Colorectal Dis 2011;13:e345–8.

40. Horiuchi A, Nakayama Y, Kajiyama M, et al. Removal of small colorectal polyps in anticoagulated patients: a prospective randomized comparison of cold snare and conventional polypectomy. Gastrointest Endosc 2014;79:417–23.

41. Monkemuller K, Neumann H, Malfertheiner P, et al. Advanced colon polypectomy. Clin Gastroenterol Hepatol 2009;7:641–52.

42. Van Gossum A, Cozzoli A, Adler M, et al. Colonoscopic snare polypectomy: analysis of 1485 resections comparing two types of current. Gastrointest Endosc 1992;38:472–5.

43. Hogan RB, Hogan RB 3rd. Epinephrine volume reduction of giant colon polyps facilitates endoscopic assessment and removal. Gastrointest Endosc 2007;66: 1018–22.

44. Lee SH, Chung IK, Kim SJ, et al. Comparison of postpolypectomy bleeding between epinephrine and saline submucosal injection for large colon polyps by conventional polypectomy: a prospective randomized, multicenter study. World J Gastroenterol 2007;13:2973–7.

45. Dobrowolski S, Dobosz M, Babicki A, et al. Prophylactic submucosal saline-adrenaline injection in colonoscopic polypectomy: prospective randomized study. Surg Endosc 2004;18:990–3.

46. Liaquat H, Rohn E, Rex DK. Prophylactic clip closure reduced the risk of delayed postpolypectomy hemorrhage: experience in 277 clipped large sessile or flat colorectal lesions and 247 control lesions. Gastrointest Endosc 2013; 77:401–7.

47. Feagins LA, Nguyen AD, Iqbal R, et al. The prophylactic placement of hemoclips to prevent delayed post-polypectomy bleeding: an unnecessary practice? A case control study. Dig Dis Sci 2014;59:823–8.

48. Katsinelos P, Fasoulas K, Chatzimavroudis G, et al. Prophylactic clip application before endoscopic resection of large pedunculated colorectal polyps in patients receiving anticoagulation or antiplatelet medications. Surg Laparosc Endosc Percutan Tech 2012;22:e254–8.

49. Parikh ND, Zanocco K, Keswani RN, et al. A cost-efficacy decision analysis of prophylactic clip placement after endoscopic removal of large polyps. Clin Gastroenterol Hepatol 2013;11:1319–24.

50. Quintanilla E, Castro JL, Rabago LR, et al. Is the use of prophylactic hemoclips in the endoscopic resection of large pedunculated polyps useful? A prospective and randomized study. J Interv Gastroenterol 2012;2:183–8.

51. Ji JS, Lee SW, Kim TH, et al. Comparison of prophylactic clip and endoloop application for the prevention of postpolypectomy bleeding in pedunculated colonic polyps: a prospective, randomized, multicenter study. Endoscopy 2014;46:598–604.

52. Di Giorgio P, De Luca L, Calcagno G, et al. Detachable snare versus epinephrine injection in the prevention of postpolypectomy bleeding: a randomized and controlled study. Endoscopy 2004;36:860–3.

53. Lee CK, Lee SH, Park JY, et al. Prophylactic argon plasma coagulation ablation does not decrease delayed postpolypectomy bleeding. Gastrointest Endosc 2009;70:353–61.

54. Bahin FF, Naidoo M, Williams SJ, et al. Prophylactic endoscopic coagulation to prevent bleeding after wide-field endoscopic mucosal resection of large sessile colon polyps. Clin Gastroenterol Hepatol 2014. [Epub ahead of print].

55. Paspatis GA, Paraskeva K, Theodoropoulou A, et al. A prospective, randomized comparison of adrenaline injection in combination with detachable snare versus adrenaline injection alone in the prevention of postpolypectomy bleeding in large colonic polyps. Am J Gastroenterol 2006;101:2805 [quiz: 2913].

56. Kouklakis G, Mpoumponaris A, Gatopoulou A, et al. Endoscopic resection of large pedunculated colonic polyps and risk of postpolypectomy bleeding with adrenaline injection versus endoloop and hemoclip: a prospective, randomized study. Surg Endosc 2009;23:2732–7.

57. Li LY, Liu QS, Li L, et al. A meta-analysis and systematic review of prophylactic endoscopic treatments for postpolypectomy bleeding. Int J Colorectal Dis 2011; 26:709–19.

58. Burgess NG, Metz AJ, Williams SJ, et al. Risk factors for intraprocedural and clinically significant delayed bleeding after wide-field endoscopic mucosal resection of large colonic lesions. Clin Gastroenterol Hepatol 2014;12: 651–61.e1–3.

59. Hong SP. How do I manage post-polypectomy bleeding? Clin Endosc 2012;45: 282–4.

60. Fahrtash-Bahin F, Holt BA, Jayasekeran V, et al. Snare tip soft coagulation achieves effective and safe endoscopic hemostasis during wide-field endoscopic resection of large colonic lesions (with videos). Gastrointest Endosc 2013;78:158–63.e1.

61. Coumaros D, Tsesmeli N. Active gastrointestinal bleeding: use of hemostatic forceps beyond endoscopic submucosal dissection. World J Gastroenterol 2010; 16:2061–4.

62. Asge Technology C, Conway JD, Adler DG, et al. Endoscopic hemostatic devices. Gastrointest Endosc 2009;69:987–96.

63. Feagins LA, Spechler SJ. Use of hemoclips and other measures to prevent bleeding during colonoscopy by gastroenterologists in Veterans Affairs hospitals. Am J Gastroenterol 2014;109:288–90.

64. Chen WC, Maru DM, Abraham SC, et al. Endoscopic clip tamponade of bleeding: a novel adjunct technique for endoscopic mucosal resection. Endoscopy 2013;45(Suppl 2 UCTN):E104–5.

65. Parra-Blanco A, Kaminaga N, Kojima T, et al. Hemoclipping for postpolypectomy and postbiopsy colonic bleeding. Gastrointest Endosc 2000;51:37–41.
66. Akahoshi K, Yoshinaga S, Fujimaru T, et al. Endoscopic resection with hypertonic saline-solution-epinephrine injection plus band ligation for large peduncu- lated or semipedunculated gastric polyp. Gastrointest Endosc 2006;63:312–6.
67. Alcaide N, Penas-Herrero I, Sancho-del-Val L, et al. Ovesco system for treat- ment of postpolypectomy bleeding after failure of conventional treatment. Rev Esp Enferm Dig 2014;106:55–8.
68. Singhal S, Changela K, Papafragkakis H, et al. Over the scope clip: technique and expanding clinical applications. J Clin Gastroenterol 2013;47:749–56.
69. Oka S, Tanaka S, Kanao H, et al. Current status in the occurrence of postoper- ative bleeding, perforation and residual/local recurrence during colonoscopic treatment in Japan. Dig Endosc 2010;22:376–80.
70. Wada Y, Kudo SE, Tanaka S, et al. Predictive factors for complications in endo- scopic resection of large colorectal lesions: a multicenter prospective study. Surg Endosc 2014. [Epub ahead of print].
71. Asge Technology Committee, Kantsevoy SV, Adler DG, et al. Endoscopic mucosal resection and endoscopic submucosal dissection. Gastrointest En- dosc 2008;68:11–8.
72. Swan MP, Bourke MJ, Moss A, et al. The target sign: an endoscopic marker for the resection of the muscularis propria and potential perforation during colonic endoscopic mucosal resection. Gastrointest Endosc 2011;73:79–85.
73. Kipple JC. Bilateral tension pneumothoraces and subcutaneous emphysema following colonoscopic polypectomy: a case report and discussion of anes- thesia considerations. AANA J 2010;78:462–7.
74. Broeders E, Al-Taher M, Peeters K, et al. Verres needle desufflation as an effec- tive treatment option for colonic perforation after colonoscopy. Surg Laparosc Endosc Percutan Tech 2014. [Epub ahead of print].
75. Iqbal CW, Cullinane DC, Schiller HJ, et al. Surgical management and outcomes of 165 colonoscopic perforations from a single institution. Arch Surg 2008;143: 701–6 [discussion: 706–7].
76. Lee DW, Jeon SW. Management of complications during gastric endoscopic submucosal dissection. Diagn Ther Endosc 2012;2012:624835.
77. Raju GS. Gastrointestinal perforations: role of endoscopic closure. Curr Opin Gastroenterol 2011;27:418–22.
78. Rutter MD, Nickerson C, Rees CJ, et al. Risk factors for adverse events related to polypectomy in the English Bowel Cancer Screening Programme. Endoscopy 2014;46:90–7.
79. Lee EJ, Lee JB, Choi YS, et al. Clinical risk factors for perforation during endo- scopic submucosal dissection (ESD) for large-sized, nonpedunculated colo- rectal tumors. Surg Endosc 2012;26:1587–94.
80. Kim ES, Cho KB, Park KS, et al. Factors predictive of perforation during endo- scopic submucosal dissection for the treatment of colorectal tumors. Endos- copy 2011;43:573–8.
81. Raju GS, Saito Y, Matsuda T, et al. Endoscopic management of colonoscopic perforations (with videos). Gastrointest Endosc 2011;74:1380–8.
82. Chukmaitov A, Bradley CJ, Dahman B, et al. Association of polypectomy tech- niques, endoscopist volume, and facility type with colonoscopy complications. Gastrointest Endosc 2013;77:436–46.
83. Lohsiriwat V, Sujarittanakarn S, Akaraviputh T, et al. What are the risk factors of colonoscopic perforation? BMC Gastroenterol 2009;9:71.

84. Lorenzo-Zuniga V, Moreno de Vega V, Domenech E, et al. Endoscopist experience as a risk factor for colonoscopic complications. Colorectal Dis 2010;12:e273–7.

85. Bielawska B, Day AG, Lieberman DA, et al. Risk factors for early colonoscopic perforation include non-gastroenterologist endoscopists: a multivariable analysis. Clin Gastroenterol Hepatol 2014;12:85–92.

86. Buchner AM, Guarner-Argente C, Ginsberg GG. Outcomes of EMR of defiant colorectal lesions directed to an endoscopy referral center. Gastrointest Endosc 2012;76:255–63.

87. Lai EJ, Calderwood AH, Doros G, et al. The Boston bowel preparation scale: a valid and reliable instrument for colonoscopy-oriented research. Gastrointest Endosc 2009;69:620–5.

88. Shergill AK, McQuaid KR, Rempel D. Ergonomics and GI endoscopy. Gastrointest Endosc 2009;70:145–53.

89. Bassan MS, Holt B, Moss A, et al. Carbon dioxide insufflation reduces number of postprocedure admissions after endoscopic resection of large colonic lesions: a prospective cohort study. Gastrointest Endosc 2013;77:90–5.

90. Holt BA, Jayasekeran V, Sonson R, et al. Topical submucosal chromoendoscopy defines the level of resection in colonic EMR and may improve procedural safety (with video). Gastrointest Endosc 2013;77:949–53.

91. Binmoeller KF, Grimm H, Soehendra N. Endoscopic closure of a perforation using metallic clips after snare excision of a gastric leiomyoma. Gastrointest Endosc 1993;39:172–4.

92. Raju GS, Gajula L. Endoclips for GI endoscopy. Gastrointest Endosc 2004;59: 267–79.

93. Raju GS. Endoscopic management of gastrointestinal leaks. Gastrointest Endosc Clin N Am 2007;17:487–503, vi.

94. Jayaraman V, Hammerle C, Lo SK, et al. Clinical application and outcomes of over the scope clip device: initial US experience in humans. Diagn Ther Endosc 2013;2013:381873.

95. Baron TH, Song LM, Ross A, et al. Use of an over-the-scope clipping device: multicenter retrospective results of the first U.S. experience (with videos). Gastrointest Endosc 2012;76:202–8.

96. Seebach L, Bauerfeind P, Gubler C. "Sparing the surgeon": clinical experience with over-the-scope clips for gastrointestinal perforation. Endoscopy 2010;42:1108–11.

97. Weiland T, Fehlker M, Gottwald T, et al. Performance of the OTSC system in the endoscopic closure of iatrogenic gastrointestinal perforations: a systematic review. Surg Endosc 2013;27:2258–74.

98. Pham BV, Raju GS, Ahmed I, et al. Immediate endoscopic closure of colon perforation by using a prototype endoscopic suturing device: feasibility and outcome in a porcine model (with video). Gastrointest Endosc 2006;64:113–9.

99. Raju GS. Endoscopic closure of gastrointestinal leaks. Am J Gastroenterol 2009; 104:1315–20.

100. Paraskeva KD, Paspatis GA. Management of bleeding and perforation after colonoscopy. Expert Rev Gastroenterol Hepatol 2014;8(8):963–72.

101. Kantsevoy SV, Bitner M, Mitrakov AA, et al. Endoscopic suturing closure of large mucosal defects after endoscopic submucosal dissection is technically feasible, fast, and eliminates the need for hospitalization (with videos). Gastrointest Endosc 2014;79:503–7.

102. Cho SB, Lee WS, Joo YE, et al. Therapeutic options for iatrogenic colon perforation: feasibility of endoscopic clip closure and predictors of the need for early surgery. Surg Endosc 2012;26:473–9.

103. Kim JS, Kim BW, Kim JI, et al. Endoscopic clip closure versus surgery for the treatment of iatrogenic colon perforations developed during diagnostic colonoscopy: a review of 115,285 patients. Surg Endosc 2013;27:501–4.
104. Kim HW. What is different between postpolypectomy fever and postpolypectomy coagulation syndrome? Clin Endosc 2014;47:205–6.
105. ASGE Standards of Practice Committee, Fisher DA, Maple JT, et al. Complications of colonoscopy. Gastrointest Endosc 2011;74:745–52.
106. Cha JM, Lim KS, Lee SH, et al. Clinical outcomes and risk factors of postpolypectomy coagulation syndrome: a multicenter, retrospective, case-control study. Endoscopy 2013;45:202–7.

Colonic Strictures
Dilation and Stents

Douglas G. Adler, MD

KEYWORDS

- Colonic stricture • Inflammatory bowel disease • Colonic stent
- Anastomotic stricture • Colon cancer • Colonic obstruction
- Large bowel obstruction

KEY POINTS

- Colonic strictures, both benign and malignant, are common.
- Dilation of benign colonic strictures, most notably caused by inflammatory bowel disease, is safe and effective, and can obviate surgery in some patients.
- Malignant colonic strictures rarely respond to dilation.
- Malignant colonic strictures are typically treated by stents and/or surgery.
- Colonic stents are safe and effective for malignant large bowel obstruction and can play a role in certain benign colonic strictures, notably anastomotic strictures.

INTRODUCTION

Colonic strictures, both benign and malignant, are commonly encountered in clinical practice by both gastroenterologists and surgeons. Benign strictures are most commonly treated by balloon dilation and less frequently with stents. The opposite is true for malignant strictures, whether they are intrinsic or extrinsic to the colon. This article reviews the endoscopic management of colonic strictures.

ENDOSCOPIC BALLOON DILATION OF BENIGN COLONIC STRICTURES

Endoscopic dilation of colonic strictures is primarily used for benign indications: anastomotic strictures, strictures from inflammatory bowel disease (IBD) (usually Crohn's disease), colopathy induced by nonsteroidal anti-inflammatory drugs, and, rarely, diverticular strictures that develop following acute diverticulitis. There is only a limited role for dilation of malignant strictures, as the duration of effect is typically short lived.

Dilation of strictures is typically performed by using through-the-scope (TTS) balloons. Passage dilators are largely reserved for very distal strictures and are uncommonly used in current practice. The technique for balloon dilation is relatively simple. The endoscope (usually a colonoscope) is advanced to the level of the colonic

Gastroenterology and Hepatology, Huntsman Cancer Center, University of Utah School of Medicine, 30 North 1900 East 4R118, Salt Lake City, UT 84312, USA
E-mail address: douglas.adler@hsc.utah.edu

Gastrointest Endoscopy Clin N Am 25 (2015) 359–371
http://dx.doi.org/10.1016/j.giec.2014.11.001
giendo.theclinics.com

stricture. It is not mandatory to traverse the stricture with the endoscope. TTS balloons are available in over-the-wire and non–guide wire based formats, and both are equally effective. TTS balloons used in this context are typically esophageal, pyloric, or colonic balloons; there are no data to support the superiority of one type over another. If the stricture is tortuous, it is recommended that a guide wire be advanced across the stricture under fluoroscopic and endoscopic guidance. Fluoroscopy can confirm the presence of the wire in the proximal large bowel. An estimate of the required balloon size can be made and a balloon selected. Most TTS balloons are available in multiple size formats (ie, 12-, 13.5-, and 15-mm diameters when inflated with varying amounts of fluid). The TTS balloon can be advanced over the wire (if a wire was used) and across the stricture. The balloon can then be inflated with saline, contrast, or a mixture thereof. Contrast is only required if fluoroscopy is to be used.

The time required to keep the balloon inflated is not standardized. Individual preferences vary, and inflation times of 30, 60, and 120 seconds are all commonly used, with no data to suggest the superiority of one specific duration. Once the balloon is deflated the stricture can be evaluated for improvement in luminal diameter, the need for further dilation, and for any complications (most notably bleeding and/or perforation).

Almost all of the currently available data on balloon dilation of benign colonic strictures come from the IBD literature, wherein the procedure has been reported for several years. The technique is recognized as being relatively safe and an alternative to surgery (or at least a temporizing measure in patients who are not surgical candidates at the time of endoscopy). Most studies have reported on patients with small and large bowel strictures, and mix pure intestinal strictures with anastomotic strictures.

A representative study was published by Foster and colleagues[1] in 2008. A variety of strictures were identified in the small and large bowel of 24 patients, most of whom had Crohn's disease (22 of 24). Overall, 71 dilations were performed in 29 strictures. Of note, 46 dilations for 17 strictures were performed with a simultaneous injection of triamcinolone to increase the duration of effect. Mean follow-up was 32 months. The investigators reported results in 1 stomal, 12 anastomotic, and 16 de novo strictures. There were no complications in 22 of 24 patients; bleeding and perforation occurred in 1 patient and rupture of a paracolonic abscess developed in another with a sigmoid stricture. Two patients failed endoscopic therapy and ultimately required surgery.

Hoffman and colleagues[2] reported their results in 25 patients with Crohn's disease who underwent TTS dilations. Thirty-nine colonoscopies with 51 dilations were performed, and 52% became asymptomatic after a single dilation while 48% needed further dilations or surgery. Mild bleeding (that did not require transfusion) occurred in 3 out of 39 colonoscopies, and there was 1 perforation. The investigators found that significant negative prognostic factors were active smoking and ulcerated strictures ($P<.05$ each).

One of the largest studies regarding endoscopic dilation for strictures in Crohn's disease comes from Gustavsson and colleagues,[3] who reported on a 22-year institutional history. Between 1987 and 2009, this group performed 776 endoscopic dilations for benign strictures (80% were for anastomotic strictures) in 178 patients (94 of whom were women) with Crohn's disease. The median age of the patients was 45 years, with median disease duration of 16 years. Technical success was achieved in 689 of 776 patients (89%), and rates of patients undergoing surgery at 1, 3, and 5 years were 13%, 28%, and 36%, respectively. Complications occurred in 41 of 776 dilations (5.3%) and included bowel perforation (n = 11, 1.4%), bleeding requiring blood transfusion (n = 8, 1.0%), minor bleeding (n = 10, 1.3%), and abdominal pain or fever (n = 12, 1.5%). Ten patients required surgery to treat complications, usually perforation.

Overall, balloon dilation for benign colonic strictures is considered to be safe and effective, but generally requires repeated treatments.

ENDOSCOPIC SELF-EXPANDING METAL STENTS FOR THE TREATMENT OF MALIGNANT COLONIC STRICTURES

Malignant strictures are largely treated in current endoscopic practice through the use of self-expanding metal stents (SEMS).[4] These devices, once only used in tertiary referral centers, are now in widespread use in both academic and general gastrointestinal practices. Stents are most commonly placed by gastroenterologists, but some surgeons and interventional radiologists also perform the procedure. SEMS are most commonly used to treat malignant large bowel obstructions.

Malignant colonic obstructions can occur as a result of primary colorectal cancer causing intrinsic obstruction, or extrinsic lesions that compress the colon. Most extrinsic lesions arise from primary pelvic malignancies such as bladder, ovarian, and uterine cancer, but can also arise from metastatic lesions to the pelvis. In general, patients with extrinsic malignant colonic obstruction usually have incurable disease and are not good candidates for surgeries beyond a decompressing colostomy. Dedicated stents for use in the large bowel are all uncovered metal mesh devices that embed in the stricture site. These devices are usually placed without intent of future endoscopic removal. Fully covered esophageal stents can be used in an off-label manner to treat colonic anastomotic strictures and diverticular strictures.

SEMS are typically used in 2 settings: preoperative (as a bridge to surgery) and palliative (in patients with primary colorectal cancers who are not candidates for surgery because of metastatic disease or overall debility).

SEMS are available as TTS and non-TTS stents. TTS stents are much more commonly used in North America, but non-TTS devices still play an important role. TTS stents can be used anywhere in the colon that can be reached by an endoscope, including the very proximal colon or across the ileocecal valve. Non-TTS stents are largely confined to use in the left colon, as they cannot be advanced more proximally because of their limited catheter length and the relatively high rigidity of these same deployment catheters.

Self-Expanding Metal Stents for Malignant Colonic Obstruction in the Preoperative Setting

Many patients with primary colon cancer will have obstruction as their presenting symptom.[5] It must be stressed that patients who present with acute malignant colonic obstruction are almost always ill. Patients tend to be dehydrated, have electrolyte abnormalities, and a distended proximal colon (full of stool), and may have respiratory compromise owing to limited diaphragmatic excursion from a distended abdomen. These patients are generally poor surgical candidates in the acute setting, and surgeons may be reluctant to take such patients for emergency surgery if other options are available.

The management of patients with acute colonic obstruction arising from colon cancer includes both surgical and endoscopic approaches. Patients can undergo placement of a colonic SEMS or surgery. The surgical options are similar to what they were in years past: surgery with creation of a loop colostomy or loop ileostomy and subsequent resection (2- or 3-staged procedure), a primary resection with end colostomy (Hartmann procedure), or a primary tumor resection with creation of an internal anastomosis at the time of the primary surgery. This last option often requires on-table lavage and, though often discussed, is rarely performed given the complexity involved.

One should pay special attention to how many of the aforementioned surgical options include a temporary or permanent ostomy creation, which most patients would prefer to avoid. The use of a SEMS for acute colonic obstruction has several advantages for patients who ultimately undergo surgery. Placement of a colonic SEMS can serve as a bridge to surgery because it allows bowel decompression via the normal route, patient stabilization, correction of electrolyte abnormalities, hydration, and proper preoperative care. Placement of a SEMS before surgery allows time for a complete oncologic evaluation and cancer staging. Of importance, patients who undergo SEMS placement in the setting of an acute colonic obstruction can undergo standard bowel preparation via ingestion of an oral purgative. Once this is accomplished, most patients who proceed to surgery can undergo a 1-stage procedure whereby the primary tumor is removed and an internal colocolonic anastomosis is created, thus avoiding the need for an ostomy.

Many high-quality prospective studies have been performed to evaluate the technical and clinical success rates for SEMS placement in the preoperative setting for acute colonic obstruction.[5–11] Technical success (defined as successful placement of 1 or more stents across the stricture) is common, occurring in 75% to 100% of patients, and clinical success (defined as successful bowel decompression and patient stabilization) is seen in 84% to 100% of patients.

The question of whether a patient with acute colonic obstruction should undergo surgery or SEMS placement is central to management, and has been evaluated in several prospective studies and high-quality meta-analyses with comparable overall results. A recent Cochrane meta-analysis of patients with acute malignant colon obstruction reviewed 5 randomized trials that included a total of 207 patients. This study compared outcomes between colonic stenting in 102 patients and emergency surgery in 105 patients.[12] With regard to SEMS, technical success was achieved in 86% of patients. The perforation rate was 5.88% and the migration rate was 2.13%. There was no statistically significant difference in the overall complication rate or 30-day mortality rate between the patients who underwent stenting or surgery. The mean hospital stay was shorter in the patients who underwent SEMS placement than in those who underwent emergency surgery (11.5 vs 17.2 days). This study can be interpreted as arguing for SEMS placement over emergency surgery in patients who are candidates for endoscopic therapy.

A 2012 meta-analysis that included 2 randomized studies and 6 retrospective studies compared outcomes between SEMS placement as a bridge to surgery with emergency surgery in patients who presented with obstruction in the setting of colon cancer.[13] Patients who underwent SEMS placement had overall lower mortality, fewer postoperative anastomotic leaks, and a lower rate of initial stoma creation in comparison with those undergoing emergency surgery.

In practice, the decision to place a SEMS or operate in a patient with acute malignant obstruction should be made by joint consultation between patients, gastroenterologists, and surgeons, with risks and benefits weighed carefully. Some patients are not candidates for endoscopy and are best treated via emergency surgery, whereas others are better treated by endoscopy with SEMS placement followed by surgery. The current environment of multidisciplinary care should foster active discussion as to what is the best option for individual patients.

Self-Expanding Metal Stents for Malignant Obstruction in Patients Who Are Not Surgical Candidates

The presence of widespread or disseminated peritoneal or solid organ metastatic disease, malignant ascites, or significant comorbidity may preclude surgery in some patients with malignant colonic obstruction. Placement of a SEMS in these patients is performed for palliation of symptoms of obstruction and improvement in their quality of life. These patients usually have short survival, and stents are often placed before a referral for hospice care to ensure bowel patency.

As previously mentioned, some patients with malignancies of nongastrointestinal origin (ie, bladder, ovarian, and uterine cancer) can develop colonic obstruction attributable to extrinsic compression from primary tumors, malignant adenopathy, or metastases. Patients with extrinsic malignant colonic obstruction will not have a visible mass in the colonic lumen in most cases, but rather a smooth-walled area of obstruction. Extrinsic colonic obstructions are more likely to occur in the left colon and are most commonly seen in the distal large bowel.

A prospective multicenter study of SEMS placement for malignant colonic obstruction in 44 nonsurgical patients showed a technical success rate of 95% with a clinical success rate of 81%.[14] There were no perforations or SEMS-related mortality. Another retrospective study of 168 palliative colon SEMS placements reported a technical success of 96%, with 99% of these patients reported to have immediate clinical success with regard to bowel decompression.[15]

A multicenter retrospective study involving 5 tertiary care centers and 201 patients evaluated the use of palliative SEMS placement for colorectal obstruction.[16] Technical success was seen in 91.5% of patients, and clinical success was achieved in 89.7%. Fully three-quarters of enrolled patients were able to avoid undergoing creation of a colostomy. Major complications occurred in 11.9% of patients: 11 migrations, 12 perforations, and 1 reobstruction. This study noted an association between the humanized monoclonal antibody/angiogenesis inhibitor bevacizumab and perforation, the risk of which was increased 19.6-fold. Other studies have noted this risk with this agent.[17]

Most of the published literature comparing surgery with SEMS placement is based in the preoperative setting. Only limited data exist to compare the use of SEMS with surgery in the palliative setting.

A retrospective cohort study of 144 patients with inoperable and/or metastatic colon cancer included 73 patients who underwent surgery and 71 who underwent SEMS placement. Patients who had SEMS placed developed early complications (15.5% vs 32.9%, respectively).[18] Overall, major complication rates were not significantly different. Fully 39.7% of patients in the surgical group had an ostomy created, again emphasizing a potential benefit of stenting when feasible.

A retrospective study of 55 patients (29 SEMS, 26 surgery) who were treated in a palliative manner for left-sided large bowel obstruction was published in 2008.[19] Hospital stay was significantly shorter for patients who underwent SEMS placement (4 vs 13.5 days, P<.0001). Four of the patients in the SEMS group eventually required surgery. Creation of a stoma was needed in 12 of 26 patients who underwent surgery and 4 of 29 patients who had a SEMS placed. Survival among patients in both groups was similar.

The only published randomized trial of SEMS placement versus surgery in the palliative setting was stopped prematurely because of an unusually high number of perforations in the stent group.[20] There were 10 patients in the surgical treatment group and 11 in the SEMS group, with 6 perforations occurring in the SEMS group. It should be noted that this is an exceptionally high perforation rate that is inconsistent with the existing colonic stent literature.

As mentioned previously in the context of stent placement in the preoperative setting, the ultimate decision on SEMS or surgery in patients with incurable disease should be made through a multidisciplinary and individualized approach.

TECHNIQUE OF SELF-EXPANDING METAL STENT PLACEMENT

The technique of SEMS placement is relatively straightforward (**Fig. 1**). Whether using TTS or non-TTS SEMS, patients with malignant colonic obstruction should have the site of obstruction directly identified and evaluated by endoscopy. An endoscope with a therapeutic channel is required for TTS SEMS placement. Fluoroscopy, though not mandatory for SEMS placement in the colon, is extremely helpful for all phases of the procedure and is almost always used.

When the site of obstruction is reached, passing the endoscope across the stricture is generally attempted, though not mandatory. Dilation of the stricture before SEMS placement is rarely required, and can increase the risk of perforation and/or tumor fracture as well as bleeding.[21] Dilation can be gently performed with TTS balloon dilators to facilitate the passage of the stent catheter across the stricture, but a more generous dilation is usually of little additional benefit.

Endoscope selection is affected by stricture location. In patients with left-sided malignant obstruction, a therapeutic esophagogastroduodenoscopy scope or a flexible sigmoidoscope can be used, as both of these devices have a 3.7-mm therapeutic channel that can accommodate a 10F TTS stent catheter. In patients with an obstruction at or proximal to the level of the splenic flexure, an adult colonoscope is required, given its longer insertion tube. Rarely, a duodenoscope may be needed if the site of obstruction is severely angulated and cannot be seen en face. The duodenoscope can allow the physician to see "around a corner" in a very angulated stricture to allow catheter and guide wire placement.

Once the endoscope reaches the site of the obstruction, the stricture can be directly inspected for the presence of an intrinsic mass or any signs of extrinsic compression (**Fig. 2**). Evaluation of the colonic lumen (which may be obvious or obscure), signs of any active blood loss, and shallow or deep ulcerations are all important findings that affect the decision of whether to proceed with stent placement. If the lesion appears to have already perforated or if the bowel at the site of the obstruction appears ischemic, stent placement is generally deferred and the patient is referred to surgery. Again, passage of the endoscope through the site of the obstruction is usually not required, but endoscope passage is not absolutely contraindicated if it can be performed easily and in a minimally traumatic manner.

The next step is the advancement of a flexible guide wire across the stenosis into the proximal large bowel. Most physicians first advance a biliary retrieval balloon or a straight biliary catheter through the working channel of the endoscope and then pass the guide wire through the catheter itself. The tip of the catheter can be used to gently probe the mass/obstruction in an attempt to identify a site for accessing the proximal large bowel. Once a possible lumen is identified, attempts at guide wire passage can be gently initiated. Passage of the guide wire is performed under both endoscopic and fluoroscopic guidance.

There is no ideal guide wire for colonic SEMS placement, and individual preferences vary. Nevertheless, a guide wire with a floppy hydrophilic tip should be selected to minimize trauma during the procedure. Some physicians believe that stiff 0.035" (0.889 mm) guide wires are best, whereas others prefer the softer, floppier

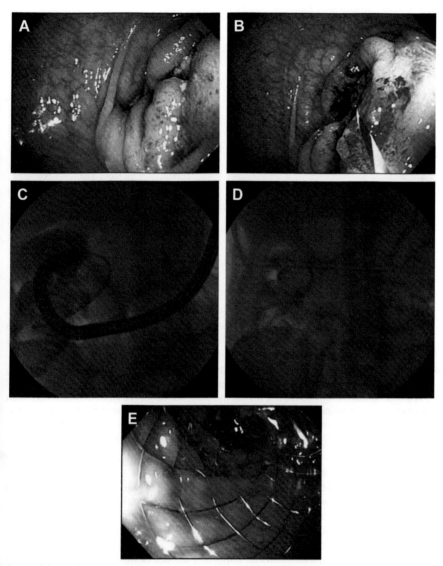

Fig. 1. (*A*) A primary, intrinsic, obstructing colon cancer. (*B*) A 0.025″ guide wire has been advanced across the malignant obstruction. (*C*) A through-the-scope (TTS) stent has been advanced through the working channel of the endoscope, over the wire, and across the stricture. (*D*) Fluoroscopic image of the fully deployed stent. Note the narrow waist in the middle of the stent; this will resolve over 24 to 48 hours, but the patient can still pass stool and gas immediately. (*E*) Endoscopic image of the stent after deployment.

0.025″ (0.635 mm) guide wires. A stiff 0.035″ guide wire may provide greater stability as the stent is advanced across the stricture, and may facilitate advancement and deployment of stents through severely angulated strictures. 0.025″ guide wires tend to more easily traverse severe stenoses, and may be advantageous for crossing strictures that are long and have a complicated geometry or a tortuous lumen.

In the only study comparing the technical success, clinical success, and complications between patients undergoing enteral SEMS placement over 0.035″ and

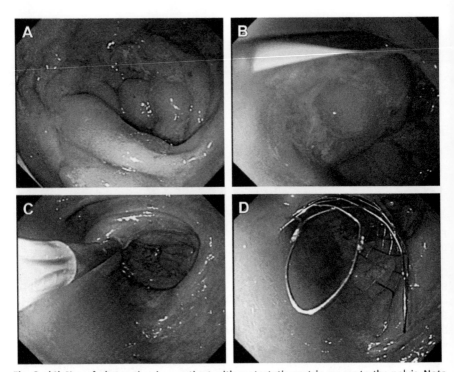

Fig. 2. (*A*) Site of obstruction in a patient with metastatic gastric cancer to the pelvis. Note that the site of obstruction has relatively normal mucosa and no sign of an intrinsic lesion. (*B*) A 0.035″ guide wire is advanced across the stenosis. (*C*) A TTS stent catheter has been advanced over the guide wire and into position across the malignant stricture. Note that the endoscope has backed away from the tumor to give better visualization during deployment in this case. (*D*) The stent immediately after deployment, showing passage of liquid stool.

0.025″ wires, both wire sizes were found to be equally safe and effective. The study included 59 patients who underwent 34 duodenal and 30 colonic stent placements. This study suggests that both wire sizes work equally well and that the choice can be left to individual operators during the procedure based on experience, personal preference, and local tumor/stricture anatomy.[22]

It should be stressed that the most important aspect of this procedure is the successful traversal of the stricture by a guide wire. If this cannot be achieved, the procedure is likely to fail or simply be aborted. Guide wire passage across a malignant colonic obstruction or stricture can be simple and straightforward or agonizingly difficult, and the technical ease of this maneuver is generally unpredictable beforehand.

If the obstruction is caused by a primary colon cancer, the tumor may cause some rotation of the bowel lumen, which can lead to a highly angulated stricture. Sometimes a clear, en face view of the stricture cannot be obtained. In such settings a duodenoscope may provide a superior view over a forward-viewing instrument. If the lumen of the stricture is angulated relative to the lumen of the bowel, use of a biliary sphincterotome may allow for additional degrees of freedom when attempting to cannulate the stricture and achieve successful guide wire passage (**Fig. 3**).[23]

Once the guide wire has traversed the stricture, it should be advanced far into the proximal bowel to provide stability for stent advancement. The catheter or

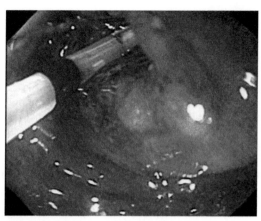

Fig. 3. An obstructing colonic mass causes a severe angulation. A biliary sphincterotome is used to achieve an optimal angle to pass a guide wire across the stricture.

sphincterotome can then be advanced over the wire and into the stricture or into the bowel beyond. This action can also provide some assessment of the tightness of the stricture. The injection of radiopaque contrast dye through the catheter under fluoroscopy will almost always demonstrate the length and geometry of the stricture, which will allow for the selection of a stent of the proper size and type. In addition, contrast injection will confirm the presence of the guide wire in the proximal bowel and will reveal any preexisting perforation. Identification of a preexisting perforation is an indication to abort the procedure and refer the patient to surgery.

The selection of an appropriate stent is based on the type and location of the colonic obstruction, operator experience, and personal preference. If a TTS stent is to be used it can simply be advanced over the wire, through the working channel of the endoscope, and across the stricture at this point. If a non-TTS stent is used, the endoscope and the biliary catheter must be removed from the patient while leaving the guide wire in place across the stricture. The non-TTS stent is then advanced over the wire and across the stricture site under fluoroscopy. At the time of writing, TTS stents are overwhelmingly preferred to non-TTS stents.

The principles of stent deployment are similar for all available colonic SEMS. The stents come supplied in a constrained configuration, preloaded on their respective delivery catheter. Once the stent is thought to be in an optimal position, it is deployed via the withdrawal or removal of some form of a restraining sheath. As the restraining sheath is withdrawn from or allowed to unravel around the stent, the stent will expand in a proximal to distal direction. Some TTS stents are reconstrainable if the deployment is proceeding poorly, and this feature can give the endoscopist a measure of security during deployment. A fluoroscopic marker delineates the "point of no return" beyond which the stent cannot be recaptured on reconstrainable systems.

As all currently available colonic stents in the United States are uncovered metal mesh devices (and as such are very difficult to remove endoscopically), the deployment of these devices should be performed in a slow, careful, and controlled manner. Interactive and clear communication between the endoscopist and his or her assistant is vital in all procedures, as often the assistant controls the actual deployment of the stent. As the assistant deploys the stent the endoscopist (who is also holding the catheter) can usually make multiple small adjustments to the overall position of the deployment catheter and the stent itself to achieve an optimal position. After stent deployment the guide wire and delivery catheter can be removed from the patient, usually without difficulty.

The final endoscopic and fluoroscopic position of the stent should then be carefully evaluated. If satisfactory, the procedure is complete. If suboptimal, the stent can be adjusted or removed using a rat-tooth forceps (which are most helpful if the stent needs to be pulled distally for a short distance). If the stent is considered to have been deployed too far distally and the proximal end of the stricture is incompletely opened, or if the stricture is longer than had been originally anticipated, a second stent is typically placed in a stent-within-stent manner to fully traverse the obstruction and allow for adequate restoration of bowel patency.

SELF-EXPANDING METAL STENTS IN PATIENTS WITH BENIGN COLONIC OBSTRUCTION

Benign obstructions are typically not treated with standard colonic SEMS, as their uncovered metal mesh may make them prone to the ingrowth of benign hyperplastic tissue, which may make removal difficult if not impossible. Nonetheless, uncovered SEMS have occasionally been used to treat benign colonic obstructions. Limited data also suggest that fully covered esophageal stents can be used in an off-label manner to treat benign colonic obstructions, most commonly those resulting from anastomotic or diverticular strictures. Fully covered esophageal stents used in this manner are very likely to migrate because their covering prevents them from embedding at the site of the obstruction.

One small case series of 3 patients demonstrated the successful use of Polyflex esophageal stents (Boston Scientific, Natick, MA, USA) for the treatment of benign postoperative colonic strictures.[24] Spontaneous migration occurred in 2 of the 3 patients. A larger retrospective study evaluated 21 patients who had a SEMS placed for benign obstruction (10 with anastomotic strictures [some of which were secondary to Crohn's disease], 10 with diverticular obstructions, and 1 with a stricture caused by radiation therapy).[25] Technical success was seen in 100% of patients and clinical success in 76%; 43% developed adverse events (including 6 perforations). Patients with diverticular disease were the most likely to develop an adverse event.

COMPLICATIONS AND THEIR MANAGEMENT

Early complications of colonic SEMS placement include perforation, hemorrhage, stent misdeployment, and cardiopulmonary complications such as aspiration. Delayed complications can include perforation, stent migration, and hemorrhage. Stent occlusion/reobstruction can occur from tumor ingrowth through the stent interstices or from overgrowth of tumor at the proximal or distal end of the stent. Stent migration is rare in patients with intrinsic colonic masses, but can be seen somewhat more frequently in patients with extrinsically obstructing lesions. If the patient has undergone stent placement low in the rectum, some patients can develop tenesmus, hematochezia, and (rarely) incontinence.

One of the largest studies to evaluate the long-term outcomes and complication rates of patients undergoing colonic SEMS placement for palliation of malignant obstruction in 168 patients noted a complication rate of 24.4%.[21] This relatively high rate includes both major and minor complications. Sixty-five patients undergoing colonic SEMS in the preoperative setting were included in this study, and 23.1% of patients in this group developed complications. Male sex, dilation of a stricture before SEMS insertion, complete large bowel obstruction, receipt (paradoxically) of smaller-diameter stents, and operator inexperience were all found to be significant risk factors for complications. The fact that operator inexperience is a risk factor is of some concern globally, as many endoscopists have relatively limited experience with colon stents, with more experience concentrated in a smaller number of individuals at tertiary referral centers.

Many of the aforementioned complications of SEMS placement can be managed without the need for surgery. Tumor ingrowth and/or overgrowth can generally be managed by the placement of 1 or more additional stents through the existing stent(s) to recanalize the lumen. Tissue overgrowth and ingrowth can be also ablated by cryotherapy, laser therapy, argon plasma coagulation, or radiofrequency ablation. Stent migration can often be addressed by removing the migrated stent (if the patient does not spontaneously pass the stent) and placement of a new stent if clinically indicated. Many perforations require surgical intervention and repair, although a growing number of colonic perforations can be closed by a variety of TTS and over-the-scope clips.

SUMMARY

Colonic strictures remain a common problem. Benign strictures can be successfully treated by dilation and the off-label use of fully covered esophageal stents. Malignant strictures are most commonly treated by stenting or surgery, with stents commonly deployed in patients with resectable and unresectable disease. Patients with resectable disease often undergo stenting as a bridge to surgery, whereas patients with unresectable disease usually have stents placed for permanent palliation. Complications are reasonable in frequency and severity, and most can be managed endoscopically.

REFERENCES

1. Foster EN, Quiros JA, Prindiville TP. Long-term follow-up of the endoscopic treatment of strictures in pediatric and patients with inflammatory bowel disease. J Clin Gastroenterol 2008;42(8):880–5. http://dx.doi.org/10.1097/MCG. 0b013e3181354440.
2. Hoffmann JC, Heller F, Faiss S, et al. Through the endoscope balloon dilation of ileocolonic strictures: prognostic factors, complications, and effectiveness. Int J Colorectal Dis 2008;23(7):689–96. http://dx.doi.org/10.1007/s00384-008-0461-9.
3. Gustavsson A, Magnuson A, Blomberg B, et al. Endoscopic dilation is an efficacious and safe treatment of intestinal strictures in Crohn's disease. Aliment Pharmacol Ther 2012;36(2):151–8. http://dx.doi.org/10.1111/j.1365-2036.2012. 05146.x.
4. Spinelli P, Dal Fante M, Mancini A. Self-expanding mesh stent for endoscopic palliation of rectal obstructing tumors: a preliminary report. Surg Endosc 1992; 6(2):72–4.
5. Ansaloni L, Andersson RE, Bazzoli F, et al. Guidelines in the management of obstructing cancer of the left colon: consensus conference of the World Society of Emergency Surgery (WSES) and Peritoneum and Surgery (PnS) Society. World J Emerg Surg 2010;5:29. http://dx.doi.org/10.1186/1749-7922-5-29.
6. Brehant O, Fuks D, Bartoli E, et al. Elective (planned) colectomy in patients with colorectal obstruction after placement of a self-expanding metallic stent as a bridge to surgery: the results of a prospective study. Colorectal Dis 2009;11(2): 178–83. http://dx.doi.org/10.1111/j.1463-1318.2008.01578.x.
7. Cheung HY, Chung CC, Tsang WW, et al. Endolaparoscopic approach vs conventional open surgery in the treatment of obstructing left-sided colon cancer: a randomized controlled trial. Arch Surg 2009;144(12):1127–32. http://dx.doi.org/ 10.1001/archsurg.2009.216.

8. Park IJ, Choi GS, Kang BM, et al. Comparison of one-stage managements of obstructing left-sided colon and rectal cancer: stent-laparoscopic approach vs. intraoperative colonic lavage. J Gastrointest Surg 2009;13(5):960–5. http://dx.doi.org/10.1007/s11605-008-0798-y.

9. Jiménez-Pérez J, Casellas J, García-Cano J, et al. Colonic stenting as a bridge to surgery in malignant large-bowel obstruction: a report from two large multinational registries. Am J Gastroenterol 2011;106(12):2174–80. http://dx.doi.org/10.1038/ajg.2011.360.

10. Fregonese D, Naspetti R, Ferrer S, et al. Ultraflex precision colonic stent placement as a bridge to surgery in patients with malignant colon obstruction. Gastrointest Endosc 2008;67(1):68–73.

11. Ng KC, Law WL, Lee YM, et al. Self-expanding metallic stent as a bridge to surgery versus emergency resection for obstructing left-sided colorectal cancer: a case-matched study. J Gastrointest Surg 2006;10(6):798–803.

12. Sagar J. Colorectal stents for the management of malignant colonic obstructions. Cochrane Database Syst Rev 2011;(11):CD007378. http://dx.doi.org/10.1002/14651858.CD007378.pub2.

13. Zhang Y, Shi J, Shi B, et al. Self-expanding metallic stent as a bridge to surgery versus emergency surgery for obstructive colorectal cancer: a meta-analysis. Surg Endosc 2012;26(1):110–9. http://dx.doi.org/10.1007/s00464-011-1835-6.

14. Repici A, Fregonese D, Costamagna G, et al. Ultraflex precision colonic stent placement for palliation of malignant colonic obstruction: a prospective multicenter study. Gastrointest Endosc 2007;66(5):920–7.

15. Baron TH, Wong Kee Song LM, Repici A. Role of self-expandable stents for patients with colon cancer (with videos). Gastrointest Endosc 2012;75(3):653–62. http://dx.doi.org/10.1016/j.gie.2011.12.020.

16. Manes G, de Bellis M, Fuccio L, et al. Endoscopic palliation in patients with incurable malignant colorectal obstruction by means of self-expanding metal stent: analysis of results and predictors of outcomes in a large multicenter series. Arch Surg 2011;146(10):1157–62. http://dx.doi.org/10.1001/archsurg.2011.233.

17. Sliesoraitis S, Tawfik B. Bevacizumab-induced bowel perforation. J Am Osteopath Assoc 2011;111(7):437–41.

18. Lee HJ, Hong SP, Cheon JH, et al. Long-term outcome of palliative therapy for malignant colorectal obstruction in patients with unresectable metastatic colorectal cancers: endoscopic stenting versus surgery. Gastrointest Endosc 2011;73(3):535–42. http://dx.doi.org/10.1016/j.gie.2010.10.052.

19. Faragher IG, Chaitowitz IM, Stupart DA. Long-term results of palliative stenting or surgery for incurable obstructing colon cancer. Colorectal Dis 2008;10(7):668–72. http://dx.doi.org/10.1111/j.1463-1318.2007.01446.x.

20. van Hooft JE, Fockens P, Marinelli AW, et al, Dutch Colorectal Stent Group. Early closure of a multicenter randomized clinical trial of endoscopic stenting versus surgery for stage IV left-sided colorectal cancer. Endoscopy 2008;40(3):184–91. http://dx.doi.org/10.1055/s-2007-995426.

21. Small AJ, Coelho-Prabhu N, Baron TH. Endoscopic placement of self-expandable metal stents for malignant colonic obstruction: long-term outcomes and complication factors. Gastrointest Endosc 2010;71(3):560–72. http://dx.doi.org/10.1016/j.gie.2009.10.012.

22. Chan J, Hilden K, Fang J, et al. Duodenal and colonic stent placement with 0.025″ and 0.035″ guidewires is equally safe and effective. Dig Dis Sci 2012;57(3):726–31. http://dx.doi.org/10.1007/s10620-011-1932-3.

23. Armstrong EM, Fox BM. Assistance of colorectal stent insertion by sphincterotome. Dis Colon Rectum 2007;50(3):399–400.
24. García-Cano J. Dilation of benign strictures in the esophagus and colon with the Polyflex stent: a case series study. Dig Dis Sci 2008;53(2):341–6.
25. Keränen I, Lepistö A, Udd M, et al. Outcome of patients after endoluminal stent placement for benign colorectal obstruction. Scand J Gastroenterol 2010;45(6): 725–31. http://dx.doi.org/10.3109/00365521003663696.

Colonoscopy Quality Assessment

Nabil F. Fayad, MD[a,b,*], Charles J. Kahi, MD, MSc[a,b]

KEYWORDS

- Colorectal cancer • Colonoscopy • Quality • Measures • Adenoma detection rate

KEY POINTS

- Colonoscopy is the cornerstone of colorectal cancer screening programs.
- There is significant variability in the quality of colonoscopy between endoscopists.
- Colonoscopy quality assessment tracks various metrics to improve the effectiveness of colonoscopy, aiming at reducing the incidence and mortality from colorectal cancer.
- Adenoma detection rate is the prime metric, because it is associated with the risk of interval cancer. Implementing processes to measure and improve the adenoma detection rate is essential to improve the quality of colonoscopy.

INTRODUCTION

Colonoscopy is the cornerstone of colorectal cancer (CRC) screening programs, whether used as a primary modality or as follow-up to another screening test.[1] Therefore, adequate prevention of CRC relies heavily on colonoscopy.

Although studies from the 1990s indicated that colonoscopy could prevent up to 90% of CRC,[2–4] more recent research suggests that the reduction in CRC incidence might be lower, particularly in the right colon.[5–9] Interval CRCs (or postcolonoscopy CRCs) account for 3.4% to 9% of all cases of CRCs and are primarily diagnosed in the right colon.[10–15]

Several factors can contribute to limited effectiveness of colonoscopy[16]; however, data suggest that endoscopist-related factors are the most important element.[17–19] In fact, 71% to 86% of interval cancers can be attributed to colonoscopist-related factors, because they represent missed lesions or result from incompletely resected lesions.[20–23]

[a] Division of Gastroenterology and Hepatology, Department of Medicine, Indiana University School of Medicine, 702 Rotary Circle, suite 225, Indianapolis, IN 46202, USA; [b] Section of Gastroenterology and Hepatology, Medicine Department, Richard L. Roudebush VA Medical Center, 1481 West 10th Street, Room 111G, Indianapolis, IN 46202, USA
* Corresponding author. Richard L. Roudebush VA Medical Center, 1481 West 10th Street, Room 111G, Indianapolis, IN 46202.
E-mail address: nfayad@iu.edu

Gastrointest Endoscopy Clin N Am 25 (2015) 373–386
http://dx.doi.org/10.1016/j.giec.2014.11.008
1052-5157/15/$ – see front matter Published by Elsevier Inc.
giendo.theclinics.com

These concerns have led to an increased emphasis on improving the quality of colonoscopy to maximize its ability to reduce CRC incidence. The Gastroenterology societies have proposed various indicators of colonoscopy quality.[24] Choosing and measuring the most appropriate metrics to assess the quality of colonoscopy for practitioners, and improving them when required, remain a work in progress. This article discusses the value and limitations of quality metrics and considerations for implementing them in practice to improve colonoscopy performance.

COLONOSCOPY QUALITY PROCESS MEASURES

The debate continues regarding the ideal quality measure for colonoscopy, because each of the indicators has advantages and drawbacks.[25,26] It is now beyond debate though that colonoscopy performance should be regularly assessed for every endoscopist.[27,28] Although adenoma detection rate (ADR) is largely viewed as the best validated practical outcome measure,[25–29] 2 other process measures warrant consideration.

Cecal Intubation Rate

The use of cecal intubation rate as a quality metric derives from the fact that colonoscopists should have the ability to perform a complete examination to the cecum in the great majority of procedures.[30] Based on established benchmarks, effective colonoscopists should be able to intubate the cecum in 90% or more of all cases, including 95% or more of screening colonoscopies in healthy adults.[24]

Although some data from the late 1990s suggested that these targets were attained by only 55% of practitioners in North America,[31] more recent evidence shows improved cecal intubation rates. A study of 10 endoscopists from the University of Maryland reported cecal intubation rates ranging between 88% and 97%, except for one endoscopist, with a rate of 63%.[32] This study highlights the importance of measuring cecal intubation rates to identify outliers.

Failure to routinely intubate the cecum is, in fact, one of the reasons that limit colonoscopy's effectiveness. A study from Japan and another from New Zealand found that interval cancers were due to failure to reach the cecum, in 27% and 54% of cases, respectively.[33,34] Furthermore, Baxter and colleagues[12] found that patients who undergo colonoscopy by endoscopists with cecal intubation rates of 95% or greater were less likely to have interval cancers compared with patients who undergo colonoscopy by endoscopists with intubation rates less than 80% (distal odds ratio [OR], 0.73; 95% confidence interval [CI], 0.54–0.97; proximal OR, 0.72; 95% CI, 0.53–0.97). Thus, evaluating cecal intubation rates is an important first step toward assessing overall colonoscopy quality.

Withdrawal Time

Spending sufficient time between intubating the cecum and removing the colonoscope from the patient is necessary to perform a thorough mucosal inspection, with a low miss rate for significant lesions.[35] The suggested benchmark for withdrawal time (WT) is an average of at least 6 minutes in examinations where no biopsies or polypectomies are performed (derived from a large number of colonoscopies in patients without prior surgical resection).[24]

The utility of WT as a quality measure has been somewhat disputed, because the evidence is inconsistent regarding its correlation with adenoma or polyp detection rate (PDR).[19,36–39] A recent large observational study from England, which included more than 31,000 colonoscopies, supports the value of WT as a quality metric.[40]

Colonoscopists with WT less than 7 minutes had significantly lower ADRs compared with those with WT of 11 minutes or longer (42.5% vs 47.1%, $P<.001$), with 50% less right-sided adenomas detected per procedure. The authors also found that there was no incremental benefit in ADR beyond 10 minutes of WT (which does not include duration of polyp removal). Data from a recent study (currently in abstract form) by Shaukat and colleagues[41] suggest that WT might be a more sensitive indicator of interval cancer than ADR. The authors analyzed records of more than 76,000 colonoscopies performed by 51 gastroenterologists in Minnesota; they found that colonoscopists' average annual WTs were inversely associated with interval cancers ($P<.0001$), whereas physicians' ADR were not ($P = .40$). Compared with WT greater than 6 minutes, the adjusted incidence rate ratio for WT less than 6 minutes was 2.3 (95% CI, 1.5–3.4; $P<.0001$).

It remains likely though that longer mean WT reflects better withdrawal technique (including cleaning of residual fluid, adequate colonic distention, and proper examination of proximal side of folds).[42] Therefore, colonoscopy experts and the American Society for Gastrointestinal Endoscopy and the American College of Gastroenterology task force recommend the use of WT mainly as a quality indicator for colonoscopists who have low ADR, rather than a stand-alone metric.[24,30]

ADENOMA DETECTION RATE

Although it would be most meaningful to measure CRC incidence and mortality, or alternatively, the incidence of interval cancers, as outcomes of colonoscopy,[2] these are not practical for timely quality interventions. Thus, ADR, or the proportion of screening colonoscopies where at least one adenoma is detected, has been proposed as the best, most reliable and practical surrogate quality metric.[24–26] Current ADR benchmarks are 25% or greater for men and 15% or greater for women.[24]

Adenoma Detection Rate Correlation with Risk of Interval Cancer

Two large studies from Poland and from the United States validated the ADR as a quality metric by showing its association with the risk of interval CRC.[43,44] The Polish study was conducted by Kaminski and colleagues[43]; the authors evaluated 45,026 subjects undergoing screening colonoscopy, performed by 186 endoscopists. The results, published in 2010, showed that patients whose endoscopists had an ADR less than 20% were at least 10 times more likely to be diagnosed with an interval CRC, compared with those whose endoscopists had ADR 20% or greater ($P = .008$). Interval cancer risk increased as ADR decreased, and there were no other factors associated with interval CRC besides age.

The US study was carried by Corley and colleagues[44]; the authors reviewed 314,872 screening colonoscopies performed between 1998 and 2010, by 136 high-volume gastroenterologists on patients in the Kaiser Permanente health plan. The results, published in 2014, showed that ADR is an independent predictor of interval CRC, with a hazard ratio of 0.52 (95% CI, 0.39–0.69) for patients whose examinations were performed by colonoscopists with ADR greater than 33.5%, compared with those whose colonoscopists had ADR less than 19%. Interval cancer risk decreased linearly with increasing endoscopist ADR, overall and separately in the proximal colon and in the distal colon, and there was no ADR threshold above which there was no further protective benefit; the risk of interval cancer decreased by 3% for each 1% increase in ADR (hazard ratio 0.97; 95% CI, 0.96–0.98). In addition, there was an inverse association between CRC mortality and ADR: patients whose colonoscopists were in the highest ADR quintile had a 62% (95% CI, 35%–88%) reduction in fatal CRC, as compared with patients whose physicians were in the lowest quintile.

Adenoma Detection Rate Measurement

Measuring the ADR of every colonoscopist is a priority for colonoscopy quality improvement.[24] It should be noted though that a reliable ADR assessment likely requires a large sample of colonoscopies per practitioner. In a mathematical model developed by Do and colleagues,[45] at least 500 procedures were needed in the ADR calculation to provide narrow 95% confidence intervals that more accurately reflect performance.

Nevertheless, ADR is relatively easy to measure, even when it requires manual chart reviews.[46] Despite a somewhat time-consuming process to periodically review pathology data, this is largely facilitated by an objective approach, limited to a binary query (ie, presence or absence of adenoma—without further characteristics or count). Serrated lesions should not be counted toward the ADR. Added strength of ADR as a quality metric is that it indirectly reflects other factors, including WT, colonoscopist technique and motivation, and bowel preparation quality.[47]

The importance of ADR measurement is underscored by the wide variability among colonoscopists, with reported rates ranging from less than 10% to more than 50%.[17,36,43,44,48] The impact of the endoscopist on ADR is substantial, accounting for up to a 10-fold difference between colonoscopists, and exceeding the effect of patient age and gender.[17] The baseline colonoscopy is decisive for effective CRC screening, because it impacts initial clearance from neoplastic lesions and also dictates subsequent surveillance intervals.[30] Therefore, colonoscopists with high ADR provide their patients with double protection: more complete baseline clearance and shorter surveillance intervals. Thus, assessing and improving ADR is at the core of a successful CRC prevention program.

Polyp Detection Rate

PDR has received some attention as a surrogate for ADR, because it is automatically collected by colonoscopists while generating procedure reports and/or billing codes, making it more practical to measure than ADR. PDR was validated as a surrogate to ADR by 2 studies by Williams and colleagues.[49,50] In the first study conducted at a single academic institution, the authors showed a strong correlation between ADR and PDR (correlation 0.86, $P<.001$).[49] In the second study, which included 60 endoscopists at multiple practice sites, they found again a high correlation between colonoscopists' PDR and ADR in both men and women (correlation 0.91, $P<.001$) as well as a correlation between PDR and advanced adenoma detection.[50]

In addition, Baxter and colleagues[12] carried out a large observational study in Ontario, Canada, that showed an association between the PDR and the incidence of interval cancers in the right colon. Patients who underwent colonoscopy by endoscopists with PDR 30% or greater were less likely to have proximal interval cancers, compared with patients whose colonoscopists had PDR less than 10% (OR, 0.61; 95% CI, 0.42–0.89, $P<.0001$).

To date, there is no prospective study that evaluates PDR as a quality measure, and there are 2 main predicaments that can hinder the use of PDR. First, there are no recommended benchmarks from the leading US Gastroenterology societies; potentially, the targets suggested by Williams and colleagues[49,50] can be used (40% for men and 30% for women based on correlation with ADR targets of 25% for men and 15% for women, respectively), but these still await validation and official endorsement. Second, PDR is more prone to corruption than ADR, because it can be inflated by resection of nonneoplastic diminutive polyps or by biopsy of normal tissue. A remedy as suggested by Williams and colleagues[49,50] could be periodic audits; however, these could negate to some extent the practicality of PDR.

ADENOMA DETECTION RATE: LIMITATIONS

Expecting colonoscopy to prevent all cases of CRC is unrealistic; however, its effectiveness is based on the ability of endoscopists to detect the vast majority of neoplastic lesions and to remove them completely. Although ADR has certainly proven to be a reliable measure of colonoscopy quality, it can be criticized for its inability to gauge if a colonoscopist is leaving behind additional adenomas, other precancerous lesions, or fragments of identified/resected adenomas.

Adenomas per Colonoscopy

ADR can overlook differences in colonoscopy quality, because endoscopists with the same ADR could be detecting highly variable numbers of adenomas per colonoscopy.[51,52] Denis and colleagues[51] analyzed more than 42,000 colonoscopies performed by 316 endoscopists in France. They evaluated the mean number of adenomas per procedure (MAP, total number of adenomas detected divided by the number of colonoscopies); for colonoscopists with ADR around 35%, the MAP varied markedly between 0.36 and 0.98. Wang and colleagues[52] compared 2 groups of endoscopists serving the same patient pool in Los Angeles, California, at a tertiary care teaching hospital and at 3 nonteaching facilities. The authors assessed the MAP as well as another suggested metric, the ADR-Plus (mean number of adenomas detected after the first adenoma, in procedures in which at least one adenoma was found). Both groups had comparable ADRs (28.8% and 25.7%; $P = .052$), but the teaching group had 23.5% higher MAP and 29.5% higher ADR-Plus.

Coupling ADR with another total adenoma metric has therefore been suggested by both previous groups to better assess colonoscopists' performance.[51,52] Similarly, Lee and colleagues[53] proposed 2 measures of total adenoma detection to complement the ADR: MAP and MAP+ (mean adenoma per positive procedure, calculated as total number of adenomas detected divided by the number of colonoscopies in which at least one adenoma was detected).

Adding a total adenoma detection metric provides a more comprehensive assessment of the thoroughness of a colonoscopic examination, provides better discrimination between endoscopists, and limits potential inclination to "gaming" (ie, a less thorough examination once a first adenoma is detected and resected). However, this makes the assessment much more labor-intensive. Furthermore, this could be an incentive to separate polyps from the same colon segment into different specimen bottles, leading to increased colonoscopy costs. In the absence of formally established benchmarks, and while adherence to measuring ADR remains far from optimal in routine practice, total adenoma detection metrics will primarily be applied in research settings in the short term.

Adenoma Detection Rate Benchmarks

The ADR targets originally defined in 2002 ($\geq$25% for men and $\geq$15% for women[24]) may be outdated. Several recent studies report ADRs in the 40% to 50% range or even higher in average-risk individuals.[40,44,48,53] Demographic features, other than gender, also affect the prevalence of adenomas[54]; this includes increasing prevalence with age and more proximal adenomas in blacks compared with whites.[55] As ADR use becomes more prevalent in clinical practice and in different populations, benchmark adjustments will be necessary based on the specific characteristics of the screened demographic group and the most recent ADRs reported in the literature that have been proven to provide cancer prevention.

Advanced Adenomas

Measuring the advanced ADR might be more clinically relevant, because advanced adenomas are more prone to progress to CRC.[56] Similar to ADR, there is significant variability in advanced ADR between colonoscopists.[17,57] Among 9 colonoscopists in Indianapolis, detection of adenomas 1 cm in size and larger varied from 1.7% to 6.2%.[17] Among 14 colonoscopists in Chicago, advanced ADR varied from 2% to 18.18%.[57]

This study[57] generated concerns, because it showed that colonoscopists' advanced ADR were independent of their nonadvanced ADR (correlation -0.42; 95% CI -0.77 to 0.14, $P = .13$). In addition, the study by Wang and colleagues[52] showed that the teaching group had a 28.7% higher advanced ADR compared with the nonteaching group, whereas ADRs were similar for both groups. These results suggest that some colonoscopists might have adequate ADRs, while missing a significant number of advanced adenomas. These findings warrant future investigation, because they could carry important implications in assessing colonoscopy quality. However, using advanced ADR as a quality metric will likely prove to be very challenging, because of variable polyp size measurement by endoscopists and large interobserver variability for villous elements among pathologists.

Serrated Polyps

An inherent limitation of the ADR is that it does not account for the detection of serrated polyps; this might be problematic as recent evidence suggests that the serrated pathway likely accounts for up to one-third of all CRCs.[58,59] Endoscopic detection of serrated polyps is more challenging than detection of adenomatous lesions, because they have a subtle, pale appearance and indistinct margins.[60] The prevalence of serrated polyps in the right colon in average-risk patients is higher than previously reported, with a mean of 13% in a recent study.[61]

The variability in detecting proximal colon serrated lesions is more striking compared with ADR, ranging from 5-fold to 18-fold among endoscopists, whereas ADR variation is typically around 3-fold to 4-fold.[38,62,63] In 2 recent studies, detection rates varied from 1% to 18% among 15 academic gastroenterologists who performed a total of 6681 screening colonoscopies,[62] and from 6% to 22% among 5 colonoscopists who completed 1354 screening examinations.[38]

Interestingly, and despite the variation in detection of proximal serrated lesions, there seems to be a strong correlation between it and ADR,[61] which was the case in both men (correlation 0.71, $P = .003$) and women (correlation 0.73, $P = .002$).[61] Therefore, although not directly capturing serrated polyps, ADR might still be valid by itself to assess the detection of both adenomatous and serrated lesions. This validity has important practical implications because of several problems impacting the use of serrated PDR as a quality metric: there are currently no endorsed benchmarks for serrated lesion detection rates; the measurement should only include lesions proximal to the sigmoid colon to avoid the confounding effect of hyperplastic polyps from the rectosigmoid (whereas it is difficult to reliably identify the junction between the sigmoid and the descending colon); and the histologic classification of serrated lesions remains challenging and variable in practice.[63]

Incomplete Adenoma Resection

Several studies evaluating interval CRCs found that these cancers can be attributed to incomplete polypectomy in about 10% to 30% of cases.[13,20,22,64,65] Because ADR is essentially geared at assessing detection and not resection, the inadequate quality in these cases would not be reflected by the ADR. Competent colonoscopists should be able to completely resect most sessile polyps up to 2 cm in size and all mucosally based pedunculated polyps.[24]

In the CARE study, Pohl and colleagues[66] assessed the completeness of resection based on 346 polypectomies performed in 269 patients by 11 colonoscopists. Polyps assessed were sessile or flat, ranged from 5 to 20 mm in size, and 59% were in the right colon. The evaluation was based on a biopsy protocol of the margins of the polypectomy site and revealed an incomplete resection in 10.1% of cases. In addition, there was a wide variability in incomplete resection rate, ranging from 6.5% to 22.7% between endoscopists. Of note, serrated lesions were more likely to be incompletely resected compared with adenomatous polyps (31% vs 7.2%, $P<.001$).

Polypectomy technique and effectiveness are key components of colonoscopy quality. Although awareness is increasing about its variability between colonoscopists, assessing resection quality is more difficult than assessing detection quality. However, this should not be an absolute deterrent. A group from the United Kingdom recently published work to develop and validate a tool to assess polypectomy skills using video reviews,[67] but this area requires further research.

IMPLEMENTATION OF QUALITY MEASUREMENT

Assessing colonoscopy quality in day-to-day practice should no longer be optional for endoscopists. It is our obligation to provide patients with the best possible prevention against CRC. Measuring competency, and when necessary improving it, can ensure that colonoscopists are held accountable to quality standards.

Process Planning

The initial step in establishing a colonoscopy quality program is to select the metric that will be assessed.[26] This metric should be measured according to clearly defined parameters, and the measurement method should be precise and consistent. Metrics with well-established benchmarks are likely more useful to gauge performance related to standards. Once the metric and the measurement method are determined, a baseline data collection can be carried out. According to the measurement results, it can be decided if improvement is required to achieve high value colonoscopy. Repeat data collection will allow assessment of progress.

For endoscopists, the first step in this process is to regularly measure ADR, and if warranted, take action to improve it.[68] Similar considerations apply at the level of an endoscopy center. Hilsden and colleagues[69] shared their process and experience in implementing a colonoscopy quality assurance program at their endoscopy facility in Calgary, Canada. Participation in the quality monitoring program was a requirement to be granted endoscopy privileges at the center. Their program included several aspects, one of which was distribution of report cards to endoscopists, reflecting measurements of their collected indicators, with comparison to the entire group of endoscopists at the center. Metrics reported in the early phase of the program were cecal intubation rate, average WT, and average PDR. Subsequently, the reports included various measures of ADR.

On a larger scale, audits can be conducted to assess the quality of colonoscopy. In the United Kingdom, the results of a 2011 nationwide audit were recently published[70] and included 2 main quality metrics: cecal intubation rate and PDR. Compared with previous audit results from 1999, the cecal intubation rate improved from 76.9% to 92.3%, and the PDR increased from 22.5% to 32.1%. These examples reflect the feasibility and benefit of implementing colonoscopy quality assessment initiatives.

Resources to Facilitate Implementation

Quality measurement for colonoscopy cannot be achieved without adequate procedure documentation. It is fundamental to have complete data to accurately measure quality metrics, and standardized electronic reports can facilitate this process. In 2007, the Quality Assurance Task Force of the National Colorectal Cancer Roundtable developed a reporting and data system for colonoscopy (CO-RADS) to facilitate quality monitoring within and across practices.[71] Several commercially available endoscopy software programs generate electronic reports that include the elements suggested in CO-RADS.

A group from the Netherlands created a structured colonoscopy reporting system (EndoALPHA) that mandates endoscopists to document various quality indicators and that automatically generates quality measurement reports.[72] The Clinical Outcomes Research Initiative (CORI) developed software that captures most of the indicators proposed in CO-RADS.[73] The CORI consortium included 73 practices from 24 states in the United States that electronically submitted their colonoscopy reports to the database for analysis to measure and improve quality.

The Gastroenterology societies have established 2 registries to assist individual endoscopists and practice groups in monitoring colonoscopy quality: GIQuIC (GI Quality Improvement Consortium; developed by the American College of Gastroenterology and the American Society of Gastrointestinal Endoscopy) and DHOR (Digestive Health Outcome Registry; developed by the American Gastroenterology Association). Submitting colonoscopy reports to these registries will generate performance reports for gastroenterologists, assessing various metrics, with ADR being the most important.

Natural language processing (NLP) is a medical informatics tool that identifies and extracts information from free-text reports, using artificial intelligence. NLP can retrieve data necessary for colonoscopy quality measurement with high accuracy, specifically adenoma detection metrics.[74] NLP can be helpful in easily quantifying quality metrics for endoscopists and awaits further study for validation and standardization.

Interventions to Improve Quality

Ideally, a colonoscopy quality improvement program should allow identifying underperformers to pursue interventions that will improve their performance. The benefit of various interventions is quite variable, and the optimal approach to ameliorate substandard effectiveness is yet to be identified.[75]

Withdrawal time interventions

Targeting a longer WT in colonoscopists with low ADR has been evaluated by several studies. Simply recording WT has not been shown to have a significant effect on increasing overall PDR.[76] Longer WT might improve serrated PDR in the proximal colon.[38] Forcing endoscopists to spend at least 7 minutes on withdrawal did not affect PDR[77]; this reflects that a forced increase in WT is not spent in effective inspection, when it is not paired with education about withdrawal and inspection techniques.

The most beneficial intervention involving WT was undertaken by Barclay and colleagues.[78] It started with a group review of optimal inspection techniques, followed by implementation of a segmental withdrawal protocol: at least 2 minutes per colonic segment, indicated by digital stopwatch beeps, with a total withdrawal duration of 8 minutes minimum, which resulted in a significant increase of the ADR from 23.5% to 34.7% (P<.0001).

Educational interventions
In the intervention by Barclay and colleagues,[78] the education component that preceded the withdrawal protocol implementation likely played an important role. The Endoscopic Quality Improvement Program (EQUIP) is a recently described educational process.[79] Endoscopists who were assigned to the training group (2 sessions: techniques of high-quality colonoscopy and polyp overview and classification) increased their ADR from 36% at baseline to 47% after training (P = .0013), whereas the untrained group ADR remained unchanged at 35%.

Adler and colleagues[19] found that the number of Continuing Medical Education meetings attended by colonoscopists correlated with their ADR (P = .012). The authors suggested that a better understanding of polyp morphology and examination techniques, taught at the meetings, resulted in better colonoscopy performance. Educational programs, whether at local or larger scales, have an important role in improving adenoma detection and resection as well as recognition and removal of serrated lesions.

Feedback methods
In the EQUIP study,[79] it should be noted that the training group also received monthly ADR feedback, possibly contributing to the observed benefit. Harewood and colleagues[80] provided quarterly feedback to a group of 58 endoscopists and noted a 19% decline in incomplete colonoscopies. Lin and colleagues[81] also reported that monitoring and feedback aided quality improvement, with increases in mean WT and polyp (but not adenoma) detection rate (33.1%–38.1%, P = .04). Implementation of a quarterly quality report card resulted in a significant increase in cecal intubation rate (98.1% vs 95.6%, P = .027) and in ADR (53.9% vs 44.7%, P = .013)[48]; the increment in adenoma detection was mostly due to increased detection of proximal adenomas.

The impact of feedback has not been consistently significant, and several other groups that used feedback interventions reported negative results.[75] Shaukat and colleagues[82] applied a series of systematic interventions over a 3-year period, including feedback and educational programs, but were not successful at improving endoscopists' ADR.

Video-monitoring
Rex and colleagues[83] assessed the impact of video recording on the quality of colonoscopy performance. Endoscopists' awareness of the recording resulted in a 49% increase of mean inspection time, and a 31% improvement in mucosal inspection technique. Whether this improves ADR remains to be seen, but Madhoun and Tierney[84] recently reported that video recording was associated with a nonsignificant increase in ADR (whereas hyperplastic polyp detection increased significantly).

Researchers at the Mayo Clinic created an Endoscopic Multimedia Information System that involves recording, monitoring, and assessing colonoscopies.[85] The system is being developed to allow real-time analysis and as-needed feedback related to routine colonoscopy maneuvers, to achieve high quality with each colonoscopy.

Video-monitoring or advanced automated assessment systems could prove valuable to complement the current interventions used to enhance colonoscopy quality, especially because many of these interventions have limited effectiveness.

REFERENCES

1. Lieberman DA, Rex DK, Winawer SJ, et al. Guidelines for colonoscopy surveillance after screening and polypectomy: a consensus update by the US Multi-Society Task Force on Colorectal Cancer. Gastroenterology 2012;143: 844–57.
2. Winawer SJ, Zauber AG, Ho MN, et al. Prevention of colorectal cancer by colonoscopic polypectomy. The National Polyp Study Workgroup. N Engl J Med 1993; 329:1977–81.
3. Thiis-Evensen E, Hoff GS, Sauar J, et al. Population-based surveillance by colonoscopy: effect on the incidence of colorectal cancer. Telemark Polyp Study I. Scand J Gastroenterol 1999;34:414–20.
4. Citarda F, Tomaselli G, Capocaccia R, et al. Efficacy in standard clinical practice of colonoscopic polypectomy in reducing colorectal cancer incidence. Gut 2001; 48:812–5.
5. Robertson DJ, Greenberg ER, Beach M, et al. Colorectal cancer in patients under close colonoscopic surveillance. Gastroenterology 2005;129:34–41.
6. Kahi CJ, Imperiale TF, Juliar BE, et al. Effect of screening colonoscopy on colorectal cancer incidence and mortality. Clin Gastroenterol Hepatol 2009;7:770–5 [quiz: 711].
7. Singh H, Nugent Z, Mahmud SM, et al. Predictors of colorectal cancer after negative colonoscopy: a population-based study. Am J Gastroenterol 2010;105: 663–73 [quiz: 674].
8. Brenner H, Chang-Claude J, Seiler CM, et al. Protection from colorectal cancer after colonoscopy: a population-based, case-control study. Ann Intern Med 2011;154:22–30.
9. Mulder SA, van Soest EM, Dieleman JP, et al. Exposure to colorectal examinations before a colorectal cancer diagnosis: a case-control study. Eur J Gastroenterol Hepatol 2010;22:437–43.
10. Bressler B, Paszat LF, Chen Z, et al. Rates of new or missed colorectal cancers after colonoscopy and their risk factors: a population-based analysis. Gastroenterology 2007;132:96–102.
11. Singh H, Nugent Z, Demers AA, et al. Rate and predictors of early/missed colorectal cancers after colonoscopy in Manitoba: a population-based study. Am J Gastroenterol 2010;105:2588–96.
12. Baxter NN, Sutradhar R, Forbes SS, et al. Analysis of administrative data finds endoscopist quality measures associated with postcolonoscopy colorectal cancer. Gastroenterology 2011;140:65–72.
13. Farrar WD, Sawhney MS, Nelson DB, et al. Colorectal cancers found after a complete colonoscopy. Clin Gastroenterol Hepatol 2006;4:1259–64.
14. Cooper GS, Xu F, Barnholtz Sloan JS, et al. Prevalence and predictors of interval colorectal cancers in medicare beneficiaries. Cancer 2012;118:3044–52.
15. Brenner H, Chang-Claude J, Seiler CM, et al. Interval cancers after negative colonoscopy: population-based case-control study. Gut 2012;61:1576–82.
16. Hewett DG, Kahi CJ, Rex DK. Does colonoscopy work? J Natl Compr Canc Netw 2010;8:67–76 [quiz: 77].
17. Chen SC, Rex DK. Endoscopist can be more powerful than age and male gender in predicting adenoma detection at colonoscopy. Am J Gastroenterol 2007;102: 856–61.
18. Ko CW, Dominitz JA, Green P, et al. Specialty differences in polyp detection, removal, and biopsy during colonoscopy. Am J Med 2010;123:528–35.

19. Adler A, Wegscheider K, Lieberman D, et al. Factors determining the quality of screening colonoscopy: a prospective study on adenoma detection rates, from 12,134 examinations (Berlin colonoscopy project 3, BECOP-3). Gut 2013;62: 236–41.
20. Robertson DJ, Lieberman DA, Winawer SJ, et al. Colorectal cancers soon after colonoscopy: a pooled multicohort analysis. Gut 2014;63:949–56.
21. Pohl H, Robertson DJ. Colorectal cancers detected after colonoscopy frequently result from missed lesions. Clin Gastroenterol Hepatol 2010;8:858–64.
22. le Clercq CM, Bouwens MW, Rondagh EJ, et al. Postcolonoscopy colorectal cancers are preventable: a population-based study. Gut 2014;63:957–63.
23. Huang Y, Gong W, Su B, et al. Risk and cause of interval colorectal cancer after colonoscopic polypectomy. Digestion 2012;86:148–54.
24. Rex DK, Petrini JL, Baron TH, et al. Quality indicators for colonoscopy. Am J Gastroenterol 2006;101:873–85.
25. Fayad NF, Kahi CJ. Quality measures for colonoscopy: a critical evaluation. Clin Gastroenterol Hepatol 2014;12:1973–80.
26. Calderwood AH, Jacobson BC. Colonoscopy quality: metrics and implementation. Gastroenterol Clin North Am 2013;42:599–618.
27. Rex DK. Can we fix colonoscopy?...Yes! Gastroenterology 2011;140:19–21.
28. Weinberg DS. Colonoscopy: what does it take to get it "right"? Ann Intern Med 2011;154:68–9.
29. Kahi CJ, Anderson JC, Rex DK. Screening and surveillance for colorectal cancer: state of the art. Gastrointest Endosc 2013;77:335–50.
30. Rex DK. Quality in colonoscopy: cecal intubation first, then what? Am J Gastroenterol 2006;101:732–4.
31. Cotton PB, Connor P, McGee D, et al. Colonoscopy: practice variation among 69 hospital-based endoscopists. Gastrointest Endosc 2003;57:352–7.
32. Aslinia F, Uradomo L, Steele A, et al. Quality assessment of colonoscopic cecal intubation: an analysis of 6 years of continuous practice at a university hospital. Am J Gastroenterol 2006;101:721–31.
33. Hosokawa O, Shirasaki S, Kaizaki Y, et al. Invasive colorectal cancer detected up to 3 years after a colonoscopy negative for cancer. Endoscopy 2003;35:506–10.
34. Leaper M, Johnston MJ, Barclay M, et al. Reasons for failure to diagnose colorectal carcinoma at colonoscopy. Endoscopy 2004;36:499–503.
35. Rex DK. Colonoscopic withdrawal technique is associated with adenoma miss rates. Gastrointest Endosc 2000;51:33–6.
36. Barclay RL, Vicari JJ, Doughty AS, et al. Colonoscopic withdrawal times and adenoma detection during screening colonoscopy. N Engl J Med 2006;355: 2533–41.
37. Imperiale TF, Glowinski EA, Juliar BE, et al. Variation in polyp detection rates at screening colonoscopy. Gastrointest Endosc 2009;69:1288–95.
38. de Wijkerslooth TR, Stoop EM, Bossuyt PM, et al. Differences in proximal serrated polyp detection among endoscopists are associated with variability in withdrawal time. Gastrointest Endosc 2013;77:617–23.
39. Moritz V, Bretthauer M, Ruud HK, et al. Withdrawal time as a quality indicator for colonoscopy - a nationwide analysis. Endoscopy 2012;44:476–81.
40. Lee TJ, Blanks RG, Rees CJ, et al. Longer mean colonoscopy withdrawal time is associated with increased adenoma detection: evidence from the Bowel Cancer Screening Programme in England. Endoscopy 2013;45:20–6.
41. Shaukat A, Rector T, Church T, et al. Withdrawal times, adenoma detection rates, and risk of interval cancer. Am J Gastroenterol 2014;109:S613.

42. Rex DK. Optimal withdrawal and examination in colonoscopy. Gastroenterol Clin North Am 2013;42:429–42.

43. Kaminski MF, Regula J, Kraszewska E, et al. Quality indicators for colonoscopy and the risk of interval cancer. N Engl J Med 2010;362:1795–803.

44. Corley DA, Jensen CD, Marks AR, et al. Adenoma detection rate and risk of colorectal cancer and death. N Engl J Med 2014;370:1298–306.

45. Do A, Weinberg J, Kakkar A, et al. Reliability of adenoma detection rate is based on procedural volume. Gastrointest Endosc 2013;77:376–80.

46. Rex DK, Eid E. Considerations regarding the present and future roles of colonoscopy in colorectal cancer prevention. Clin Gastroenterol Hepatol 2008;6: 506–14.

47. Bretagne JF, Ponchon T. Do we need to embrace adenoma detection rate as the main quality control parameter during colonoscopy? Endoscopy 2008;40: 523–8.

48. Kahi CJ, Ballard D, Shah AS, et al. Impact of a quarterly report card on colonoscopy quality measures. Gastrointest Endosc 2013;77:925–31.

49. Williams JE, Le TD, Faigel DO. Polypectomy rate as a quality measure for colonoscopy. Gastrointest Endosc 2011;73:498–506.

50. Williams JE, Holub JL, Faigel DO. Polypectomy rate is a valid quality measure for colonoscopy: results from a national endoscopy database. Gastrointest Endosc 2012;75:576–82.

51. Denis B, Sauleau EA, Gendre I, et al. The mean number of adenomas per procedure should become the gold standard to measure the neoplasia yield of colonoscopy: a population-based cohort study. Dig Liver Dis 2014;46:176–81.

52. Wang HS, Pisegna J, Modi R, et al. Adenoma detection rate is necessary but insufficient for distinguishing high versus low endoscopist performance. Gastrointest Endosc 2013;77:71–8.

53. Lee TJ, Rutter MD, Blanks RG, et al. Colonoscopy quality measures: experience from the NHS Bowel Cancer Screening Programme. Gut 2012;61:1050–7.

54. Lieberman DA, Holub J, Eisen G, et al. Prevalence of polyps greater than 9 mm in a consortium of diverse clinical practice settings in the United States. Clin Gastroenterol Hepatol 2005;3:798–805.

55. Corley DA, Jensen CD, Marks AR, et al. Variation of adenoma prevalence by age, sex, race, and colon location in a large population: implications for screening and quality programs. Clin Gastroenterol Hepatol 2013;11:172–80.

56. Brenner H, Hoffmeister M, Stegmaier C, et al. Risk of progression of advanced adenomas to colorectal cancer by age and sex: estimates based on 840,149 screening colonoscopies. Gut 2007;56:1585–9.

57. Greenspan M, Rajan KB, Baig A, et al. Advanced adenoma detection rate is independent of nonadvanced adenoma detection rate. Am J Gastroenterol 2013; 108:1286–92.

58. Snover DC. Update on the serrated pathway to colorectal carcinoma. Hum Pathol 2011;42:1–10.

59. Rex DK, Ahnen DJ, Baron JA, et al. Serrated lesions of the colorectum: review and recommendations from an expert panel. Am J Gastroenterol 2012;107: 1315–29 [quiz: 1314, 1330].

60. Sweetser S, Smyrk TC, Sinicrope FA. Serrated colon polyps as precursors to colorectal cancer. Clin Gastroenterol Hepatol 2013;11:760–7 [quiz: e54–5].

61. Kahi CJ, Li X, Eckert GJ, et al. High colonoscopic prevalence of proximal colon serrated polyps in average-risk men and women. Gastrointest Endosc 2012;75: 515–20.

62. Kahi CJ, Hewett DG, Norton DL, et al. Prevalence and variable detection of prox-
    imal colon serrated polyps during screening colonoscopy. Clin Gastroenterol
    Hepatol 2011;9:42–6.
63. Hetzel JT, Huang CS, Coukos JA, et al. Variation in the detection of serrated
    polyps in an average risk colorectal cancer screening cohort. Am J Gastroenterol
    2010;105:2656–64.
64. Leung K, Pinsky P, Laiyemo AO, et al. Ongoing colorectal cancer risk despite sur-
    veillance colonoscopy: the polyp prevention trial continued follow-up study.
    Gastrointest Endosc 2010;71:111–7.
65. Pabby A, Schoen RE, Weissfeld JL, et al. Analysis of colorectal cancer occur-
    rence during surveillance colonoscopy in the dietary polyp prevention trial.
    Gastrointest Endosc 2005;61:385–91.
66. Pohl H, Srivastava A, Bensen SP, et al. Incomplete polyp resection during
    colonoscopy-results of the complete adenoma resection (CARE) study. Gastroen-
    terology 2013;144:74–80.e1.
67. Gupta S, Anderson J, Bhandari P, et al. Development and validation of a novel
    method for assessing competency in polypectomy: direct observation of poly-
    pectomy skills. Gastrointest Endosc 2011;73:1232–9.e2.
68. Hewett DG, Kahi CJ, Rex DK. Efficacy and effectiveness of colonoscopy: how do
    we bridge the gap? Gastrointest Endosc Clin N Am 2010;20:673–84.
69. Hilsden RJ, Rostom A, Dube C, et al. Development and implementation of a
    comprehensive quality assurance program at a community endoscopy facility.
    Can J Gastroenterol 2011;25:547–54.
70. Gavin DR, Valori RM, Anderson JT, et al. The national colonoscopy audit: a nation-
    wide assessment of the quality and safety of colonoscopy in the UK. Gut 2013;62:
    242–9.
71. Lieberman D, Nadel M, Smith RA, et al. Standardized colonoscopy reporting and
    data system: report of the Quality Assurance Task Group of the National Colo-
    rectal Cancer Roundtable. Gastrointest Endosc 2007;65:757–66.
72. van Doorn SC, van Vliet J, Fockens P, et al. A novel colonoscopy reporting system
    enabling quality assurance. Endoscopy 2014;46:181–7.
73. Lieberman DA, Faigel DO, Logan JR, et al. Assessment of the quality of colonos-
    copy reports: results from a multicenter consortium. Gastrointest Endosc 2009;
    69:645–53.
74. Imler TD, Morea J, Kahi C, et al. Natural language processing accurately catego-
    rizes findings from colonoscopy and pathology reports. Clin Gastroenterol
    Hepatol 2013;11:689–94.
75. Corley DA, Jensen CD, Marks AR. Can we improve adenoma detection rates?
    A systematic review of intervention studies. Gastrointest Endosc 2011;74:
    656–65.
76. Taber A, Romagnuolo J. Effect of simply recording colonoscopy withdrawal time
    on polyp and adenoma detection rates. Gastrointest Endosc 2010;71:782–6.
77. Sawhney MS, Cury MS, Neeman N, et al. Effect of institution-wide policy of colo-
    noscopy withdrawal time > or = 7 minutes on polyp detection. Gastroenterology
    2008;135:1892–8.
78. Barclay RL, Vicari JJ, Greenlaw RL. Effect of a time-dependent colonoscopic
    withdrawal protocol on adenoma detection during screening colonoscopy. Clin
    Gastroenterol Hepatol 2008;6:1091–8.
79. Coe SG, Crook JE, Diehl NN, et al. An endoscopic quality improvement program
    improves detection of colorectal adenomas. Am J Gastroenterol 2013;108:
    219–26 [quiz: 227].

80. Harewood GC, Petersen BT, Ott BJ. Prospective assessment of the impact of feedback on colonoscopy performance. Aliment Pharmacol Ther 2006;24:313–8.
81. Lin OS, Kozarek RA, Arai A, et al. The effect of periodic monitoring and feedback on screening colonoscopy withdrawal times, polyp detection rates, and patient satisfaction scores. Gastrointest Endosc 2010;71:1253–9.
82. Shaukat A, Oancea C, Bond JH, et al. Variation in detection of adenomas and polyps by colonoscopy and change over time with a performance improvement program. Clin Gastroenterol Hepatol 2009;7:1335–40.
83. Rex DK, Hewett DG, Raghavendra M, et al. The impact of videorecording on the quality of colonoscopy performance: a pilot study. Am J Gastroenterol 2010;105:2312–7.
84. Madhoun MF, Tierney WM. The impact of video recording colonoscopy on adenoma detection rates. Gastrointest Endosc 2012;75:127–33.
85. de Groen PC. Advanced systems to assess colonoscopy. Gastrointest Endosc Clin N Am 2010;20:699–716.

Colon Capsule Endoscopy

Cristiano Spada, MD*, Cesare Hassan, MD,
Guido Costamagna, MD, FACG

KEYWORDS

- Colon capsule endoscopy • Incomplete colonoscopy • Regimen of preparation
- Accuracy • Fields of application

KEY POINTS

- Colon capsule endoscopy (CCE) is a minimally invasive, painless endoscopic tool that allows colonic investigation without requiring intubation, insufflation or sedation.
- CCE is not an alternative to colonoscopy, but a complementary test for average-risk patients unwilling or unable to undergo colonoscopy, and cases of incomplete colonoscopy.
- For such indications, CCE is advantageous because it is minimally invasive and allows direct visualization of the colonic mucosa with good accuracy, without radiation exposure.
- CCE bowel preparation must be exhaustive because fecal remains cannot be removed by CCE. It also needs to promote capsule propulsion through the entire small bowel and then through the colon to the rectum.
- The second generation of CCE is an accurate tool for colonic evaluation.

INTRODUCTION

Colorectal cancer (CRC) is a leading cause of cancer death around the world, being the second most common cause of cancer-related death in developed countries with 500,000 deaths per year worldwide.[1] The procedure of choice for CRC prevention is colonoscopy, which allows the identification and removal of premalignant adenomatous polyps.[2,3] Although the risk of colonoscopy-related severe complications is small, conventional colonoscopy is perceived as an invasive and potentially painful procedure, which requires conscious or deep sedation and takes place in an unpleasant setting.[4,5]

Colon capsule endoscopy (CCE) was initially released in 2006 by Given Imaging (Yoqneam, Israel).[6,7] More recently the technology has been implemented, and a

Author Contributions: C. Spada and C. Hassan made the literature search and the analysis of the results; C. Spada, C. Hassan and G. Costamagna wrote the article and were involved in the revision process, and approved the final article.
Digestive Endoscopy Unit, Catholic University, Rome, Italy
* Corresponding author. Digestive Endoscopy Unit, Catholic University, Largo A Gemelli, 8, Rome 00168, Italy.
E-mail address: cristianospada@gmail.com

second generation of CCE is now available.[8–10] CCE allows a minimally invasive, painless colonic investigation without requiring intubation, insufflation, or sedation, allowing the pursuit of normal daily activities during the procedure.

According to the European Society of Gastrointestinal Endoscopy (ESGE) guidelines, CCE can be used in average-risk patients, in patients with a previous incomplete colonoscopy, in those unwilling to undergo conventional colonoscopy, or in those for whom colonoscopy is not possible or contraindicated.[10]

PILLCAM COLON CAPSULE SYSTEM

The Given Imaging diagnostic system is composed of 3 main subsystems: the ingestible capsule endoscope (second-generation colon capsule), the Data Recorder, and the RAPID workstation. The second-generation CCE (PCC-2) is 11.6 × 31.5 mm in size.[8,9] It has been endowed with a battery lasting about 10 hours and has 2 cameras, one at each end, with an angle of view of 172° for each camera, allowing a near full visual coverage of the colon. To enhance colon visualization and to save battery energy and video reading, the capsule is equipped with an adaptive frame rate (AFR), which alternates from 35 images per second while in motion to 4 images per second when virtually stationary. At the moment of the ingestion the capsule begins working, using AFR allowing proper visualization of the esophagus, then slows down to 14 images per minute. When small bowel images are detected, the system switches the capsule to the AFR mode. This advanced system for control of capsule image rate is the result of a bidirectional communication between the capsule and the Data Recorder. The new Data Recorder (Data Recorder 3 [DR3]) not only stores the capsule's incoming images but also analyzes them in real time to control the capsule capture rate of images. When DR3 recognizes that the capsule is virtually stationary, it sets the image capture rate to 4 frames per second. When the DR3 recognizes that the capsule is in motion, it sets the image capture rate to 35 frames per second. The DR3 also assists and guides patients and physicians by means of visual and audio signals throughout the procedure activities. It buzzes, vibrates, and displays instructions on its liquid crystal diode screen to alert the patient to continue the preparation protocol. In practice, when the video capsule has detected intestinal villi, the patient is informed and invited to orally ingest the "booster," according to the preparation regimen.[11] On completion of the examination, data from the Recorder are downloaded to the Workstation that is provided with dedicated software (RAPID) for video viewing and processing. The new RAPID software has an integrated tool to estimate polyp size. To make the examination interpretations easier, the new RAPID software has flexible spectral intelligent color enhancement to improve image quality and pathologic visualization.

BOWEL PREPARATION

The current ESGE guidelines for CCE preparation recommend 4 L polyethylene glycol (PEG) solution administered in split doses (2 L the day before the examination and 2 L on the day of the examination, before capsule ingestion) combined with oral low-volume sodium phosphate (NaP) boosters to assist capsule propulsion and excretion (**Table 1**).[10]

In contrast to conventional colonoscopy, it is not possible to clean the colon during the CCE procedure. Therefore colonic preparation is crucial, as even a small amount of debris could interfere with colon capsule capability in identifying colonic polyps, and ultimately compromise the outcome of the procedure (**Fig. 1**). Colonic preparation for CCE is not limited to achieving an adequate cleansing level, but is also aimed at distending the colonic wall, filling the lumen with clean liquids, and promoting capsule

Table 1		
Regimen of preparation for colon capsule endoscopy (CCE)		
	Schedule	**Intake**
Day −2	Bedtime	Senna, 4 tablets (48 mg)
Day −1	All day	Clear liquid diet
	Evening (7–9 PM)	2 L PEG
Examination day	7–9 AM	2 L PEG
	10 AM (∼1 h after last intake of PEG)	**Capsule ingestion**[a]
	After small bowel detection	**First boost**
		30 mL NaP + 1 L water
	3 h after first boost	**Second boost**
		[b]15 mL NaP + 0.5 L water
	2 h after second boost	**Suppository**
		[b]10 mg bisacodyl

Abbreviations: NaP, sodium phosphate; PEG, polyethylene glycol.
[a] 10 mg metoclopramide tablet if capsule delayed in stomach longer than 1 hour.
[b] Only if capsule not excreted yet.
From Spada C, Hassan C, Galmiche JP, et al. Colon capsule endoscopy: European Society of Gastrointestinal Endoscopy (ESGE) guideline. Endoscopy 2012;44:527–36; with permission.

propulsion and excretion, ensuring that the journey is completed within the battery's lifetime.[12,13] Because preliminary studies using the same preparation as colonoscopy (PEG solution) showed low excretion rates (20%), a protocol combining PEG (4 L) and boosts with NaP (75 mL) was adopted, and was demonstrated to allow a complete colon examination in most cases.[7,14,15] Subsequent studies proposed modifications in the timing and doses of the components, the inclusion of dietary recommendations (low-residue diet, liquid diet the day before) and suppositories (in case of delayed capsule excretion), prokinetics (for delayed stomach emptying), and different kinds of boosters. In particular, because of concerns related to the administration of NaP, other boosters have been investigated. Caution should be exercised when NaP is administered to the elderly, patients with dehydration or renal disease, and those receiving angiotensin-converting enzyme inhibitors. Unfortunately, studies that tried to replace NaP resulted in unsatisfactory outcomes, namely significant reduction of capsule excretion and completion rate. When considering that cecal intubation rates of higher than 90% and 95% are recommended for routine and screening colonoscopies, respectively,[16] CCE could not be considered an efficient option if only 75% of patients achieve a complete examination, as observed when administering a PEG instead of an NaP booster.[12] Moreover, an incomplete capsule examination, in contrast to an incomplete colonoscopy, tends to leave the left colon uninvestigated. Recently, Rex[17] reported the results of a United States trial in which NaP was replaced by Suprep (sodium sulfate, potassium sulfate, and magnesium sulfate) (Braintree Laboratories Inc, Braintree, MA, USA), maintaining the split dose of PEG. The 91% of capsule excretion rate within 10 hours is comparable with the results of trials in which NaP was adopted. Results of different regimens of preparation are listed in **Table 1**. Collectively these studies lead to 2 important conclusions: (1) split regimens of PEG (2 L + 2 L) are recommended to improve the cleansing level; and (2) effective boosters (to date most of the evidence applies to NaP boosters) should be recommended to achieve a reasonable capsule excretion rate. When NaP was included in the preparation regimen, low doses (45–55 mL) were shown to achieve an adequate capsule excretion rate with the advantage of decreasing the risk of NaP toxicity (acute nephropathy, electrolyte imbalance, kidney failure).[10] The role of low-volume–based

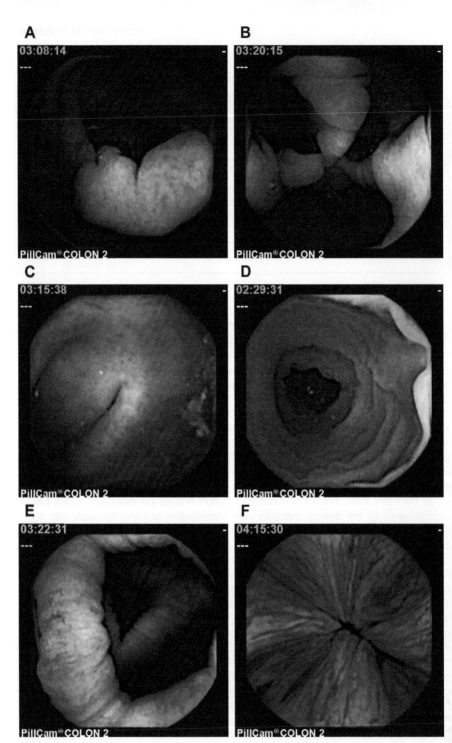

Fig. 1. Capsule endoscopy images of normal colon. (*A*, *B*) Ileocecal valve. (*C*) Appendiceal orifice. Colonic preparation for colon capsule endoscopy (CCE) is not limited to achievement of an adequate cleansing level, but is also aimed at distending the colonic wall filling the lumen of clean liquids. The capsule transits like a submarine through the distended colon (*D*, *E*). Colon capsule endoscopy is defined as complete when the capsule is excreted or when the anal verge is visualized (*F*).

preparation regimens is not well studied. Preliminary results show that low-volume regimens (2 L of PEG + ascorbic acid) are at least as effective as a 4-L PEG regimen in terms of both cleansing level and excretion rate.[18,19] If such results are confirmed by further trials, the low-volume regimen of preparation would be an effective alternative that could improve compliance to CCE.

ACCURACY

Second-generation CCE (CCE-2) was demonstrated to be a feasible and reliable tool to detect colonic lesions, such as polyps and tumors (**Fig. 2**).[8,9,17,20] Results of

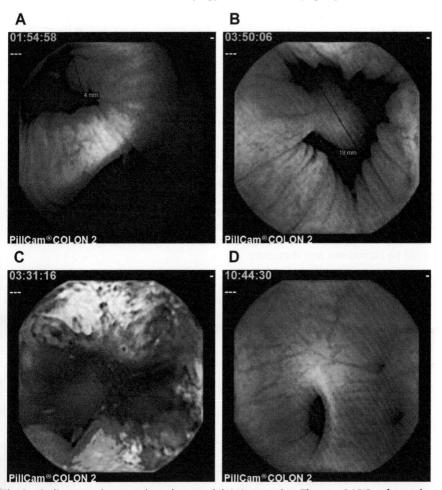

Fig. 2. Findings at colon capsule endoscopy. (*A*) A 4-mm polyp. The new RAPID software has a tool integrated to estimate the polyp size. The video reviewer places the mouse cursor on one end of the polyp displayed on the monitor and then drags the cursor to the other end of the polyp. The RAPID software calculates the distance and instantly displays the estimated polyp size in millimeters. A 4-mm polyp is considered a nonsignificant finding. Only patients with a polyp of 6 mm or larger at CCE, in addition to those with 3 polyps or more irrespective of size, should be sent to post-CCE colonoscopy for polypectomy.[10] (*B*) An 18-mm pedunculated polyp. (*C*) Colonic carcinoma. (*D*) Diverticula. Colonic diverticula do not represent a contraindication for CCE.

published studies are shown in **Table 2**. Overall more than 1100 were involved in comparative trials that used standard colonoscopy as gold standard. The relatively low number of patients studied is a clear limitation, and further data are needed. However, it should be emphasized that these studies show comparable results in terms of accuracy, cleanliness, excretion rate, and safety, suggesting that they accurately represent the actual performance characteristics of CCE-2. The low specificity observed in the European[8] and Israeli[9] trials was mainly related to a consistent number of false-positive cases generated by size mismatching between standard colonoscopy and CCE. Only a minority of false positives was related to findings visualized by CCE and not confirmed by colonoscopy, it being not possible to exclude the risk of missed polyps by colonoscopy (ie, falsely negative at colonoscopy). To date 10 cancers have been detected by conventional colonoscopy in comparative trials: CCE-2 identified cancers in all cases, suggesting a potential 100% sensitivity.[8,9,17,21]

CLINICAL INDICATIONS
Patients Without Alarm Symptoms

Based on the available evidence CCE-2 cannot replace conventional colonoscopy, but it should be considered a complementary test in specific settings. According to the ESGE guidelines,[10] CCE can be used in average-risk subjects who do not appear to be at increased risk of colorectal neoplasia. In this setting a noninvasive test may be considered, and CCE might be preferred over nonimaging tests (ie, fecal tests) because of its ability to detect nonneoplastic conditions that may be regarded as clinically useful (eg, vascular malformations). On the other hand, patients with alarm symptoms (because of symptoms or signs, or a family or personal history of CRC) are at increased risk of colorectal neoplasia. These patients should be referred to colonoscopy. For patients who are not compliant with colonoscopy, the use of CCE should be considered and discussed.

Incomplete Colonoscopy

To date, most of the evidence for CCE applies to patients with a previous incomplete colonoscopy.[22–28] According to the US Multi-Society Task Force (USMSTF) on Colorectal Cancer, gastroenterologists performing colonoscopy should be able to achieve

Authors,[Ref.] Year	Sample Size (N)	Adequate Cleansing (%)	Excretion Rate (%)	Polyp ≥6 mm		Polyp ≥10 mm	
				Sensitivity (%)	Specificity (%)	Sensitivity (%)	Specificity (%)
Eliakim et al,[9] 2009	98	78	81[a]	89	76	88	89
Spada et al,[8] 2011	117	85	81[a]	84	64	88	95
Rex,[17] 2013	884	80	91[b]	88	82	92	95
Hagel et al,[20] 2014	24	90.1	71[c]	72.2	90.9	75	100
Holleran et al[21]	62	92	73[c]	95	65	89	96

Table 2
Accuracy of PillCam COLON 2

[a] Within 8 hours.
[b] Within 10 hours postingestion.
[c] Within battery life span.

cecal intubation in 90% of all cases and in 95% of screening colonoscopies.[16] In the literature, incomplete colonoscopy rates range from 5% to 15%.[29] The most frequent causes of incomplete colonoscopy include left-sided angulations caused by diverticular disease or postsurgical adhesions, extensive looping or stenosing colorectal cancer, or patient intolerance.[30] At present, following an incomplete colonoscopy patients are usually referred for additional tests, given the risk of missed neoplasia in the non-visualized colon. Options include radiologic imaging (computed tomographic colonography [CTC] or barium enema), colonoscopy using different endoscopes (pediatric or variable-stiffness colonoscopes, balloon-assisted enteroscopes, cap-assisted or water-immersion technique) or with anesthetist assistance.[31] CTC,[32,33] also known as virtual colonoscopy, has been shown to be substantially more effective than double-contrast barium enema for the detection of large colorectal polyps and colorectal cancer. CTC is now recommended by the American Gastroenterological Society as the imaging modality of choice in cases of incomplete colonoscopy.[3] When compared with other endoscopic modalities, CCE has the unique characteristic of examining the colon in a proximal to distal direction. Colonic segments that are not explored because of an incomplete colonoscopy (the right colon) are the ones visualized first with CCE. Several studies[22-24,26-28,34,35] have shown that CCE can allow visualization of colonic segments not visualized by previous incomplete conventional colonoscopy in 83–98% of cases. In this setting, CCE can detect additional findings that would have been missed, as they were localized in unexamined segments (**Table 3**). European studies suggest that CCE yields significant findings and guides further workup in 23–45% of cases. The optimal timing of CCE after an incomplete colonoscopy, and how to proceed with the preparation if CCE is performed immediately after colonoscopy, are not known. This issue is important because it affects whether patients are asked to perform an additional preparation. CCE immediately after an incomplete colonoscopy would also allow the endoscopist to complete an examination of the colon on the same day without rescheduling or referring the patient to other physicians. To date, only one prospective trial from Greece[23] that used the first generation of colon capsule showed that CCE can be performed effectively and safely immediately after incomplete colonoscopy, thus minimizing patient burden. Patients who underwent same-day CCE received the second part of the bowel preparation as described by Schoofs and colleagues.[36]

When compared with CTC (the first-choice imaging technique in case of incomplete colonoscopy), CCE was demonstrated to have a significantly higher diagnostic yield for polyps 6 mm or larger,[24] and was better tolerated.[37] Of interest is that lesions

Table 3
Results of CCE in incomplete conventional colonoscopy

Authors,[Ref.] Year	Sample Size (N)	Completeness (%)	CCE Complementary Findings (%)
Pioche et al,[22] 2012	107	83	34[a]
Alarcon-Fernandez et al,[26] 2013	34	85	23.5[a]
Triantafyllou et al,[23] 2014	75	90.7	44[a]
Nogales et al,[28] 2013	96	93	45[b]
Baltes et al,[27] 2014	74	95	28[b]
Spada et al,[24] 2014	100	98	24[b]

[a] Any finding.
[b] Significant findings (Polyp ≥6 mm or more than 3 polyps).

missed by CTC were mainly flat and/or sessile lesions, less than 10 mm in size, located in the right colon.[24] Further confirmatory studies are awaited.

Worthy of note is that all published CCE studies have several methodological limitations that can affect the generalizability of their findings, such as the inclusion of relatively selected study populations, heterogeneous preparation regimens, and differences in the expertise available at medical centers. Moreover, uncertainty regarding the documentation of successful colonoscopy after CCE, relatively small sample sizes, and lack of a reference procedure that could serve as a gold standard are issues that should be addressed by ongoing studies.

In summary, the management of patients with an incomplete colonoscopy depends on several issues, including the setting of the examination and the available expertise. If CCE is available, capsule could be potentially offered immediately after an incomplete colonoscopy or, alternatively, patients could be maintained on a liquid diet with additional bowel preparation and CCE administered the following day. The most cost-effective approach in this scenario warrants further study.[34] CCE adds another diagnostic option for the gastroenterologist faced with a patient with an incomplete colonoscopy, with the advantage that patients could be safely and accurately managed "internally" without the need for referral to other centers.

Patients Unable or Unwilling to Undergo Colonoscopy

Patients with alarm symptoms (eg, rectal bleeding, anemia, weight loss) are at increased risk for colorectal neoplasia; specifically, at a 5- to 10-fold increased risk of malignancy.[38] Patients with a positive fecal blood test are also at increased risk for CRC and advanced neoplasia.[3,39–41] In this setting, a test with very high sensitivity is desirable and, therefore, colonoscopy is the primary option.[42] However, in patients not compliant with colonoscopy, CCE can be considered. The accuracy of CCE in high-risk patients who are unable or unwilling to undergo colonoscopy was recently assessed.[35] In a series of 70 patients, CCE-2 yielded findings in 34% of patients. Six patients were diagnosed with tumors: 4 with colon cancer, 1 with gastric cancer, and 1 with small bowel cancer. The capsule findings were confirmed after surgery in all patients. A prospective multicenter study confirmed these results by assessing the diagnostic yield of CCE in patients with colonoscopy failure or contraindication for anesthesia. CCE yielded findings in 33.6% of patients who subsequently underwent therapeutic intervention. Although the evidence is still very limited and awaits confirmation in larger trials, CCE seems to be a reasonable alternative option for patients who are unable or unwilling to undergo colonoscopy.[22,35]

Inflammatory Bowel Disease

To date, there are insufficient data to support the use of CCE in the diagnostic workup or in the surveillance of patients with suspected or known inflammatory bowel disease (IBD) (see **Fig. 1**).[10] The few articles evaluating the role of CCE in patients with ulcerative colitis (UC) report discordant results[43] and are difficult to compare because they differ significantly in terms of technology (first/second generation of CCE), methodology, and measured outcomes (**Table 4**). The overall results show that the accuracy of CCE for assessment of mucosal inflammation in UC appears comparable with that of colonoscopy. Consensus guidelines issued by the ESGE state that CCE-2 may be useful to monitor inflammation in UC, which may help to guide therapy.[10]

Several studies have shown good correlation between CCE and conventional colonoscopy. The largest was a multicenter study carried out by Sung and colleagues[44] involving 100 suspected or known UC patients. The aim was to determine whether mucosal appearance reported by CCE can be used to differentiate active from inactive

Table 4
Performance of CCE in inflammatory bowel disease

Authors,[Ref.] Year	Sample Size (N)	Outcomes
Sung et al,[44] 2012	100	Sens: 89% Spec: 75% PPV: 93% NPV: 65%
Oliva et al,[45] 2014	30	Sens: 95% Spec: 100% PPV: 100% NPV: 85%
Ye et al,[46] 2013	26	Good correlation in severity and extent between OC and CCE
Hosoe et al,[47] 2013	40	Good correlation in severity between OC and CCE
San Juan-Acosta et al,[48] 2014	42	79% agreement for disease activity 71% agreement for extent of inflamation
Kobayashi,[49] 2013	49	Good correlation in severity between OC and CCE
Meister et al,[50] 2013	13	Poor correlation in severity and extent between OC and CCE
Singeap et al,[51] 2013	15	60% correlation between OC and CCE
Manes et al,[52] 2013	20	Poor correlation in severity and extent between OC and CCE

Abbreviations: CCE, colon capsule endoscopy; NPV, negative predictive value; OC, optical colonoscopy; PPV, positive predictive value; Sens, sensitivity; Spec, specificity.

UC, with conventional colonoscopy as the gold standard. The sensitivity of CCE in detecting active colonic inflammation was 89% and the specificity was 75%, with positive and negative predictive values of 93% and 65%, respectively. The investigators concluded that CCE could be indicated to monitor mucosal healing in UC but that it could not replace conventional colonoscopy. Studies conducted by Hosoe and colleagues[47] and Kobayashi and colleagues[49] evaluated the endoscopic score for each colon section (i.e. cecum, ascending colon, transverse colon, proximal left-sided colon, distal left-sided colon). These investigators found a strong correlation for disease activity between CCE and colonoscopy in the cecum and ascending, transverse, and left-sided proximal colon (r range 0.765–0.906), and moderate correlation in the distal colon ($r = 0.673$). Overall, there was a strong correlation between CCE and colonoscopy in all segments (average $r = 0.797$). Ye and colleagues[46] found a significant correlation ($P<.001$) in terms of severity and extent of UC between CCE and colonoscopy. San Juan-Acosta and colleagues[48] reported that the agreement in determining severity and extent of UC between CCE and colonoscopy was 79% and 71%, respectively. By contrast, other studies have shown lower agreement between CCE and colonoscopy findings (see **Table 4**). Manes and colleagues,[52] in a study of 20 UC subjects, reported that the complete agreement between CCE and colonoscopy in assessing mucosal activity and disease extent was 56% and 61%, respectively. Singeap and colleagues[51] reported a similarly low concordance (60%) of findings between CCE and colonoscopy in 15 IBD subjects. Meister and colleagues[50] recommended the preferential use of colonoscopy in the assessment of inflammation in UC patients, because the severity and extent of disease were both underestimated by CCE in comparison with conventional colonoscopy. These studies have all been conducted in adults. Recently, the potential role of CCE (ie, CCE-2) in pediatric IBD was evaluated in 30 consecutive children with UC.[45] The sensitivity of CCE for disease activity was 96% and the specificity was 100%, while the positive and negative predictive values were 100% and 85%, respectively. In the same trial, CCE had a higher overall tolerability than colonoscopy, and interobserver agreement was excellent ($\geq$0.86).[45]

Additional aspects regarding CCE and IBD are important. Although CCE is specifically designed to explore the colon, it can also offer excellent imaging of the small bowel, which may be of benefit for some IBD patients. Although colonoscopy remains the gold standard for disease diagnosis and monitoring, new noninvasive tools such as CCE, which allow exploration of the small bowel and colon without the need for sedation, intubation, and gas insufflation, represent an appealing complementary option. In one study,[51] which reported low concordance (60%) between CCE and colonoscopy, half of the discordance reflected the diagnostic impact of CCE. In patients diagnosed as unclassified colitis by colonoscopy, CCE contributed to a change of diagnosis from ulcerative pancolitis to Crohn disease, based on finding lesions in the small bowel.[28]

Colorectal Cancer Screening

The potential role of CCE in colorectal cancer screening programs is unknown because specific trials in this setting are unavailable. A recent article from the American Society of Gastrointestinal Endoscopy stated that the use of CCE in the colon was limited at the time of publication.[53] Current USMSTF or American College of Gastroenterology guidelines for CRC screening have not included CCE in their recommendations.[3,54] More studies regarding sensitivity and patient compliance are needed. Although the sensitivity and specificity of CCE for detecting polyps and cancers in patients with suspected or known colonic lesions are good, it should be emphasized that data in average-risk screening populations are scant. The most common screening strategy in Europe involves a 2-stage population-based approach. In this model, individuals who are identified as at risk, by either fecal occult blood test or fecal immunologic test (FIT), are referred for colonoscopy. However, whereas these tests select out a population at higher risk for colon cancer and adenomas, most individuals who undergo colonoscopy do not harbor neoplasia. This anomaly represents a major burden on screening resources and places screening participants at increased risk for significant, albeit infrequent, colonoscopy-related adverse events. In a recent trial, Holleran and colleagues,[21] aiming to reduce the number of colonoscopies without relevant findings, evaluated whether CCE could constitute a screening "filter" for people who have positive FIT results. In a total of 62 FIT-positive participants, optical colonoscopy detected at least 1 polyp in 36 participants (58%), significant lesions in 18 (29%), and cancer in 1 (2%). The investigators found a good correlation between CCE and optical colonoscopy for any lesion and for significant lesions ($r =$ 0.62 and 0.84, respectively). The negative predictive value of CCE was high for both any polyp (90%) and significant lesions (96%). These results suggest that CCE is an effective means of detecting cancer and polyps in a positive FIT cohort. In particular, if the capsules are used as a filter test, as the investigators proposed, the negative predictive values for any polyp and significant lesions are excellent at 90% and 96%, respectively, and could reduce the demand for optical colonoscopy by up to one-third.[21] A cost-effective analysis using a Markov model showed that FIT repeated every year is the most cost-effective strategy, and although CCE every 5 years is as effective as annual FIT, it is not a cost-effective alternative.[55]

Although CCE is not a cost-effective option when assuming equal adherence, it may become an efficient option when assuming that adherence to CCE was higher in comparison with screening colonoscopy, a feature that as yet has not been demonstrated. In the screening setting, the possibility of performing a colonoscopy immediately after a "positive" CCE is very appealing because it allows conventional colonoscopy to be performed using the same bowel regimen used for CCE. This scenario has not been explored, and may be feasible only with a certain set of circumstances. First, the video of CCE should be evaluated in a relatively short time, without running the risk of decreasing the overall accuracy of CCE. In this sense, the QuickView (a tool in the RAPID software to decrease reading time) may offer the opportunity to review the colonic video within a few minutes.[56] However, the accuracy of QuickView for significant findings is not well evaluated.[56] Second, the preparation regimen should provide a CCE colon transit time sufficiently short to meet logistic constraints. Bowel preparation is no longer a major hurdle in terms of cleansing, as regimens now allow procurement of an adequate cleansing level in more than 80% of patients. Nevertheless, colonic transit time is still difficult to predict when a CCE is performed, with some patients with a very short transit time and others without capsule excretion at the end of battery life. A preparation regimen that allows for an adequate cleansing level with a homogeneous and relatively short CCE colonic transit time is highly desirable. CCE might also play a role in increasing the compliance to colonoscopy. No colorectal imaging test may be performed on an out-of-clinic basis, a major drawback in comparison with fecal tests. CCE has the potential to become the first colorectal imaging test to be performed outside of the clinic. The out-of-clinic aspect (CCE as a home procedure), in combination with the noninvasiveness of CCE, are attractive and relevant features that might increase compliance to colonoscopy. Adler and colleagues[11] evaluated the feasibility and efficiency of CCE when offered as an out-of-clinic procedure, and showed that CCE is feasible and easily performed outside of the clinic. However, it remains unknown as to whether a home-based procedure may be associated with better acceptability and compliance to colonoscopy, and, therefore, increased adherence to colorectal cancer screening.

In summary, although appealing, the role of CCE in CRC screening programs is largely undefined. To date the only information available comes from a single-center trial, which reported that CCE effectively detects cancer and polyps in FIT-positive patients, making CCE a useful filter test to select patients for conventional colonoscopy. Two large trials are under way in Europe to evaluate the potential role of CCE in CRC screening programs. One Italian trial (CCANDY trial) that will enroll approximately 400 FIT-positive patients is aimed at assessing the sensitivity, specificity, and positive and negative predictive values in detecting CRC and advanced adenomas. The second study, conducted in the Netherlands (ORCA trial), will enroll up to 1000 patients with the aim of determining the uptake and diagnostic yield of primary population screening for CRC by means of CCE. The results of these 2 trials are eagerly awaited because they will clarify: (1) if CCE accuracy in CRC screening programs is sufficiently high for CCE to be included in the menu of screening options; and (2) if the uptake is adequate enough to ensure equal or even higher participation in CRC screening programs.

It is also important to know whether CCE can capture those FIT-positive patients who are unwilling to undergo conventional colonoscopy. In such cases, 2 scenarios might arise: (1) CCE detects significant findings, which might convince the patient to undergo therapeutic colonoscopy; and (2) CCE will not detect any finding, and patients will be referred for a screening colonoscopy after 3 years.[10]

SUMMARY

The second generation of colon capsule represents an accurate tool for colonic evaluation. CCE is not an alternative to colonoscopy. Rather, it is a complementary test for average-risk patients unwilling or unable to undergo colonoscopy, and cases of incomplete colonoscopy. For such indications, CCE is advantageous because it is minimally invasive, and allows direct visualization of the colonic mucosa with good accuracy and without radiation exposure.

REFERENCES

1. Jemal A, Siegel R, Ward E, et al. Cancer statistics, 2009. CA Cancer J Clin 2009; 59:225–49.
2. Winawer SJ, Zauber AG, Ho MN, et al. Prevention of colorectal cancer by colonoscopic polypectomy. The National Polyp Study Workgroup. N Engl J Med 1993; 329:1977–81.
3. Levin B, Lieberman DA, McFarland B, et al. Screening and surveillance for the early detection of colorectal cancer and adenomatous polyps, 2008: a joint guideline from the American Cancer Society, the US Multi-Society Task Force on Colorectal Cancer, and the American College of Radiology. Gastroenterology 2008;134:1570–95.
4. Edwards BK, Ward E, Kohler BA, et al. Annual report to the nation on the status of cancer, 1975-2006, featuring colorectal cancer trends and impact of interventions (risk factors, screening, and treatment) to reduce future rates. Cancer 2010;116: 544–73.
5. Ferlay J, Autier P, Boniol M, et al. Estimates of the cancer incidence and mortality in Europe in 2006. Ann Oncol 2007;18:581–92.
6. Eliakim R, Fireman Z, Gralnek IM, et al. Evaluation of the PillCam Colon capsule in the detection of colonic pathology: results of the first multicenter, prospective, comparative study. Endoscopy 2006;38:963–70.
7. Van Gossum A, Munoz-Navas M, Fernandez-Urien I, et al. Capsule endoscopy versus colonoscopy for the detection of polyps and cancer. N Engl J Med 2009;361:264–70.
8. Spada C, Hassan C, Munoz-Navas M, et al. Second-generation colon capsule endoscopy compared with colonoscopy. Gastrointest Endosc 2011;74:581–9.
9. Eliakim R, Yassin K, Niv Y, et al. Prospective multicenter performance evaluation of the second-generation colon capsule compared with colonoscopy. Endoscopy 2009;41:1026–31.
10. Spada C, Hassan C, Galmiche JP, et al. Colon capsule endoscopy: European Society of Gastrointestinal Endoscopy (ESGE) Guideline. Endoscopy 2012;44: 527–36.
11. Adler SN, Hassan C, Metzger Y, et al. Second-generation colon capsule endoscopy is feasible in the out-of-clinic setting. Surg Endosc 2014;28:570–5.
12. Spada C, Riccioni ME, Hassan C, et al. PillCam colon capsule endoscopy: a prospective, randomized trial comparing two regimens of preparation. J Clin Gastroenterol 2011;45:119–24.
13. Spada C, Hassan C, Ingrosso M, et al. A new regimen of bowel preparation for PillCam colon capsule endoscopy: a pilot study. Dig Liver Dis 2011;43:300–4.
14. Sieg A, Friedrich K, Sieg U. Is PillCam COLON capsule endoscopy ready for colorectal cancer screening? a prospective feasibility study in a community gastroenterology practice. Am J Gastroenterol 2009;104:848–54.

15. Sacher-Huvelin S, Coron E, Gaudric M, et al. Colon capsule endoscopy vs. colonoscopy in patients at average or increased risk of colorectal cancer. Aliment Pharmacol Ther 2010;32:1145–53.

16. Rex DK, Petrini JL, Baron TH, et al. Quality indicators for colonoscopy. Am J Gastroenterol 2006;101:873–85.

17. Rex D, Adler SN, Aisenberg J, et al. Accuracy of PillCam Colon 2 for Detecting Subjects With Adenomas > 6 mm. Gastrointest Endosc 2013;77:AB703.

18. Arguelles-Arias F, San-Juan-Acosta M, Belda A, et al. Preparations for colon capsule endoscopy. Prospective and randomized comparative study between two preparations for colon capsule endoscopy: PEG 2 liters + ascorbic acid versus PEG 4 liters. Rev Esp Enferm Dig 2014;106:312–7.

19. Fernandez-Urien I, Valdivielso E. Low-volume cleansing regimens for colon capsule endoscopy: the answer to the million-dollar question? Rev Esp Enferm Dig 2014;106:301–4.

20. Hagel AF, Gabele E, Raithel M, et al. Colon capsule endoscopy: detection of colonic polyps compared with conventional colonoscopy and visualization of extracolonic pathologies. Can J Gastroenterol Hepatol 2014;28:77–82.

21. Holleran G, Leen R, O'Morain C, et al. Colon capsule endoscopy as possible filter test for colonoscopy selection in a screening population with positive fecal immunology. Endoscopy 2014;46:473–8.

22. Pioche M, de LA, Filoche B, et al. Prospective multicenter evaluation of colon capsule examination indicated by colonoscopy failure or anesthesia contraindication. Endoscopy 2012;44:911–6.

23. Triantafyllou K, Viazis N, Tsibouris P, et al. Colon capsule endoscopy is feasible to perform after incomplete colonoscopy and guides further workup in clinical practice. Gastrointest Endosc 2014;79:307–16.

24. Spada C, Hassan C, Barbaro B, et al. Colon capsule versus CT colonography in patients with incomplete colonoscopy: a prospective, comparative trial. Gut 2015;64:271–81.

25. Van GA. Wireless capsule endoscopy of the large intestine: a review with future projections. Curr Opin Gastroenterol 2014;30:472–6.

26. Alarcon-Fernandez O, Ramos L, Adrian-de-Ganzo Z, et al. Effects of colon capsule endoscopy on medical decision making in patients with incomplete colonoscopies. Clin Gastroenterol Hepatol 2013;11:534–40.

27. Baltes P, Bota M, Albert J, et al. PillCam Colon2 after incomplete colonoscopy - First preliminary results of a multicenter study. United European Gastroenterol J 2013;1(Suppl 1):A190.

28. Nogales O, Lujan M, Nicolas D, et al. Utility of colon capsule endoscopy after an incomplete colonoscopy. Multicentric Spanish study. United European Gastroenterol J 2013;1(Suppl 1):A344.

29. McCoy E, Gerson LB. Is colon capsule endoscopy ready for prime time? Gastroenterology 2014;147:709–11.

30. Hanson ME, Pickhardt PJ, Kim DH, et al. Anatomic factors predictive of incomplete colonoscopy based on findings at CT colonography. AJR Am J Roentgenol 2007;189:774–9.

31. Rex DK. Achieving cecal intubation in the very difficult colon. Gastrointest Endosc 2008;67:938–44.

32. Laghi A, Rengo M, Graser A, et al. Current status on performance of CT colonography and clinical indications. Eur J Radiol 2013;82:1192–200.

33. Spada C, Stoker J, Alarcon O, et al. Clinical indications for computed tomographic colonography: European Society of Gastrointestinal Endoscopy (ESGE)

and European Society of Gastrointestinal and Abdominal Radiology (ESGAR) guideline. Endoscopy 2014;46:897–915.

34. Triantafyllou K, Beintaris I, Dimitriadis GD. Is there a role for colon capsule endoscopy beyond colorectal cancer screening? a literature review. World J Gastroenterol 2014;20:13006–14.

35. Negreanu L, Babiuc R, Bengus A, et al. PillCam Colon 2 capsule in patients unable or unwilling to undergo colonoscopy. World J Gastrointest Endosc 2013;5:559–67.

36. Schoofs N, Deviere J, Van GA. PillCam colon capsule endoscopy compared with colonoscopy for colorectal tumor diagnosis: a prospective pilot study. Endoscopy 2006;38:971–7.

37. Rondonotti E, Borghi C, Mandelli G, et al. Accuracy of capsule colonoscopy and computed tomographic colonography in individuals with positive results from the fecal occult blood test. Clin Gastroenterol Hepatol 2014;12:1303–10.

38. Goulston KJ, Cook I, Dent OF. How important is rectal bleeding in the diagnosis of bowel cancer and polyps? Lancet 1986;2:261–5.

39. Haug U, Hundt S, Brenner H. Quantitative immunochemical fecal occult blood testing for colorectal adenoma detection: evaluation in the target population of screening and comparison with qualitative tests. Am J Gastroenterol 2010;105: 682–90.

40. Hundt S, Haug U, Brenner H. Comparative evaluation of immunochemical fecal occult blood tests for colorectal adenoma detection. Ann Intern Med 2009;150: 162–9.

41. Lieberman DA. Clinical practice. screening for colorectal cancer. N Engl J Med 2009;361:1179–87.

42. Appropriate use of gastrointestinal endoscopy. American Society for Gastrointestinal Endoscopy. Gastrointest Endosc 2000;52:831–7.

43. Shi HY, Ng SC, Tsoi KK, et al. The role of capsule endoscopy in assessing mucosal inflammation in ulcerative colitis. Expert Rev Gastroenterol Hepatol 2015;9:47–54.

44. Sung J, Ho KY, Chiu HM, et al. The use of Pillcam Colon in assessing mucosal inflammation in ulcerative colitis: a multicenter study. Endoscopy 2012;44: 754–8.

45. Oliva S, Di NG, Hassan C, et al. Second-generation colon capsule endoscopy vs. colonoscopy in pediatric ulcerative colitis: a pilot study. Endoscopy 2014;46: 485–92.

46. Ye CA, Gao YJ, Ge ZZ, et al. PillCam colon capsule endoscopy versus conventional colonoscopy for the detection of severity and extent of ulcerative colitis. J Dig Dis 2013;14:117–24.

47. Hosoe N, Matsuoka K, Naganuma M, et al. Applicability of second-generation colon capsule endoscope to ulcerative colitis: a clinical feasibility study. J Gastroenterol Hepatol 2013;28:1174–9.

48. San Juan-Acosta M, Caunedo-Álvarez A, Argüelles-Arias F, et al. Colon capsule endoscopy is a safe and useful tool to assess disease parameters in patients with ulcerative colitis. Eur J Gastroenterol Hepatol 2014;26:894–901.

49. Kobayashi T, Hosoe N, Matsuoka K, et al. Feasibility of the second-generation colon capsule endoscopy in patients with ulcerative colitis with a reduced preparation regimen. J Crohns Colitis 2013;7(Suppl 1):S105.

50. Meister T, Heinzow HS, Domagk D, et al. Colon capsule endoscopy versus standard colonoscopy in assessing disease activity of ulcerative colitis: a prospective trial. Tech Coloproctol 2013;17:641–6.

51. Singeap AM, Trifan A, Cojocariu C, et al. Colonoscopy and colon capsule endo-scopy in inflammatory large bowel disease: concordant or discordant results, alternative or complementary methods? J Crohns Colitis 2013;7(Suppl 1):S117–8.
52. Manes G, Ardizzone S, Cassinotti A. PillCam Colon and ulcerative colitis: what do physicians need to know? Endoscopy 2013;45:325.
53. Wang A, Banerjee S, Barth BA, et al. Wireless capsule endoscopy. Gastrointest Endosc 2013;78:805–15.
54. Rex DK, Johnson DA, Anderson JC, et al. American College of Gastroenterology guidelines for colorectal cancer screening 2009 [corrected]. Am J Gastroenterol 2009;104:739–50.
55. Hassan C, Benamouzig R, Spada C, et al. Cost effectiveness and projected national impact of colorectal cancer screening in France. Endoscopy 2011;43: 780–93.
56. Farnbacher MJ, Krause HH, Hagel AF, et al. QuickView video preview software of colon capsule endoscopy: reliability in presenting colorectal polyps as compared to normal mode reading. Scand J Gastroenterol 2014;49:339–46.

The Big Picture
Does Colonoscopy Work?

David G. Hewett, MBBS, MSc, PhD, FRACP[a,b,*], Douglas K. Rex, MD[c]

KEYWORDS

- Colorectal cancer screening • Colonoscopy • Colorectal cancer
- Adenoma detection • Interval cancer

KEY POINTS

- Colonoscopy is the dominant colorectal screening strategy in the United States, yet its use is not supported by randomized controlled trials.
- Observational data do support a protective effect of colonoscopy and polypectomy on colorectal cancer incidence and mortality, but the level of protection in the proximal colon is variable and operator-dependent.
- Reducing operator dependence and developing new technical improvements in colonoscopy are and will remain priorities in colorectal cancer prevention.
- Ongoing quality improvement initiatives should consider regulatory factors that motivate changes in physician behavior.

Colonoscopy was first endorsed in the United States as a screening strategy for colorectal cancer in 1997.[1] This followed the publication of several observational studies of screening colonoscopy, highlighting the prevalence of adenomas in asymptomatic volunteers.[2–5] Screening recommendations prior to this centered on structural examination of the distal colon and rectum with flexible sigmoidoscopy and noninvasive stool tests.[6] At the time, colonoscopy was the logical extension to sigmoidoscopic screening, as it allowed complete and direct visualization of the whole colon and combined diagnosis and therapy in a single session, compared with noninvasive, two-stage screening strategies.

Disclosure Statement: Dr D.G. Hewett receives consulting fees from Olympus Medical Systems Corporation, Tokyo, Japan. Dr D.K. Rex receives consulting fees and research support from Olympus America Inc, and Boston Scientific and consulting fees from Endochoice.
a School of Medicine, The University of Queensland, Brisbane, QLD 4006, Australia; b Department of Gastroenterology, Queen Elizabeth II Jubilee Hospital, Brisbane, QLD 4108, Australia; c Division of Gastroenterology/Hepatology, Department of Medicine, Indiana University School of Medicine, 550 North University Boulevard, Indiana University Hospital #4100, Indianapolis, IN 46202, USA
* Corresponding author. PO Box 372, Grange QLD 4051, Brisbane, Australia.
E-mail address: d.hewett@uq.edu.au

Gastrointest Endoscopy Clin N Am 25 (2015) 403–413
http://dx.doi.org/10.1016/j.giec.2014.12.002
1052-5157/15/$ – see front matter © 2015 Elsevier Inc. All rights reserved.

Two multi-center studies in 2000 definitively established the safety and feasibility of screening colonoscopy, while highlighting the prevalence of proximal neoplasia in patients without any findings in the distal colon and rectum.[7,8] These results, combined with academic[9] and media attention,[10,11] provided support for lobbying efforts by professional societies with the US Congress, which passed legislation mandating coverage for screening colonoscopy every 10 years in Medicare beneficiaries aged 50 years and older from July 1, 2001.

This law heralded the transformation of gastroenterology practice in the United States. Colonoscopy was adopted by endoscopists and patients, and in the ensuing years, it has become the dominant colorectal cancer screening strategy in the United States.[12] Screening colonoscopy is now recommended by 95% of primary care physicians,[13] and it is estimated that approximately 12 million colonoscopies are performed each year in the United States.[14]

However, the position of colonoscopy as a colorectal cancer screening strategy has not been evaluated in randomized controlled trials. Detractors of screening colonoscopy highlight this lack of clinical trial evidence, together with concerns about lack of cost-effectiveness.[15,16] In contrast, programmatic screening with flexible sigmoidoscopy is supported by high-level evidence. Four randomized controlled trials have now been performed of flexible sigmoidoscopy, all showing a reduction in distal colorectal cancer incidence and mortality.[17–20] The challenge for colonoscopy is whether it offers any additional benefit in screening the proximal colon.

There is ample indirect evidence of a protective effect for colonoscopy on colorectal cancer. For example, population-level cancer statistics show that coincident with the establishment of screening colonoscopy in the United States, colorectal cancer incidence and mortality have progressively fallen over recent decades. A report from the US Centers for Disease Control and Prevention described an overall 30% reduction in colorectal cancer incidence between 2001 and 2010 (3.4% per year), with the greatest impact in the screening-eligible age group (3.9% per year).[21] Colorectal cancer mortality has been falling in the United States since 1975, and this has been attributed to improvements in treatment (12%) and risk factor profiles (32%) and increases in screening (53%).[22]

Other indirect evidence comes from the original study of the fecal occult blood test (FOBT). The Minnesota randomized controlled trial of FOBT was the first to establish a role for screening for colorectal cancer.[23] Although not a trial of screening colonoscopy, colonoscopy was performed in patients with positive tests, and polyps were removed. Subsequent long-term follow-up showed 17% to 20% reductions in colorectal cancer incidence compared with those who were not screened, and 22% to 32% reductions on colorectal cancer mortality at 30 years.[24,25]

THE PROXIMAL COLON

However, the incremental benefit of colonoscopy over flexible sigmoidoscopy depends on extending the protection against colorectal cancer to the proximal colon. In the early days of screening colonoscopy, it was assumed that proximal colon protection would naturally extend from a structural examination of the whole colon. Here are reviewed the data on colorectal cancer protection from colonoscopy, focusing on protection in the proximal colon.

By definition, flexible sigmoidoscopy is a screening test of the distal colon and rectum, so any impact on the incidence of proximal cancer in sigmoidoscopy trials is attributable to colonoscopy, performed following the detection of sentinel lesions on initial index sigmoidoscopy. For example, in the US study (Prostate, Lung

Colorectal and Ovarian Cancer Screening Trial),[18] a 14% reduction in the incidence of proximal colorectal cancer was seen. This reduction is consistent with exposure to colonoscopy in 21.9% of participants, either from referral for colonoscopy for sigmoidoscopy findings, or colonoscopy outside the study protocol. In contrast, the UK flexible sigmoidoscopy trial showed no impact on proximal cancer risk.[17] However, these studies differed in participant recruitment and in criteria for referral for colonoscopy, with only 5% of participants in the UK trial referred for colonoscopy (compared with 21.9% in the US trial[18]).

During the initial lobbying for introduction of screening colonoscopy in the United States, observational data on the protective effect of colonoscopy on colorectal cancer incidence were derived from studies in adenoma-bearing cohorts. The first and most widely quoted of these studies was the US National Polyp Study, in which patients were initially randomized to different colonoscopic surveillance intervals.[26] Findings showed a 76% to 90% reduction in colorectal cancer incidence compared with reference cohorts. A related Italian study with comparable methodology also demonstrated a 76% reduction in cancer incidence after colonoscopic polypectomy.[27]

These studies, showing high levels of cancer protection, were widely cited as evidence of the effectiveness of colonoscopy. Colonoscopy was regarded as preventing approximately 80% of colorectal cancer, and the National Polyp Study was extensively utilized in lobbying of the US Congress for coverage of screening colonoscopy. Long-term follow-up from the National Polyp Study was published in 2012, showing a sustained reduction in colorectal cancer mortality of 53% at a mean of 15.8 years in the adenoma-bearing cohort.

Other adenoma cohort studies have not shown such high levels of colorectal cancer protection.[28-32] Several studies were not able to demonstrate any reduction in colorectal cancer incidence compared with the general population.[30,31] Methodologic variation makes direct comparison of these cohort studies difficult,[33] although an analysis of the cancers detected in these other studies indicated the occurrence of early interval (often proximal) cancers may explain variable levels of cancer protection after colonoscopy.[33]

The incidence of colorectal cancer has also been studied in long-term follow-up of patients who had colonoscopy performed in the original screening studies.[34,35] Colorectal cancer incidence reductions of up to 67% were documented. However, further analysis of the interval cancers found during follow-up, which represent a failure of colonoscopic protection, showed that most were located in the proximal colon and found within 3 to 5 years of the index colonoscopy.

The highest protective effect of colonoscopy comes when the index baseline examination is negative. In 2 prospective cohort US studies of average-risk screening patients with a negative baseline colonoscopy, no cancers were found at 5 years in either group.[36,37] Two retrospective Canadian studies of large cohorts of patients with negative, complete colonoscopies (n = 32,203[38] and n = 111,402[39]) in which colorectal cancer incidence was compared with the general population, showed incidence ratios of 0.66 to 0.80 at 1 to 2 years respectively, and 0.25 to 0.28 at 10 to 14 years. However, cancers that occurred during follow-up were more likely proximal,[38] and the reduction in risk for proximal cancers was less.[39]

More recently, analysis of large US cohorts from the Nurses Health Study and the Health Professionals Follow-up Study (n = 88,902) showed a reduction in risk of colorectal cancer after colonoscopy.[40] Specifically, adjusted hazard ratios were 0.57 (95% confidence interval [CI] 0.45–0.72) after colonoscopy with adenoma removal and 0.44 (95% CI 0.38–0.52) after negative colonoscopy. Again, risk reductions were greater for distal than proximal cancers, and colonoscopy with polypectomy was not associated with a significant reduction in the incidence of proximal colon cancer. The proportion of incident cases prevented with colonoscopy was 40% overall, 22% for proximal cancers, and 61% of distal colorectal cancer.

Multiple case–control studies have examined the association between colonoscopy exposure and colorectal cancer occurrence. Initial studies from Canada in nonscreening populations failed to show any protection against colorectal cancer in the proximal colon.[41,42] Complete colonoscopy was associated with a 47% to 67% reduced risk of death from left-sided colorectal cancer but no reduction in right-sided colorectal cancer mortality. However, these data are influenced by the Canadian context, where colonoscopy is typically performed by nongastroenterologists, who are known to be less effective than gastroenterologists in preventing colorectal cancer.[43–45]

In contrast, subsequent data from Germany and the United States have shown a beneficial impact from colonoscopy on proximal colon cancer incidence and mortality. In 2011, a German population-based study showed a 77% reduction in overall colorectal cancer risk, with reductions in both the right (odds ratio [OR] 0.44, 95% CI 0.35–0.55) and left colon (0.16, 95% CI 0.12–0.20).[46] In the United States, a case–control study of screening colonoscopy showed a reduced risk of colorectal cancer overall of 70%, with reductions in both left-sided (OR 0.26, 95%CI 0.06–0.11) and right-sided colorectal cancers (0.37, 0.16–0.82).[47] In the most recent German population-based study, there was a substantial reduction in cancer risk after screening colonoscopy (OR 0.09, 95% CI 0.07–0.13), with a 78% incidence reduction in the right colon (0.22, 95% CI 0.14–0.33).[48]

In summary, despite a lack of randomized trials, substantial observational data indicate that colonoscopy offers protection against colorectal cancer incidence and death. Colonoscopy does offer an incremental benefit over flexible sigmoidoscopy by extending the protection to the whole colon, even though its impact on proximal cancer incidence and mortality can be lower. Factors contributing to this inconsistent protection in the proximal colon are now considered.

FACTORS INFLUENCING THE EFFECTIVENESS OF COLONOSCOPY

Consistent with the variable colorectal cancer protection following screening colonoscopy, it is clear that, unlike many other screening tests, the performance characteristics of colonoscopy are not fixed, and vary with operator, patient, technical, and system factors (Box 1).[33,49]

Arguably the most significant factor is the operator dependence of colonoscopy, which likely underlies much of the variation in cancer protection arising from observational data. Adenoma detection varies widely between endoscopists, from 2.5-fold to eightfold,[50–55] and it is known that adenoma detection is strongly associated with postcolonoscopy colorectal cancer.[56,57] Furthermore, endoscopist specialty is an important determinant of cancer protection after colonoscopy, with gastroenterologists known to be more effective than nongastroenterologists[43–45] and more likely to detect adenomas.[58] In the proximal colon specifically, variation in protection is similarly endoscopist dependent; protection against proximal colorectal cancer is assured by some endoscopists but not others.[59] Further, those endoscopists are typically nongastroenterologists[41] and those with lower cecal intubation rates.

Patient factors include the unique tumor biology that is associated with cancers in the proximal colon. Specific insights into the patient factors involved in variable cancer can be gained from studies of cancers occurring after colonoscopy. Approximately 6% of colorectal cancer occurs within 5 years of colonoscopy.[60] These interval or postcolonoscopy cancers are more likely to occur in the proximal colon and are

---

Box 1
Potential factors influencing colorectal cancer protection after colonoscopy

Patient

- Poor bowel preparation
- Tumor biology
- Environmental factors (such as diet/smoking)

Colonoscopist

- Procedural/motor skill deficits (eg, incomplete colonoscopy, incomplete/inadequate polypectomy, inspection technique)
- Perceptual factors (eg, variation in color and depth perception)
- Personality characteristics (including conscientiousness, obsessiveness, impulsivity)
- Knowledge and attitude deficits (eg, awareness and appearance of colorectal cancer (CRC) precursor lesions)
- Fatigue

System

- Financial factors (eg, reimbursement disincentives)
- Organizational factors (eg, production pressure, procedure scheduling)

Technical

- Inadequate equipment
- Adjunctive technologies to improve detection (eg, cap-fitted colonoscopy, image-enhancement)

Adapted from Hewett DG, Kahi CJ, Rex DK. Does colonoscopy work? J Natl Compr Canc Netw 2010;8(1):73; with permission.

---

associated with higher rates of baseline adenomas, and a family history of colorectal cancer.[60] Tumor biology is also implicated in cancers not detected at colonoscopy, with interval cancers more frequently having the characteristic molecular signature of the serrated pathway of colorectal neoplasia,[61–63] specifically the CpG island methylator phenotype (CIMP), and microsatellite instability indicating a loss of function of DNA mismatch repair genes.[40,64,65]

There is likely significant interaction between operator and patient factors in the detection of serrated neoplasia and other flat or depressed lesions, all of which tend to occur in the proximal colon.[63,66] In fact, it is known that variation in the detection of serrated pathway lesions is far greater than that of conventional adenomas.[54,55] Some endoscopists are therefore more likely to detect serrated lesions and protect against cancer in the proximal colon, and these endoscopists are probably also those with high levels of conventional adenoma detection.[57] Other patient factors include bowel preparation, which must be adequate to facilitate lesion detection. The quality of mucosal cleansing is typically worse in the proximal colon when bowel preparation is not split and not completed within 3 to 5 hours of the procedure time,[67] and this reduces detection.[68]

Technical factors relate to use of modern endoscopic technologies that are known to improve lesion detection at colonoscopy (eg,, use of high-definition colonoscopes[69] or adjunctive technologies such as cap-fitted colonoscopy[70] and image-enhancement,[71,72] which may supplement or compensate for operator-dependent factors). High-definition instruments are particularly relevant for the detection of subtle lesions that occur in the proximal colon. Recently, a new colonoscope platform with a 330° angle of view (Full Spectrum Endoscopy, Endochoice Incorporated, Alpharetta, Georgia) was shown to produce substantial detection gains relative to older-generation Olympus colonoscopes.[73] Substantial gains in detection were also produced with external colonoscope attachments that straighten colonic folds, including Endocuff[74,75] (Arc Medical Design Ltd, Leeds, United Kingdom) and EndoRings[76] (Endo-Aid Ltd, Caesarea, Israel). Further research is warranted on exploiting the interaction between technical and operator factors, by requiring low-level detectors to use adjunctive detection technologies to achieve required detection standards.

Finally, system factors influence the context within which colonoscopy is performed. For example, reimbursement structures for colonoscopy have typically rewarded volume rather than quality[77] and motivated a one and done[78] approach to polyp detection and resection. Again, these system factors interact with operator factors. In particular, surveillance recommendations exacerbate the impact of low-level adenoma detection on the timing of the surveillance examination. Surveillance intervals do not consider the quality of the baseline examination, such that low-level detectors with a low adenoma detection rate (which is associated with interval cancer rates) will assign a longer time frame for surveillance. In contrast, high-level detectors, finding more adenomas and clearing the colon more completely of neoplasia, will recommend earlier interval surveillance colonoscopy. High-level detectors therefore provide a double level of protection due to surveillance recommendations, while low-level detectors provide false reassurance for their patients, who are doubly unprotected.

Ensuring that Colonoscopy Works

Improving the effectiveness of colonoscopy requires particular attention to the factors that influence physician behavior. Addressing operator variation remains the most worthwhile quality improvement target, albeit the most challenging.[53] Participation in quality audit and feedback programs[79] and external review of performance (via video recording)[80] are known to motivate operator improvement. Likewise, training in lesion recognition and mucosal inspection techniques can improve performance.[55,56] However, despite publication of quality improvement targets[81] and development of registries to systematically collect performance data,[82] mandatory enforcement of quality standards has not been readily achievable in US practice. More could be achieved through provider regulation as has been adopted in other countries.[77,83,84]

The variable protection afforded by colonoscopy is a major disadvantage of colonoscopy as a screening strategy. However, proximal colon protection is clearly achievable and interval cancers preventable.[85] Continued international effort to reduce the variation in colonoscopy effectiveness must be a priority to realize the full potential of colonoscopy as a colorectal cancer screening test and maintain its dominance for screening in the United States. Regardless of whether colonoscopy remains in use as a screening test, it will continue to play a critical role in surveillance, and as the diagnostic imaging test of choice for evaluation of symptoms and other positive screening tests. Reducing operator dependence and developing new technical improvements in colonoscopy are and will remain priorities in colorectal cancer prevention.

REFERENCES

1. Winawer S, Fletcher R, Miller L, et al. Colorectal cancer screening: clinical guidelines and rationale. Gastroenterology 1997;112:594–642.

2. Rex DK, Lehman GA, Hawes RH, et al. Screening colonoscopy in asymptomatic average-risk persons with negative fecal occult blood tests. Gastroenterology 1991;100(1):64–7.
3. Johnson DA, Gurney MS, Volpe RJ, et al. A prospective study of the prevalence of colonic neoplasms in asymptomatic patients with an age-related risk. Am J Gastroenterol 1990;85(8):969–74.
4. Lieberman DA, Smith FW. Screening for colon malignancy with colonoscopy. Am J Gastroenterol 1991;86(8):946–51.
5. Foutch PG, Mai H, Pardy K, et al. Flexible sigmoidoscopy may be ineffective for secondary prevention of colorectal cancer in asymptomatic, average-risk men. Dig Dis Sci 1991;36(7):924–8.
6. US Preventive Services Task Force. Chapter 8: screening for colorectal cancer. Guide to clinical preventive services. 2nd edition. Washington, DC: US Government Printing Office; 1996. p. 89–103.
7. Lieberman DA, Weiss DG, Bond JH, et al. Use of colonoscopy to screen asymptomatic adults for colorectal cancer. N Engl J Med 2000;343(3):162–8.
8. Imperiale T, Wagner D, Lin C, et al. Risk of advanced proximal neoplasms in asymptomatic adults according to the distal colorectal findings. N Engl J Med 2000;343:169–74.
9. Podolsky DK. Going the distance—the case for true colorectal-cancer screening. N Engl J Med 2000;343(3):207–8.
10. Grady D. More extensive test needed for colon cancer, studies say. New York Times 2000;A1 A20.
11. Cram P, Fendrick AM, Inadomi J, et al. The impact of a celebrity promotional campaign on the use of colon cancer screening: the Katie Couric effect. Arch Intern Med 2003;163(13):1601–5.
12. Kahi CJ, Anderson JC, Rex DK. Screening and surveillance for colorectal cancer: state of the art. Gastrointest Endosc 2013;77(3):335–50.
13. Klabunde CN, Lanier D, Nadel MR, et al. Colorectal cancer screening by primary care physicians: recommendations and practices, 2006–2007. Am J Prev Med 2009;37(1):8–16.
14. Peery AF, Dellon ES, Lund J, et al. Burden of gastrointestinal disease in the united states: 2012 update. Gastroenterology 2012;143(5):1179–87.e1–3.
15. Ransohoff DF. Colon cancer screening in 2005: status and challenges. Gastroenterology 2005;128(6):1685–95.
16. Pignone M, Rich M, Teutsch SM, et al. Screening for colorectal cancer in adults at average risk: a summary of the evidence for the U.S. Preventive Services Task Force. Ann Intern Med 2002;137(2):132–41.
17. Atkin WS, Edwards R, Kralj-Hans I, et al. Once-only flexible sigmoidoscopy screening in prevention of colorectal cancer: a multicentre randomised controlled trial. Lancet 2010;375(9726):1624–33.
18. Schoen RE, Pinsky PF, Weissfeld JL, et al. Colorectal-cancer incidence and mortality with screening flexible sigmoidoscopy. N Engl J Med 2012;366(25):2345–57.
19. Holme O, Loberg M, Kalager M, et al. Effect of flexible sigmoidoscopy screening on colorectal cancer incidence and mortality: a randomized clinical trial. JAMA 2014;312(6):606–15.
20. Segnan N, Armaroli P, Bonelli L, et al. Once-only sigmoidoscopy in colorectal cancer screening: follow-up findings of the italian randomized controlled trial–score. J Natl Cancer Inst 2011;103(17):1310–22.
21. Siegel R, Desantis C, Jemal A. Colorectal cancer statistics, 2014. CA Cancer J Clin 2014;64(2):104–17.

22. Edwards BK, Ward E, Kohler BA, et al. Annual report to the nation on the status of cancer, 1975–2006, featuring colorectal cancer trends and impact of interventions (risk factors, screening, and treatment) to reduce future rates. Cancer 2010;116(3):544–73.

23. Mandel JS, Bond JH, Church TR, et al. Reducing mortality from colorectal cancer by screening for fecal occult blood. Minnesota colon cancer control study. N Engl J Med 1993;328(19):1365–71.

24. Mandel JS, Church TR, Bond JH, et al. The effect of fecal occult-blood screening on the incidence of colorectal cancer. N Engl J Med 2000;343(22):1603–7.

25. Shaukat A, Mongin SJ, Geisser MS, et al. Long-term mortality after screening for colorectal cancer. N Engl J Med 2013;369(12):1106–14.

26. Winawer SJ, Zauber AG, Ho MN, et al. Prevention of colorectal cancer by colonoscopic polypectomy. N Engl J Med 1993;329(27):1977–81.

27. Citarda F, Tomaselli G, Capocaccia R, et al. Efficacy in standard clinical practice of colonoscopic polypectomy in reducing colorectal cancer incidence. Gut 2001; 48:812–5.

28. Alberts DS, Martinez ME, Roe DJ, et al. Lack of effect of a high-fiber cereal supplement on the recurrence of colorectal adenomas. N Engl J Med 2000;342(16): 1156–62.

29. Schatzkin A, Lanza E, Corle D, et al. Lack of effect of a low-fat, high-fiber diet on the recurrence of colorectal adenomas. N Engl J Med 2000;342(16): 1149–55.

30. Jorgensen OD, Kronborg O, Fenger C. The funen adenoma follow-up study. Incidence and death from colorectal carcinoma in an adenoma surveillance program. Scand J Gastroenterol 1993;28(10):869–74.

31. Robertson DJ, Greenberg ER, Beach M, et al. Colorectal cancer in patients under close colonoscopic surveillance. Gastroenterology 2005;129(1):34–41.

32. Loberg M, Kalager M, Holme O, et al. Long-term colorectal-cancer mortality after adenoma removal. N Engl J Med 2014;371(9):799–807.

33. Hewett DG, Kahi CJ, Rex DK. Does colonoscopy work? J Natl Compr Canc Netw 2010;8(1):67–77.

34. Lieberman DA, Weiss DG, Harford WV, et al. Five-year colon surveillance after screening colonoscopy. Gastroenterology 2007;133(4):1077–85.

35. Kahi CJ, Imperiale TF, Juliar BE, et al. Effect of screening colonoscopy on colorectal cancer incidence and mortality. Clin Gastroenterol Hepatol 2009;7(7): 770–5.

36. Rex DK, Cummings OW, Helper DJ, et al. 5-year incidence of adenomas after negative colonoscopy in asymptomatic average-risk persons. Gastroenterology 1996;111(5):1178–81.

37. Imperiale TF, Glowinski EA, Lin-Cooper C, et al. Five-year risk of colorectal neoplasia after negative screening colonoscopy. N Engl J Med 2008;359(12): 1218–24.

38. Singh H, Turner D, Xue L, et al. Risk of developing colorectal cancer following a negative colonoscopy examination: evidence for a 10-year interval between colonoscopies. JAMA 2006;295(20):2366–73.

39. Lakoff J, Paszat LF, Saskin R, et al. Risk of developing proximal versus distal colorectal cancer after a negative colonoscopy: a population-based study. Clin Gastroenterol Hepatol 2008;6(10):1117–21.

40. Nishihara R, Wu K, Lochhead P, et al. Long-term colorectal-cancer incidence and mortality after lower endoscopy. N Engl J Med 2013;369(12):1095–105.

41. Singh H, Nugent Z, Demers AA, et al. The reduction in colorectal cancer mortality after colonoscopy varies by site of the cancer. Gastroenterology 2010;139(4): 1128–37.
42. Baxter NN, Goldwasser MA, Paszat LF, et al. Association of colonoscopy and death from colorectal cancer. Ann Intern Med 2009;150(1):1–8.
43. Baxter NN, Warren JL, Barrett MJ, et al. Association between colonoscopy and colorectal cancer mortality in a us cohort according to site of cancer and colonoscopist specialty. J Clin Oncol 2012;30(21):2664–9.
44. Rabeneck L, Paszat LF, Saskin R. Endoscopist specialty is associated with incident colorectal cancer after a negative colonoscopy. Clin Gastroenterol Hepatol 2010;8(3):275–9.
45. Hassan C, Rex DK, Zullo A, et al. Loss of efficacy and cost-effectiveness when screening colonoscopy is performed by nongastroenterologists. Cancer 2012; 118(18):4404–11.
46. Brenner H, Chang-Claude J, Seiler CM, et al. Protection from colorectal cancer after colonoscopy: a population-based, case-control study. Ann Intern Med 2011;154(1):22–30.
47. Doubeni CA, Weinmann S, Adams K, et al. Screening colonoscopy and risk for incident late-stage colorectal cancer diagnosis in average-risk adults: a nested case-control study. Ann Intern Med 2013;158(5 Pt 1):312–20.
48. Brenner H, Chang-Claude J, Jansen L, et al. Reduced risk of colorectal cancer up to 10 years after screening, surveillance, or diagnostic colonoscopy. Gastroenterology 2014;146(3):709–17.
49. Hewett DG, Kahi CJ, Rex DK. Efficacy and effectiveness of colonoscopy: how do we bridge the gap? Gastrointest Endosc Clin N Am 2010;20(4):673–84.
50. Rex DK, Cutler CS, Lemmel GT, et al. Colonoscopic miss rates of adenomas determined by back-to-back colonoscopies. Gastroenterology 1997;112:24–8.
51. Chen SC, Rex DK. Endoscopist can be more powerful than age and male gender in predicting adenoma detection at colonoscopy. Am J Gastroenterol 2007; 102(4):856–61.
52. Imperiale TF, Glowinski EA, Juliar BE, et al. Variation in polyp detection rates at screening colonoscopy. Gastrointest Endosc 2009;69(7):1288–95.
53. Shaukat A, Oancea C, Bond JH, et al. Variation in detection of adenomas and polyps by colonoscopy and change over time with a performance improvement program. Clin Gastroenterol Hepatol 2009;7(12):1335–40.
54. Kahi CJ, Hewett DG, Norton DL, et al. Prevalence and variable detection of proximal colon serrated polyps during screening colonoscopy. Clin Gastroenterol Hepatol 2011;9(1):42–6.
55. Hetzel JT, Huang CS, Coukos JA, et al. Variation in the detection of serrated polyps in an average risk colorectal cancer screening cohort. Am J Gastroenterol 2010;105(12):2656–64.
56. Kaminski MF, Regula J, Kraszewska E, et al. Quality indicators for colonoscopy and the risk of interval cancer. N Engl J Med 2010;362(19):1795–803.
57. Corley DA, Jensen CD, Marks AR, et al. Adenoma detection rate and risk of colorectal cancer and death. N Engl J Med 2014;370(14):1298–306.
58. Ko CW, Dominitz JA, Green P, et al. Specialty differences in polyp detection, removal, and biopsy during colonoscopy. Am J Med 2010;123(6):528–35.
59. Baxter NN, Sutradhar R, Forbes SS, et al. Analysis of administrative data finds endoscopist quality measures associated with postcolonoscopy colorectal cancer. Gastroenterology 2011;140(1):65–72.

60. Samadder NJ, Curtin K, Tuohy TM, et al. Characteristics of missed or interval colorectal cancer and patient survival: a population-based study. Gastroenterology 2014;146(4):950–60.

61. Rosty C, Hewett DG, Brown IS, et al. Serrated polyps of the large intestine: current understanding of diagnosis, pathogenesis, and clinical management. J Gastroenterol 2012;48(3):287–302.

62. Leggett B, Whitehall V. Role of the serrated pathway in colorectal cancer pathogenesis. Gastroenterology 2010;138(6):2088–100.

63. Rex DK, Ahnen DJ, Baron JA, et al. Serrated lesions of the colorectum: review and recommendations from an expert panel. Am J Gastroenterol 2012;107(9):1315–29.

64. Arain MA, Sawhney M, Sheikh S, et al. Cimp status of interval colon cancers: another piece to the puzzle. Am J Gastroenterol 2010;105(5):1189–95.

65. Sawhney MS, Farrar WD, Gudiseva S, et al. Microsatellite instability in interval colon cancers. Gastroenterology 2006;131(6):1700–5.

66. Bianco M, Cipolletta L, Rotondano G, et al. The cooperative flat lesions italian network (flin): prevalence of non-polypoid colorectal neoplasia. A multicentre observational study. Endoscopy 2010;42:279–85.

67. Seo EH, Kim TO, Park MJ, et al. Optimal preparation-to-colonoscopy interval in split-dose peg bowel preparation determines satisfactory bowel preparation quality: an observational prospective study. Gastrointest Endosc 2012;75(3):583–90.

68. Gurudu SR, Ramirez FC, Harrison ME, et al. Increased adenoma detection rate with system-wide implementation of a split-dose preparation for colonoscopy. Gastrointest Endosc 2012;76(3):603–8.

69. Buchner AM, Shahid MW, Heckman MG, et al. High-definition colonoscopy detects colorectal polyps at a higher rate than standard white-light colonoscopy. Clin Gastroenterol Hepatol 2010;8(4):364–70.

70. Hewett DG, Rex DK. Cap-fitted colonoscopy: a randomized, tandem colonoscopy study of adenoma miss rates. Gastrointest Endosc 2010;72(4):775–81.

71. Pohl J, Lotterer E, Balzer C, et al. Computed virtual chromoendoscopy versus standard colonoscopy with targeted indigocarmine chromoscopy: a randomised multicentre trial. Gut 2009;58(1):73–8.

72. Leung WK, Lo OS, Liu KS, et al. Detection of colorectal adenoma by narrow band imaging (hq190) vs. High-definition white light colonoscopy: a randomized controlled trial. Am J Gastroenterol 2014;109(6):855–63.

73. Gralnek IM, Siersema PD, Halpern Z, et al. Standard forward-viewing colonoscopy versus full-spectrum endoscopy: an international, multicentre, randomised, tandem colonoscopy trial. Lancet Oncol 2014;15(3):353–60.

74. Floer M, Biecker E, Fitzlaff R, et al. Higher adenoma detection rates with endocuff-assisted colonoscopy - a randomized controlled multicenter trial. PLoS One 2014;9(12):e114267.

75. Biecker E, Floer M, Heinecke A, et al. Novel endocuff-assisted colonoscopy significantly increases the polyp detection rate: a randomized controlled trial. J Clin Gastroenterol 2014. [Epub ahead of print].

76. Dik VK, Gralnek IM, Segol O, et al. Comparing standard colonoscopy with endorings colonoscopy: a randomized, multicenter tandem colonoscopy study – interim results of the clever study. Gastroenterology 2014;146(5 Suppl 1):S160.

77. Hewett DG, Rex DK. Improving colonoscopy quality through health-care payment reform. Am J Gastroenterol 2010;105(9):1925–33.

78. Wang HS, Pisegna J, Modi R, et al. Adenoma detection rate is necessary but insufficient for distinguishing high versus low endoscopist performance. Gastrointest Endosc 2013;77(1):71–8.

79. Kahi CJ, Ballard D, Shah AS, et al. Impact of a quarterly report card on colono-scopy quality measures. Gastrointest Endosc 2013;77(6):925–31.
80. Rex DK, Hewett DG, Raghavendra M, et al. The impact of video recording on the quality of colonoscopy performance: a pilot study. Am J Gastroenterol 2010; 105(11):2312–7.
81. Rex DK, Schoenfeld PS, Cohen J, et al. Quality indicators for colonoscopy. Gastrointest Endosc 2015;110(1):31–53.
82. Cohen J, Pike IM. Defining and measuring quality in endoscopy. Am J Gastro-enterol 2015;110(1):1–2.
83. Gavin DR, Valori RM, Anderson JT, et al. The national colonoscopy audit: a nation-wide assessment of the quality and safety of colonoscopy in the UK. Gut 2013; 62(2):242–9.
84. Australian Government. Improving colonoscopy services in Australia: report from the National Bowel Cancer Screening Program Quality Working Group. Canberra (Australia): Department of Health and Ageing; 2009.
85. le Clercq CM, Bouwens MW, Rondagh EJ, et al. Postcolonoscopy colorectal cancers are preventable: a population-based study. Gut 2014;63(6):957–63.

Moving?

Make sure your subscription moves with you!

To notify us of your new address, find your **Clinics Account Number** (located on your mailing label above your name), and contact customer service at:

Email: journalscustomerservice-usa@elsevier.com

800-654-2452 (subscribers in the U.S. & Canada)
314-447-8871 (subscribers outside of the U.S. & Canada)

Fax number: 314-447-8029

Elsevier Health Sciences Division
Subscription Customer Service
3251 Riverport Lane
Maryland Heights, MO 63043

*To ensure uninterrupted delivery of your subscription, please notify us at least 4 weeks in advance of move.

Printed and bound by CPI Group (UK) Ltd, Croydon, CR0 4YY

21/10/2024

01777262-0003